I0110466

What Color Are Your Scrubs?

Finding Your True Fit in Healthcare

Mason Preddy

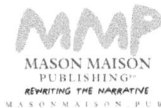

MASON MAISON
PUBLISHING™
REWRITING THE NARRATIVE
MASONMAISON PUB

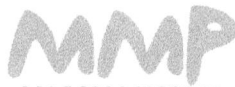

MMP

MASON MAISON
PUBLISHING™
REWRITING THE NARRATIVE
M A S O N M A I S O N . P U B

© 2026 Mason Maison® Publishing. All rights reserved.

No part of this book may be reproduced, stored, or transmitted in any form or by any means without prior written permission of the publisher, except for brief quotations used in reviews or critical articles.

This book is for informational and educational purposes only and is not medical, legal, or financial advice. Always consult qualified professionals regarding your specific circumstances.

All examples, characters, and scenarios are illustrative. The Pivot Playbook™, SCRUBfit™ Healthcare Career Assessment, the SCRUBfit™ Squad, and related character profiles are original works of the author. StaySm:)in'! is a signature mark of the author.

Mason's Alignment Theory™ (MAT), PACES™ — The Five Pillars of Career Alignment — and CARESET™ are proprietary frameworks presented for educational purposes.

Masters Series: Expert Voices on Healthcare Alignment includes real contributions from respected leaders; attribution appears where quotes or essays are used.

Early in my career, I co-chaired the Inova Health Leadership Institute, where we studied performance-improvement concepts including those popularized by organizations such as the Studer Group. That work shaped my approach to leadership and culture, and this book builds on that foundation through the lens of career alignment.

For permissions or inquiries:

Mason Maison® Publishing

www.masonmaison.pub

Printed in the United States of America.

Dedication

In memory of **Gail Boylan, RN**, **Beth Keane**, and **Jeanne Martin**—three extraordinary women whose leadership and light forever changed my path.

What began as collaboration became mentorship, and what began as mentorship became friendship—threaded with laughter, honesty, and moments that still echo in my heart.

Their influence shaped the leader I became and the person I continue to grow into. Their legacy—of courage, vision, and boundless heart—lives within every page of this book, and in every life they touched.

"Some people burn out not because they're weak, but because they're lit in the wrong place."

— *Anonymous Healthcare Proverb*

Foreword

FOREWORD

I've known Mason Preddy for more than twenty years, and to describe him best, I'd frame him around four words: trust, excellence, dogged determination, and genuine. Mason isn't just the author of this book—he's the soul of its contents. He has personally lived the lessons he's distilled onto these pages and, without even realizing it, has become one of the most authentic life coaches you may ever meet. In short, he's the real deal: someone who has captured years of experience and wisdom and, from the heart, shaped them into a valuable tool for others to learn from and share.

If you're holding this book, chances are you're standing at one of life's biggest crossroads—deciding what you want to do with your time, your energy, your talents, and ultimately, your life. Maybe you're fresh out of school and curious about healthcare. Maybe you've been working in the field for years and are starting to wonder if you're in the right role. Or maybe you've always felt called to help others but aren't sure how to turn that instinct into a sustainable, rewarding career.

Wherever you are on your journey, you're in the right place. Healthcare is a field like no other—vast, complex, and constantly evolving. It can be demanding, but it can also be deeply meaningful. And contrary to popular belief, it's not just about becoming a doctor or a nurse. This book reveals a landscape of more than three hundred roles—clinical and non-clinical, patient-facing and behind-the-scenes—that collectively keep our healthcare systems running and our communities healthy.

What sets this guide apart is that it doesn't simply list job titles and salary ranges. It walks you through the process of truly matching who you are with what healthcare needs. It offers grounded, real-world advice—from navigating interviews to earning your license to managing burnout—while also inviting you to ask the bigger questions: What kind of impact do I want to have? What environment brings out my best? How do I define success?

This isn't a book of empty motivation or one-size-fits-all answers. It's a practical toolkit for anyone ready to take ownership of their career and build a future that feels purposeful, not just productive.

So whether you're just beginning to explore your options or reevaluating your current path, take a deep breath. The journey to a fulfilling healthcare career starts here—with curiosity, clarity, and the courage to act. Now is the time to begin.

Rod Huebbers

Hospital & System Transformation Leader | Pharmacist-Turned-Executive | Culture, Strategy & Growth Architect

Preface

When I first began in healthcare recruiting, I thought my job was about filling hard-to-recruit clinical roles. Over time, I realized it was about something deeper — helping people find where they truly belonged.

Again and again, I watched bright, capable professionals walk away — not because they lacked skill or dedication, but because the role didn't align with who they were. I also saw others thrive in positions few would envy, simply because those roles matched their values, temperament, and personal rhythm of care. That realization changed everything for me.

After twenty-four years — and more interviews than I could ever count (enough to earn every gray hair I have, and maybe a few I've lost) — I've spoken with nurses, physicians, therapists, allied health professionals, leaders, and students at every career stage. Some were thriving. Some were struggling. Some were on the edge of walking away.

Those conversations gave me something better than any spreadsheet or recruitment metric — they gave me a new lens. A way of seeing that alignment between a person and their work isn't a luxury; it's the key to purpose, longevity, and joy in healthcare.

Here's what my job is *not*: convincing anyone to stay in healthcare who doesn't belong there. Healthcare needs bright, compassionate, and resilient people — but it also needs the *right* people, in the *right* roles. My job is to help you find that fit.

And if you realize through this process that healthcare isn't your path? That's okay too. Consider this your permission slip to step off the treadmill — especially if you're here because someone else always pictured you in a white coat.

Because here's the truth: when you're misaligned in healthcare, it doesn't just affect you. It ripples outward — to your coworkers, your patients, your organization, and even the people waiting for you at home. Those pre-shift gut alarms that start buzzing the night before work? The dread that builds before your next shift, your next chart, your next code? That's not weakness. That's your system warning you that something's off.

The exciting thing is this: healthcare careers come in every shape and speed imaginable. There are countless ways to use your skills and your compassion. But if you were never drawn to healthcare in the first place, you can't fake your way into fulfillment. My goal is to help you realize that *before* you invest years — and a small fortune in tuition — chasing someone else's dream.

To stop you from spending a career under constant internal alarms.

To guide you toward work that energizes you instead of empties you.

That's what this book is about.

What Color Are Your Scrubs? is the culmination of decades spent listening — and noticing patterns. It's both a mirror for individuals and a manual for organizations: a way to understand why some teams thrive while others burn out, and how to build workplaces that bring people alive instead of wearing them down.

When roles and people truly match, that's not just success — that's what I call a **SCRUB*fit*™**.

I've heard stories of burnout that nearly broke people, and stories of purpose so fierce it carried them through impossible nights. Both matter. Both belong here.

This isn't a book of shortcuts or secret formulas. The only compass that matters is *you*.

What follows is a framework to help you think differently, see more clearly, and move forward with purpose.

I'm glad you're here.

Shall we begin?

Acknowledgements

To my family—especially my mom, my constant grounding force—thank you for your patience, encouragement, and reminders that the work of caring starts at home.

A book is never written alone. **What Color Are Your Scrubs?** was born from nearly a thousand conversations with nurses, physicians, allied health professionals, advanced practice providers, and healthcare leaders who trusted me with their stories. To every clinician who sat across from me—whether in person, online, or over the phone—and shared why you stayed or why you left: thank you. Your honesty gave me both the lens of alignment and the insight I needed.

And for the record (and publishing reasons), I couldn't include every colorful word many of you used to describe your former workplaces. Let's just say your "feedback" on staffing ratios, documentation systems, and break-room coffee lives forever in my unedited notes—exactly where it belongs. I only hope your passion still shines through here, carried by my words and gratitude.

To my mentors and thought partners—David S. Goldberg; Rodney N. "Rod" Huebbers; Patricia (Patty) Mook; Joy B. Solomita; and Quint Studer—thank you. Your wisdom, generosity, and belief in alignment gave this project its depth and credibility.

To the Masters Series leaders whose essays, insights, and perspectives appear in these pages—including Diane Adams; Michael J. Avaltroni; Scott Becker; Peter Cappelli; Susan Carroll; David S. Goldberg; Rod Huebbers; Jon Macaskill; Marco Scarci; M. Maureen Lal; Patricia (Patty) Mook; Stephanie O'Bryon; Patti Rager; Chip Taunt; Knox Singleton; Joy B. Solomita; Quint Studer; and Jean Watson—thank you for trusting this project with your stories and your names. Your chapters and reflections bring alignment to life through real-world healthcare leadership and offer readers a chorus of experience far beyond my own.

I am grateful to Cathy Christopher; Ellen Menard; JoAnn Neufer; Billy Mullins; Jennifer Mosedale; and Joanna Robertson for the powerful quotes and perspectives they contributed to this book. Their words add texture, honesty, and lived experience to the themes of alignment, advocacy, education, and leadership that run through these pages.

And to Jennifer Mosedale and Joanna Robertson, whose authenticity helped inspire **SCRUB***fit*™ Jen-Jen Codedale, RN, BSN, and **SCRUB***fit*™ Anna Remedy, DNP, FNP-BC, PMHNP—and to Vera Preddy, whose leadership and example helped inspire **SCRUB***fit*™ Vera Vines, MBA, MHA, MSN, FACHE—and, in loving memory, Billy Harper (RIP), whose spirit helped inspire **SCRUB***fit*™ Harper Helpwell, CMA (AAMA)—thank you for helping shape the heart of the **SCRUB***fit*™ universe in ways that will continue to resonate with readers.

To my colleagues and friends in healthcare: thank you for proving that alignment isn't theory—it's the difference between people thriving in their careers or leaving them behind.

To my friends beyond healthcare: thank you for reminding me there's more to life than work, and for standing with me through this long journey. Your laughter, patience, and encouragement carried me farther than you know.

To my English Bulldog, JoJo—my favorite Hoya—for staying by my feet and always rooting me on. From Hoya Saxa to Roll Wave, she never misses a cheer. She rocks.

And finally, to you—the one holding these pages—thank you for opening this book. Whether you're exploring a healthcare career, rediscovering your fit, or leading others toward alignment, you are the reason this book exists.

Thanks again — and StaySm:)in'!.

Masters Series Contributors

A Note of Gratitude to the Masters Series Contributors

To the leaders, thinkers, mentors, and deeply generous human beings who make up the Masters Series:

Thank you. This project—this book, this movement, this reimagining of how people find their place in healthcare—would not exist in its current form without you. Each of you brought not only your expertise, but your stories, your integrity, and the lessons you earned through years of work, challenge, and service.

Your voices form a chorus of perspectives that stretch across the entire healthcare landscape—education, operations, workforce strategy (gl), policy (gl), nursing excellence, rehabilitation, pharmacy, patient advocacy, and clinical mastery. You offered your time and insight with real generosity, helping ground this work in reality rather than theory. What makes the Masters Series so powerful is not that it represents a single viewpoint or agenda, but that it reflects the complexity of healthcare itself—different vantage points, shared purpose, and an unwavering commitment to making the work better for the people inside it.

You strengthened this work and, more importantly, you strengthened the readers who will build their futures with it. Each of you contributed far more than a chapter—you contributed conviction. You helped build a book that tells the truth about healthcare work while still offering a path toward something better. My hope is that when readers see your names, they feel the encouragement, generosity, and integrity you brought to this project.

Thank you for lending your voice to a work designed to help people find where they fit, where they thrive, and where they can build a life filled with purpose. Your contributions will shape careers. Your generosity will shape lives.

A Note to the Reader

It's never too soon to start learning—or to see if any of this even resonates with you. You don't need to be in scrubs yet to begin exploring who you are, where you might fit, or whether healthcare truly feels like your calling. That's what this journey is for: to help you start discovering your alignment before the world decides it for you.

Throughout this book, you'll notice certain terms marked with (gl). Those are glossary terms you'll find woven through the stories and dialogue. Healthcare speaks its own language— one built on abbreviations, acronyms, and shorthand that can sound like code until you're part of it. To help you get started, I've also included *The 100 Words Every Healthcare Professional Should Know*—a companion list to help you follow the conversations, build confidence, and begin seeing the world through a clinician's eyes.

Healthcare is its own language, but I'm here to help you learn to speak it.

Introduction

THE GREAT HEALTHCARE AWAKENING: WHY NOW IS YOUR TIME

Everyone talks about a "healthcare shortage." But don't let that headline hook you—there's more to the story.

The truth? We don't have a shortage of people who care. We have an epidemic (gl) of misalignment (gl).

Bright, compassionate students and professionals are walking into the wrong roles every single day, and it's burning them out before they ever get the chance to thrive.

I've watched it for over two and a half decades:

• Brilliant clinicians (gl) who love the science but loathe the night shifts.

• Techs (gl) who live for patient interaction but wind up in the basement with the centrifuges (gl).

- Physicians (gl) whose personalities (gl) were built for problem-solving (gl), not wrestling with six logins (gl) and a copier from 1998.

That's not a shortage. That's misalignment (gl).

And misalignment (gl) is the real epidemic (gl) choking our healthcare workforce (gl).

There's no "baby shortage," and there never has been. We've never lacked people who care—we've lacked systems that know what to do with them. When values (gl) and environments (gl) don't line up, talent drains out. Not because the pipeline (gl) is empty, but because the purpose is.

You can always tell the most misaligned (gl) units (gl) in a hospital. About thirty minutes before shift change, it sounds like someone shook a pocketful of wind chimes—badges, keys, and morale (gl) all clinking at once. That's not just fatigue (gl); that's disconnection (gl) ringing in unison.

When the system is misaligned (gl), even the most passionate professionals start to disengage (gl).

The nurse who once stayed late to comfort families now counts the minutes until shift change like it's a rocket launch. The physician (gl) who once taught with joy now teaches out of obligation (gl)—and caffeine (gl). The new graduate (gl) who should feel called feels cornered instead, already Googling (gl), "What else can I do with this degree?"

Alignment (gl) doesn't ask for perfection—it asks for connection (gl).

When organizations prioritize meaning alongside metrics (gl), people don't just stay; they come alive. The future of healthcare won't be built by frantically filling vacancies (gl). It will be built by restoring alignment (gl)—by putting people where their wiring and the work actually match.

This book is here to flip the script.

It's not just about filling positions. It's about fitting people.

For the first time, healthcare careers are being designed (gl) to fit your life, instead of forcing your life to sit quietly in the break room while your career runs the show.

That's what this book is about: helping you discover where you belong before misalignment (gl) drains you of joy, purpose, and passion.

"We don't have a workforce shortage (gl). We have an alignment (gl) epidemic (gl)."

Table of Contents

Foreword   vii
Preface   xi
Acknowledgements   xv

Masters Series Contributors   1
A Note to the Reader   3
Introduction   5
Glossary   13
1. Let Your Journey Begin...   67
2. Hopewell Hospital for Tomorrow   77
3. Between Next and Now 2024-2026   86
4. A High-Schooler's Guide to This Book   93
5. Welcome, Second-Career Seekers   95
6. Welcome, Healthcare Insiders   97
7. Mason's Alignment Theory (MAT)   99
8. PACES™ and CARESET™   107
9. Misalignment: Live from the Floor—The Shape
   of Misalignment in Real Life   113
10. The Misalignment Epidemic   116
11. The Alignment Blueprint: Rebuilding Healthcare
    Through Alignment   124
12. The Alignment Revolution   131
13. Alignment & Reflection   142
14. Out of Alignment: The Human Cost   147
15. Why Alignment Matters   151
16. Mini SCRUBfit Healthcare Career Assessment   154
17. Scrubbed In and Ready: 171
18. Obstacles, Nuances & Realities   174
19. Bravo Zulu   177
20. SCRUBfit Squad: The Adrenaline Team   184
21. SCRUBfit Squad: The Compassion Corps   207
22. SCRUBfit Squad: The Diagnostic Division   236
23. SCRUBfit Squad: The Med Heads   257

24. SCRUBfit Squad: The Recovery Regimen   284

25. SCRUBfit Squad: The Prevention Pact   306

26. SCRUBfit Squad: The Leadership League   327

27. SCRUBfit Squad: The Power Panel   336

28. SCRUBfit Squad: The Vital Link   348

29. SCRUBfit Squad: The Care Crew   361

30. Recalibration Is Inevitable. Alignment Is a Choice.   372

31. Mason's Alignment Theory (MAT)   376

32. Alignment: The Missing Link in Healthcare   386

33. Education and Training Pathways   392

34. Alphabet Soup: Decoding the Letters After the Name   397

35. Professional Associations & Local Chapters   406

36. Masters Series Introduction: 412
Expert Voices on Healthcare Alignment

37. Masters Series: Learning as the Operating System of Alignment   414

38. Masters Series: Educating Humans in a Digital Healthcare World: Humanics as the Foundation of the Workforce of Tomorrow   419

39. Masters Series: Private Equity in Healthcare— The Good, The Bad and the Ugly   431

40. Masters Series: Preventing the Little Slights   438

41. Masters Series: Your 5-Year Alignment Map: From Milestones to Momentum   445

42. Masters Series: Physician Alignment: The Power of Purpose Over Position   454

43. Masters Series: The Path I Didn't Plan   465

44. Masters Series: Magnet® and the Alignment Advantage: How ANCC's Gold Standard Shapes Healthcare Careers   472

45. Masters Series: Aligning the Future of Nursing — From Bedside to Virtual   480

46. Masters Series: Breaking the Silence — Why Safety Must Be Part of Your Scrubs   488

47. Masters Series: Finding Your Path in a Profession with a Thousand Doorways   496

48. Masters Series: The Moment I Almost Walked Away   502

49. Masters Series: Aligning Hospitals, Aligning Careers: A Journey Through Mission, Merger & Meaning   507

50. Masters Series: Working with a Lifelong Vision for Quality & Safety   514

51. Masters Series: Caring Science as a Pathway to Career Alignment   524

52. Masters Series: Your Surgical Tribe: The Alignment No One Talks About   531

53. Healthcare Career Hotlist   539

54. Field of 185 Careers   551

55. 85 Careers of the Future   659

56. 50 Healthcare Side Hustles   686

57. The Pivot Playbook™   711

58. Conclusion
By Quint Studer   750

59. The Never End   756

About the Author   759
More from Mason Maison™   761

Glossary

How to Use This Glossary

You're soon going to be walking through the heart of healthcare: the people, the purpose, and the pursuit of alignment. This glossary is here to keep that journey practical.

Throughout **What Color Are Your Scrubs? (WCAYS)**, you'll notice small tags like **(gl)** beside certain words or phrases. Those tags mean the term is defined here in plain language—no jargon, no decoding required. Whether you're a nursing student, a future physician, a healthcare leader, or simply someone curious about the world behind the scrubs, this glossary is your companion.

You'll find everything from equipment and documentation shortcuts to leadership philosophies and cultural references.

Each term includes:

• A definition written for clarity (not complexity).

- A category that shows where it fits—Clinical, Process, People, Device, or Style.

- A first appearance or context to help you remember where you saw it in the book.

- A status (Active, Deprecated, or Style) showing whether the concept is in current practice or legacy use.

The goal is simple: to make healthcare language human again. Because understanding the words is the first step toward understanding the work—and yourself within it.

So take your time, flip through, and don't worry about memorizing every acronym. You're not being tested. You're being invited—to explore, to learn, and to see how each piece fits into the bigger story of care.

And who knows? One of these terms might just help you discover your own **SCRUB*fit*™**.

Here we go . . .

A

ABG (Arterial Blood Gas)

A blood test that measures oxygen, carbon dioxide, and pH levels to assess how well the lungs and metabolism are working. (Clinical / First Appearance: Ginger Gauge — Day in the Life / Active)

Acute Care

A fast-paced environment that treats patients with sudden, severe, or rapidly changing conditions, commonly found in emergency departments, intensive care units, and trauma units. (Clinical / Settings & Acuity / Active)

Adaptive Noise-Shielding

Technology that wraps around moving equipment (like drones) to cancel or soften their sound so they can operate in patient areas without adding noise. (Device / Hopewell Hospital for Tomorrow / Active)

Adaptive Smart Glass

Glass panels that automatically adjust tint, brightness, or color temperature to reduce glare, protect privacy, and support circadian rhythm. (Device / Hopewell Hospital for Tomorrow / Active)

ADC (Automated Dispensing Cabinet)

A secure, computerized medication storage system used to track and control medication access on hospital units. (Device / Polly Pillcount / Active)

AeroPrime HealthGrid™

An in-hospital drone network that moves medications, blood products, and lab specimens along ceiling tracks so supplies arrive quickly and consistently without staff running them by hand. (Device / Hopewell Hospital for Tomorrow / Active)

Alignment Debt

The accumulated emotional, financial, and cultural cost of allowing misalignment to persist within teams, departments, or health systems, which grows larger the longer it is ignored. (Concept / Alignment & Workforce Economics / Active)

Alignment Economy

The measurable financial impact that alignment—matching people to roles and environments where they can thrive—has on retention, quality, safety, and system performance. (Concept / Alignment & Workforce Economics / Active)

Alignment Inflection Point

The moment a clinician realizes that something must change in their work life—often triggered by burnout, a major life event, or a new sense of clarity about what matters most. (Concept / Mason's Alignment Theory (MAT) / Active)

Alignment Load

The total effort required for a clinician to stay functional and effective inside a misaligned environment, like carrying extra emotional weight through every shift. (Concept / Mason's Alignment Theory (MAT) / Active)

Alignment Promise

A guiding declaration that individuals deserve work that matches who they are. It emphasizes that burnout stems not from caring, but from operating in roles that contradict one's identity, and calls for shared responsibility between individuals, educators, and healthcare leaders. (Identity / Workforce Themes / Active)

Alignment Safety Net

The leaders, structures, resources, and cultural practices that help clinicians course-correct before they burn out or leave, catching them early and guiding them back toward alignment. (Concept / Organizational Design & Support / Active)

Alignment Scan

A **SCRUB*fit*™** reflection exercise helping readers evaluate whether their personality and work values match the culture of a given healthcare role. (Process / **SCRUB*fit*™** Reflection Sections / Active)

Alaris Smart Pump

A networked IV infusion pump that uses software "guardrails" to prevent medication errors by enforcing dosage limits. (Device / Polly Pillcount / Active)

Antimicrobial Stewardship

A coordinated effort to ensure antibiotics are used only when necessary, at the right dose and duration, to reduce resistance. (Process / Polly Pillcount / Active)

Anna Remedy, DNP, FNP-BC, PMHNP

A **SCRUB*fit*™** character symbolizing integrated primary care. Practical, grounded, and patient-focused; part of The Med Heads. (People / **SCRUB*fit*™** World / Active)

APP (Advanced Practice Provider)

A licensed clinician with advanced education and training who provides many of the same diagnostic, treatment, and prescriptive services as a physician. This group includes Nurse Practitioners (NPs), Physician Assistants (PAs), Certified Registered Nurse Anesthetists (CRNAs), and Clinical Nurse Specialists (CNSs). (People / Throughout book / Active)

Assessment

The clinician's ongoing collection and interpretation of data about a patient's condition; central to clinical decision-making and care planning. (Clinical / Throughout book / Active)

Archetypes

Universal role patterns representing how people naturally think, feel, and act within a care environment. In the **SCRUB***fit*™ world, each illustrated character embodies a healthcare archetype—a living example of how personality, purpose, and alignment shape care delivery. (Style / **SCRUB***fit*™ Results Section / Active)

ASHP (American Society of Health-System Pharmacists)

Professional body setting practice and safety standards for hospital pharmacists. (People / Polly Pillcount / Active)

B

Boarding (Admitted Patients)

Patients who have been admitted but remain in the Emergency Department awaiting an inpatient bed—a critical safety and throughput issue. (Process / Jen-Jen Codedale / Active)

Badge Out

To officially end one's shift by scanning an ID badge; symbolizes completion, accountability, and work-life boundaries. (Process / Clara Chartcheck / Active)

Bair Hugger

A forced-air warming blanket system that prevents hypothermia during surgery. (Device / Brad Bovie / Active)

Barcode Scanning

A safety step requiring medication and patient-armband scans before administration to ensure the "five rights": right patient, drug, dose, route, and time. (Process / Polly Pillcount / Active)

Baseline Vitals

The first set of temperature, pulse, respiration, and blood-pressure readings taken on a patient; used for comparison. (Clinical / Throughout / Active)

Bedside Recommendation (RN-to-APP)

A real-time clinical suggestion from a nurse to a prescriber or advanced practice provider, based on observation or data trend. (Process / Team Communication / Active)

Biophilic Healing

A design approach that brings natural elements like daylight, plants, water textures, and warm materials into healthcare spaces to lower stress and support physical and emotional recovery. (Design / Hopewell Hospital for Tomorrow / Active)

Biowall

A vertical living wall made of plants and integrated filtration that helps clean the air and soften the look and sound of clinical spaces. (Device / Hopewell Hospital for Tomorrow / Active)

Bloodborne Pathogens

Infectious microorganisms in blood that can cause disease in humans; prevented through standard precautions. (Clinical / Safety Foundations / Active)

Bone Conduction Headset

Device that transmits sound through skull vibrations, allowing those with certain hearing losses to perceive audio. (Device / QS Institute for Hearing & Communication / Active)

Brad Bovie, BSN, RN, CNOR

A **SCRUB*fit*™** character representing the OR circulator nurse. Precise, vigilant, and collaborative in high-stakes settings; part of The Adrenaline Team. (People / **SCRUB*fit*™** World / Active)

Bright Spots and Barriers

Hopewell Hospital's Feedback Flow Board shorthand for celebrating what's working ("bright spots") and identifying obstacles ("barriers"). (Process / Clara Chartcheck / Active)

Burnout

A state of physical, emotional, and mental exhaustion caused by chronic mismatch between a person's identity, preferred work patterns, and the demands of their role, often emerging when work contradicts an individual's strengths or values. (Workforce Themes / Wellness / Active)

Burnout Barrier

A metaphor and tool in **SCRUB*fit*™** reflection exercises that prompts users to identify early warning signs of compassion fatigue. (Process / Reflection & Self-Protection / Active)

C

CalmBoard Display

A wall-integrated, low-glare digital screen that stays blank until needed, then shows a patient's plan of care, education, and messages in simple language. (Device / Hopewell Hospital for Tomorrow / Active)

Career Micro-Pivots

Small, strategic changes in a clinician's job, schedule, specialty, or setting that can significantly improve alignment without requiring a full career change. (Concept / Career Design & Alignment / Active)

CARESET™

A proprietary alignment framework created by Mason Preddy that defines the external conditions that shape whether healthcare professionals can thrive in a role. CARESET™ stands for Culture, Autonomy, Resources, Expectations, Structure, Environment, and Team. (Framework / Mason's Alignment Theory (MAT) / Active)

Caritas Garden

A multisensory healing space within Hopewell Hospital's Watson Corridor, inspired by Jean Watson's Caritas Processes®. (People & Process / Hopewell Hospital for Tomorrow / Active)

CDI (Clinical Documentation Integrity)

Program ensuring patient records accurately reflect the care provided, linking clinical data to quality metrics and reimbursement. (Process / Clara Chartcheck / Active)

Chain-of-Custody Kit

Secure forensic evidence-collection set used by SANE nurses to document, seal, and track samples. (Device / Justice Jules / Active)

Charting

The act of documenting care in the medical record; central to communication and legal protection. (Process / Throughout / Active)

Clinical Confession

A personal, reflective quote included in each **SCRUB*fit*™** profile revealing a moment of humility, humor, or learning. (Style / **SCRUB*fit*™** Template / Active)

Clinical Decision Support

Electronic prompts within an EHR that guide safe, evidence-based choices (for example, drug-interaction alerts). (Process / Polly Pillcount / Active)

Clara Chartcheck, RHIA

A **SCRUB*fit*™** character representing the Health Information Management Director. Analytical, organized, and ethically grounded; the data conscience of The Vital Link. (People / **SCRUB*fit*™** World / Active)

Closed-Loop Communication

Safety technique where team members repeat back critical information to confirm accuracy. (Process / Team Safety / Active)

Command Bridge

A real-time operations center in Hopewell Hospital for Tomorrow that visualizes live clinical and operational metrics to support rapid, informed decisions. (Process / Hopewell Hospital for Tomorrow / Active)

Compassion Fatigue

Emotional exhaustion from sustained empathy and patient care, often mitigated through recovery practices, support, and reflection. (Workforce Themes / Compassion Corps / Active)

COPN (Certificate of Public Need)

A regulatory approval process used in several U.S. states to determine whether new healthcare services, facilities, or major equipment purchases are needed in a community. (Regulatory / Leadership League / Active)

Cultural Competence

The ability to deliver care that respects and integrates a patient's cultural beliefs, language, and values. (Process / Education Themes / Active)

Curbside Consult

An informal, quick exchange of clinical advice between colleagues outside formal documentation channels. (Process / Clinical Collaboration / Active)

Crimson Quest, MD

A **SCRUB*fit*™** character representing the physician's drive for discovery. Analytical, intense, and relentless in pursuit of better outcomes; part of The Med Heads. (People / **SCRUB*fit*™** World / Active)

D

DAR Note (Data, Action, Response)

A focused documentation format used by nurses to record

concise patient information, interventions, and outcomes. (Process / Nursing Education / Active)

Dashboard (Clinical)

A real-time digital display showing patient data, performance metrics, or safety indicators for quick situational awareness. (Device & Process / Hopewell Hospital for Tomorrow / Active)

Darcy Heplock, MLS(ASCP)

A **SCRUB*fit*™** character representing the Medical Laboratory Scientist. Exacting, detail-oriented, and indispensable behind the scenes; part of The Diagnostic Division. (People / **SCRUB*fit*™** World / Active)

Data Integrity

The accuracy and consistency of health information across systems; protected through auditing, encryption, and validation processes. (Process / The Vital Link / Active)

De-escalation

Calming techniques used to safely reduce agitation in patients, often part of crisis-prevention training. (Clinical / Compassion Corps / Active)

DEA Schedule

Federal classification system ranking controlled substances by medical use and abuse potential. (Process / Polly Pillcount / Active)

Defibrillator

Emergency device that delivers an electric shock to restore

normal heart rhythm in cardiac arrest or certain life-threatening rhythms. (Device / Adrenaline Team / Active)

Diagnostics

Healthcare roles focused on identifying conditions, gathering clinical data, and supporting medical decisions through imaging, laboratory analysis, or specialized testing. (People & Process / Career Categories / Active)

Digital Twin Studio™

A simulation tool that creates a detailed digital copy of a patient's anatomy and condition so clinicians can practice and refine treatments or procedures in advance. (Device / Hopewell Hospital for Tomorrow / Active)

Discrepancy (Medication)

Any mismatch between ordered, dispensed, administered, or documented medications; investigated to prevent diversion or error. (Process / Polly Pillcount / Active)

Diversion Prevention

Systems and monitoring processes that detect and prevent misuse or theft of controlled medications. (Process / Polly Pillcount / Active)

DNFB (Discharged Not Final Billed)

Hospital billing status indicating charts awaiting coding or documentation before claim submission. (Process / Clara Chartcheck / Active)

Documentation Amendment

The process of correcting or adding information to a medical record while preserving the integrity of the original entry. (Process / Clara Chartcheck / Active)

DVI-STAT

DVI-STAT — A bedside cognitive support system that verifies medication and clinical steps in real time, helping reduce errors caused by stress, interruption, and cognitive bias without replacing human clinical judgment. (Patient safety technology / Cognitive support / Near-future innovation)

E

EHR (Electronic Health Record)

The digital version of a patient's paper chart containing medical history, test results, medications, and treatment plans. (Device & Process / Throughout / Active)

EHR Downtime

Planned or unplanned periods when electronic systems are unavailable; teams revert to paper workflows to maintain safety and continuity of care. (Process / The Vital Link / Active)

Electrolytes

Minerals in the body (like sodium, potassium, and calcium) that help nerves, muscles, and the heart function properly. (Clinical / Throughout / Active)

Emotional GPS

The inner signals—intuition, energy level, fulfillment, and tension—that help clinicians sense whether a role or setting is moving them toward better alignment or deeper misalignment. (Concept / Mason's Alignment Theory (MAT) / Active)

Environment–Identity Clash

A specific kind of misalignment where the setting, culture, or pace of a workplace contradicts how a clinician is wired to thrive, often becoming a precursor to burnout or rapid turnover. (Concept / Mason's Alignment Theory (MAT) / Active)

Epic Circuit, MS, CPHIMS

A **SCRUB*fit*™** character representing the Healthcare IT Engineer. Systems-savvy, adaptable, and mission-critical; connects clinical teams through technology in The Power Panel. (People / **SCRUB*fit*™** World / Active)

Epinephrine (Adrenaline)

Life-saving medication used to treat anaphylaxis and cardiac arrest; works by constricting blood vessels and opening airways. (Clinical / Adrenaline Team / Active)

Evidence-Based Practice (EBP)

Integrating the best research, clinical expertise, and patient preferences to guide care decisions. (Process / Education & Training / Active)

Evidence Transfer (Forensic)

The official handoff of sealed evidence from a healthcare facility to law enforcement or a regional crime lab. (Process / Justice Jules / Active)

Exemplar

A reflective story used in nursing portfolios or Magnet applications to demonstrate professional practice excellence. (Style / Leadership League / Active)

Exposure Response Plan

A safety protocol outlining steps to take after potential contact with infectious material, including reporting, testing, and follow-up care. (Process / Compassion Corps / Active)

F

Feedback Flow Board

Hopewell Hospital's continuous-improvement dashboard using color codes (Green = Approved, Yellow = Under Review, Red = Not Approved) to visualize project progress and staff input. (Process / Hopewell Hospital for Tomorrow / Active)

FiO_2 (Fraction of Inspired Oxygen)

The concentration of oxygen in the air mixture delivered to a patient; adjusted for those on ventilators or supplemental oxygen. (Clinical / Ginger Gauge / Active)

The Fillin' Station

Hopewell's retro-themed diner and staff hub blending nostalgia, comfort food, and community. (People & Style / Hopewell Hospital for Tomorrow / Active)

Florence Lonergan Heart & Vascular Institute

A Hopewell Hospital institute focusing on cardiac prevention, genomics, and hybrid procedures; features The Living Heart installation. (People & Process / Hopewell Hospital for Tomorrow / Active)

Forensic Light Source

Specialized lighting used by SANE nurses to detect biological evidence on skin or clothing. (Device / Justice Jules / Active)

Forensic Nurse Examiner (FNE / SANE)

A registered nurse trained to care for survivors of sexual assault and trauma, blending clinical care with evidence collection. (People / Compassion Corps / Active)

Flow Restrictor (Oxygen)

A small mechanical device that limits oxygen flow from a wall outlet or tank to ensure precise delivery. (Device / Compassion Corps / Active)

Full Code / DNR

Indicates a patient's resuscitation status: "Full Code" for all life-saving measures; "DNR" (Do Not Resuscitate) for comfort-focused care without resuscitation. (Process / Adrenaline Team / Active)

Future Readiness Index

Hopewell's internal benchmark tracking how innovations align with safety, satisfaction, and sustainability goals. (Process / Hopewell Hospital for Tomorrow / Active)

G

Gait Belt

A sturdy strap placed around a patient's waist to provide support and stability during transfers or assisted walking. (Device / Compassion Corps / Active)

GE Definium 656 HD

A digital X-ray system with wireless detectors used for imaging across emergency, surgical, and inpatient units. (Device / Ray Beam / Active)

Gesture-Based Interaction

A way for clinicians to work with large displays or data by using hand movements instead of touching screens or keyboards. (Device / Hopewell Hospital for Tomorrow / Active)

Ginger Gauge, RRT

A **SCRUB*fit*™** character representing the Respiratory Therapist. Known for precision, compassion, and calm leadership on Hopewell's respiratory team; part of The Compassion Corps. (People / **SCRUB*fit*™** World / Active)

Glasgow Coma Scale (GCS)

An assessment scoring system measuring eye, verbal, and motor responses to evaluate level of consciousness. (Clinical / Adrenaline Team / Active)

Green Status (Feedback Flow Board)

Indicates that an initiative or practice change has been fully approved and assigned a go-live or arrival date. (Process / Hopewell Hospital for Tomorrow / Active)

Guardrails (Medication Safety)

Software limits programmed into infusion pumps or EHR systems to prevent unsafe dosing and reduce medication errors. (Process / Polly Pillcount / Active)

Guided Magnetic Docking

A connection system that uses magnets to automatically align and attach equipment—like mobility platforms to beds—for safer, more precise transfers. (Device / Hopewell Hospital for Tomorrow / Active)

H

Handoff Communication

The transfer of essential patient information and responsibility between caregivers during shift changes, admissions, discharges, or transfers. (Process / Throughout / Active)

Hamilton-G5 Ventilator

An advanced mechanical ventilator offering adaptive support and lung-protective modes. (Device / Ginger Gauge / Active)

Hand Hygiene

The single most effective action to prevent infection; performed before and after every patient contact. (Process / Compassion Corps / Active)

Harper Helpwell, CMA (AAMA)

A **SCRUB*fit*™** character representing the Certified Medical Assistant. Empathetic, dependable, and bridge-building; embodies connection within The Care Crew. (People / **SCRUB*fit*™** World / Active)

HCAHPS

A national survey measuring patient perceptions of hospital care quality and experience. (Process / Leadership League / Active)

Healthcare DNA

The natural patterns in how a person thinks, communicates, reacts to pressure, solves problems, and moves through the world—tendencies that influence which healthcare environments feel energizing versus draining. (Identity / Personal Traits / Active)

Health Information Management (HIM)

The field specializing in data accuracy, privacy, and information governance within healthcare organizations. (People & Process / The Vital Link / Active)

HomeSuite Halo Kits™

Compact home-care kits that include vitals monitors, small infusion pumps, supplies, and a connection back to the hospital so some patients can safely receive hospital-level care at home. (Device / Hopewell Hospital for Tomorrow / Active)

Hope Fulle, RN, BSN

A **SCRUB*fit*™** character representing the oncology nurse—endurance, advocacy, and steady compassion as part of The Compassion Corps. (People / **SCRUB*fit*™** World / Active)

Hopewell Hospital for Tomorrow

A futuristic, integrated care campus designed by Mason Preddy as a model for alignment, inclusion, and innovation in healthcare. (People & Process / Hopewell Hospital for Tomorrow / Active)

Hospital-Acquired Infection (HAI)

An infection patients acquire during hospitalization that was not present on admission. (Clinical / Compassion Corps / Active)

Human Capital Drift

The slow loss of talent from a unit, organization, or region caused by misalignment, weak support, or unsustainable working conditions—often noticed only after vacancies and burnout spike. (Concept / Workforce Strategy / Active)

I

ICU (Intensive Care Unit)

A specialized hospital unit providing continuous monitoring and advanced life support for critically ill or unstable patients. (Clinical / Adrenaline Team / Active)

Identity Footprint

A person's unique combination of values, wiring, strengths, and needs that shapes how they experience different roles and environments in healthcare. (Concept / Mason's Alignment Theory (MAT) / Active)

IMAX Conversion (Kinzie Gallery)

An architectural feature allowing the Kinzie Gallery to transform between theater, ballroom, and expo hall through hydraulic reconfiguration. (Process / Hopewell Hospital for Tomorrow / Active)

Informatics Nurse

A clinician who integrates data science, systems design, and workflow optimization to improve care delivery and usability of digital tools. (People / The Vital Link / Active)

Inline Suction

A closed respiratory system that allows airway suctioning without disconnecting a patient from the ventilator. (Device / Ginger Gauge / Active)

Injection Safety

Practices that prevent infection during injections, including sterile technique, proper disposal, and single-use vials when required. (Process / Compassion Corps / Active)

Informed Consent

A legal and ethical process ensuring patients understand and agree to the risks, benefits, and alternatives of a treatment or procedure. (Process / Compassion Corps / Active)

Inpatient

Care delivered in settings where patients stay overnight or longer, often involving higher acuity, continuous monitoring, and interdisciplinary coordination. (Clinical / Operations / Active)

Integrity Loop (Data)

A continuous review system within Hopewell's Vital Link that ensures data accuracy, privacy compliance, and corrective action when issues are detected. (Process / Hopewell Hospital for Tomorrow / Active)

Interdisciplinary Team (IDT)

A group of professionals from multiple disciplines collaborating to provide comprehensive, coordinated patient care. (People & Process / Throughout / Active)

ISMP (Institute for Safe Medication Practices)

An organization dedicated to researching medication errors and promoting best practices for medication safety. (People / Polly Pillcount / Active)

J

Jen-Jen Codedale, RN, BSN

A **SCRUB*fit*™** character representing the Emergency Department nurse—quick-thinking, team-driven, and centered under pressure as part of The Adrenaline Team. (People / **SCRUB*fit*™** World / Active)

JCAHO (Joint Commission on Accreditation of Healthcare Organizations)

The former name still commonly used to refer to The Joint Commission, the national accrediting body that conducts unannounced surveys of healthcare organizations. (Regulatory / Leadership League / Active)

Justice Jules, RN, SANE-A

A **SCRUB*fit*™** character representing the Forensic Nurse Examiner—purpose-driven, meticulous, and fiercely protective of patient dignity within The Compassion Corps. (People / **SCRUB*fit*™** World / Active)

Just Culture

A leadership philosophy that balances accountability and learning by distinguishing between human error, risky behavior, and reckless conduct. (Process / Leadership League / Active)

K

Kinzie Gallery

A transformative space inside Hopewell Hospital for Tomorrow that functions as an auditorium, ballroom, or learning hub through adaptive architecture. (People & Process / Hopewell Hospital for Tomorrow / Active)

Krashlyn Riggs, EMT-P

A SCRUB*fit*™ character representing the paramedic—bold, resourceful, and unstoppable in the field as part of The Adrenaline Team. (People / SCRUB*fit*™ World / Active)

KSA (Knowledge, Skills, Abilities)

A framework used to evaluate workforce competency, readiness, and role fit in healthcare education and hiring. (Process / Education & Training / Active)

L

Lab Values

Numeric results from diagnostic tests that guide diagnosis, treatment decisions, and monitoring of patient status. (Clinical / Diagnostic Division / Active)

Laser Safety Protocol

Guidelines designed to protect staff and patients during laser use in surgical, dermatologic, or ophthalmologic procedures. (Process / Adrenaline Team / Active)

Leadership League

A SCRUB*fit*™ category representing executive and managerial professionals who drive vision, safety, culture, and alignment. (People / SCRUB*fit*™ World / Active)

Lead-Lined Doors

Protective doors constructed with internal lead shielding to block ionizing radiation in imaging and nuclear medicine areas. (Device / Ray Beam — Day in the Life / Active)

Lean Process Improvement

A methodology focused on reducing waste and improving efficiency while preserving safety and quality in healthcare workflows. (Process / Leadership League / Active)

Lilac Lift, DPT

A SCRUB*fit*™ character representing the Physical Therapist—supportive, restorative, and movement-focused within The Recovery Regimen. (People / SCRUB*fit*™ World / Active)

Living Heart (Installation)

A large biomechanical heart installation at the Florence Lonergan Heart & Vascular Institute displaying real-time rhythms and data. (Device & Style / Hopewell Hospital for Tomorrow / Active)

Liv Well, OTR/L

A SCRUB*fit*™ character representing the Occupational Therapist—creative, adaptive, and independence-focused within The Recovery Regimen. (People / SCRUB*fit*™ World / Active)

LPN (Licensed Practical Nurse)

A nurse who provides basic bedside care under the supervision of a registered nurse or physician. (People / Education Pathways / Active)

LucentBio Atmos™

An ambient environment system that subtly adjusts lighting, tone, and sensory cues in patient rooms to promote rest and reduce stress. (Device / Hopewell Hospital for Tomorrow / Active)

Lung Recruitment Maneuver

A ventilator technique used to reopen collapsed alveoli and improve oxygenation. (Clinical / Ginger Gauge / Active)

LVN (Licensed Vocational Nurse)

The equivalent credential to LPN in certain U.S. states. (People / Education Pathways / Active)

M

Macro-Alignment

The foundational decision of choosing a healthcare identity, credential, or professional ecosystem that best matches a person's natural patterns, motivations, and long-term needs. (Career Development / Identity Fit / Active)

Magnet Recognition Program®

A credential awarded by the American Nurses Credentialing Center recognizing excellence in nursing practice, leadership, and patient outcomes. (Process / Leadership League / Active)

Manual Restraint

A last-resort physical intervention used to prevent harm when a patient is violent or unsafe; requires strict documentation and debriefing. (Process / Compassion Corps / Active)

Masimo Oximetry

Pulse oximetry technology that provides continuous readings of oxygen saturation and perfusion status. (Device / Ginger Gauge / Active)

Max Volt, BMET

A SCRUB*fit*™ character representing the Biomedical Equipment Technician—innovative, dependable, and essential to hospital operations within The Power Panel. (People / SCRUB*fit*™ World / Active)

Medication Reconciliation

The formal process of verifying a patient's complete medication list at every transition of care to prevent errors. (Process / Polly Pillcount / Active)

MedMotion Dynamics™ Mobility Platform

An autonomous transport unit that docks to hospital beds and assists with safe patient movement, reducing physical strain on staff. (Device / Hopewell Hospital for Tomorrow / Active)

Meso-Alignment

Mid-level career adjustments made within a credential—such as switching specialties, settings, or patient populations—to refine fit without changing professions. (Career Development / Identity Fit / Active)

Micro-Alignment

Small day-to-day changes that improve fit within a role, such as adjusting pace, shift type, communication style, or team dynamics. (Career Development / Identity Fit / Active)

Micro-Haptic Feedback

Subtle vibration cues built into devices or controls that confirm actions without visual or auditory interruption. (Device / Hopewell Hospital for Tomorrow / Active)

Mindfulness Pause

A brief moment taken before critical tasks to center attention, reduce error, and support emotional regulation. (Process / Compassion Corps / Active)

Mini SCRUB*fit*™ Healthcare Career Assessment

A short introductory assessment that highlights pace preference, interaction style, task focus, and pressure response to guide early alignment insights. (Career Tools / Assessment / Active)

Minty Mary, RDH

A SCRUB*fit*™ character representing the Registered Dental Hygienist—prevention-focused, detail-oriented, and proactive within The Prevention Pact. (People / SCRUB*fit*™ World / Active)

Mission Drift

When an organization's actions, incentives, or culture move away from its stated purpose, often weakening alignment and morale. (Process / Leadership League / Active)

Mode (Ventilation)

The control setting on a ventilator that determines how breaths are delivered and supported. (Device / Ginger Gauge / Active)

Mouth-to-Mask Ventilation

A resuscitation technique delivering breaths through a barrier device to protect both patient and provider. (Clinical / Adrenaline Team / Active)

N

Naloxone (Narcan)

A medication that rapidly reverses opioid overdose by restoring normal breathing. (Clinical / Polly Pillcount / Active)

Near Miss

An event that could have caused harm but did not, either by chance or timely intervention; used for learning and prevention. (Process / Safety & Quality / Active)

Neutral Zone (Surgery)

A designated area where sharps are placed and retrieved without hand-to-hand passing to reduce injury risk. (Process / Brad Bovie / Active)

Non-Negotiables (Alignment)

Core personal values or conditions that must be met for a role to be sustainable and aligned. (Process / Alignment Evaluation / Active)

Non-Verbal Cues

Body language, eye contact, posture, and tone that influence communication effectiveness in care settings. (Process / Compassion Corps / Active)

Nurse Navigator

A clinician who guides patients through complex care pathways, coordinating services and providing education and emotional support. (People / Compassion Corps / Active)

O

Obi

A robotic self-feeding assistive device that helps individuals with upper-extremity mobility impairments eat more independently by adapting to user motion, pacing, and tremor. (Rehabilitation Technology / Assistive Robotics / Active)

On-Call Rotation

A scheduled period during which staff must be available to respond to urgent needs outside regular hours. (Process / Compassion Corps / Active)

Open Disclosure

Transparent communication with patients and families following an adverse event or error. (Process / Leadership League / Active)

Operating Room (OR)

A controlled surgical environment where sterile technique is maintained and operative procedures are performed. (Clinical / Adrenaline Team / Active)

Opioid Stewardship

A coordinated initiative ensuring opioids are prescribed and monitored responsibly to reduce misuse and harm. (Process / Polly Pillcount / Active)

Outpatient

Care delivered in settings where patients are evaluated, treated, and discharged the same day, often with more predictable schedules. (Clinical / Operations / Active)

Oxygen Concentrator

A device that filters nitrogen from ambient air to deliver purified oxygen to patients. (Device / Compassion Corps / Active)

Oxygen Saturation (SpO$_2$)

A measure of how much oxygen the blood is carrying compared to its maximum capacity. (Clinical / Ginger Gauge / Active)

P

PACS (Picture Archiving and Communication System)

A digital imaging platform used to store, retrieve, and share radiology studies. (Device / Ray Beam / Active)

Passive Biosensor Patch

A thin wearable sensor that continuously tracks vital signs without requiring patient interaction. (Device / Hopewell Hospital for Tomorrow / Active)

Patient-Centered Care

A care model that prioritizes patient preferences, values, and needs in all clinical decisions. (Process / Compassion Corps / Active)

Patient Safety Event

Any occurrence that did or could have resulted in patient harm, used for reporting, learning, and prevention. (Process / Leadership League / Active)

People Investment Gap

The difference between what healthcare organizations should invest in their workforce to reduce burnout and turnover and what they actually invest. (Concept / Alignment & Workforce Economics / Active)

Perfusion

The flow of blood through tissue, delivering oxygen and nutrients necessary for cellular function. (Clinical / Adrenaline Team / Active)

Personal Protective Equipment (PPE)

Items such as gloves, gowns, masks, and eye protection that reduce exposure to infectious or hazardous materials. (Device / Compassion Corps / Active)

Pharmacokinetics

The study of how the body absorbs, distributes, metabolizes, and excretes medications. (Clinical / Polly Pillcount / Active)

Polly Pillcount, PharmD

A **SCRUB*fit*™** character representing the Hospital Pharmacist

—methodical, safety-driven, and systems-oriented within The Med Heads. (People / SCRUB*fit*™ World / Active)

Power Panel

A **SCRUB*fit*™** category representing biomedical and IT professionals who keep healthcare systems running behind the scenes. (People / SCRUB*fit*™ World / Active)

Privacy Byte

Hopewell's daily micro-training on confidentiality and data protection delivered through the EHR login banner. (Process / Hopewell Hospital for Tomorrow / Active)

Pulse Oximeter

A device that measures blood oxygen saturation using light sensors placed on a fingertip or earlobe. (Device / Compassion Corps / Active)

Pulse Picture Wall

A digital mural inside The Fillin' Station replaying cultural, educational, and healthcare media. (Device & Style / Hopewell Hospital for Tomorrow / Active)

Q

Quality Improvement (QI)

A systematic approach to measuring, analyzing, and improving healthcare processes, outcomes, and safety. (Process / Leadership League / Active)

Quiet Superpowers

Subtle strengths—such as listening, intuition, steadiness, and emotional awareness—that help healthcare professionals succeed but are often overlooked. (Style / **SCRUB*fit*™** Profiles / Active)

Quint Studer Influence

A reference to leadership and culture-building principles that inform Hopewell's alignment-focused design and workforce philosophy. (People / Leadership League / Active)

R

Radiometer ABL90

A blood-gas analyzer that provides rapid results for oxygenation, ventilation, and acid–base balance. (Device / Ginger Gauge / Active)

Ray Beam, RT(R)

A **SCRUB*fit*™** character representing the Radiologic Technologist—technically precise and quietly confident within The Diagnostic Division. (People / **SCRUB*fit*™** World / Active)

Recovery Regimen

A **SCRUB*fit*™** category uniting rehabilitation, therapy, and recovery-focused professionals who guide patients back to function. (People / **SCRUB*fit*™** World / Active)

Red Rules (Safety)

Non-negotiable safety behaviors that must always be followed to prevent catastrophic errors. (Process / Leadership League / Active)

Red Status (Feedback Flow Board)

Indicates that an initiative has been halted or not approved, with reasons documented for transparency and learning. (Process / Hopewell Hospital for Tomorrow / Active)

Reflective Practice

The habit of examining experiences to improve clinical judgment, self-awareness, and professional growth. (Process / Education Themes / Active)

Respiratory Therapist (RT)

A clinician specializing in airway management, mechanical ventilation, and cardiopulmonary support. (People / Compassion Corps / Active)

ROI (Release of Information)

The regulated process of providing medical records to authorized individuals while protecting patient privacy. (Process / Clara Chartcheck / Active)

Role–Reality Gap

The difference between expectations about a healthcare career and the actual day-to-day demands once in the role. (Concept / Career Expectations / Active)

Rounds

Scheduled interdisciplinary discussions reviewing patient progress, plans of care, and coordination needs. (Process / Throughout / Active)

Rounding for Outcomes

Rounding for Outcomes — A structured leadership practice developed by the Studer Group in which leaders conduct regular, purposeful rounds with staff and patients to identify barriers, reinforce best practices, recognize good work, and improve clinical, operational, and experiential outcomes through real-time feedback and follow-up. (Leadership Practice / Healthcare Operations / Active)

Route to the Role

A section in each **SCRUB*fit*™** profile outlining educational pathways, credentials, and entry points into a career. (Style / **SCRUB*fit*™** Templates / Active)

Rural Health Clinic (RHC)

A federally certified outpatient facility designed to improve access to care in underserved or rural communities. (People & Process / Prevention Pact / Active)

S

Safety Callout

A dedicated section within **SCRUB*fit*™** chapters highlighting key lessons from real clinical cases. (Style / **SCRUB*fit*™** Templates / Active)

Safety Culture

Shared values, beliefs, and behaviors that make safety a system priority rather than an individual burden. (Process / Leadership League / Active)

Sage Engage, MPH

A **SCRUB*fit*™** character representing the Community Health Educator—prevention-focused and proactive within The Prevention Pact. (People / **SCRUB*fit*™** World / Active)

SANE Kit (Sexual Assault Nurse Examiner Kit)

An evidence-collection kit containing swabs, documentation materials, and containers used during forensic exams. (Device / Justice Jules / Active)

SBAR (Situation, Background, Assessment, Recommendation)

A structured communication framework for concise, effective clinical handoffs and updates. (Process / Adrenaline Team / Active)

SCD (Sequential Compression Device)

A pneumatic sleeve system that inflates rhythmically to promote blood flow and reduce clot risk in immobile patients. (Device / Brad Bovie / Active)

Scope of Practice

The tasks and responsibilities a healthcare professional is legally authorized to perform based on licensure and training. (Process / Education Themes / Active)

SCRUB*fit*™

A healthcare identity model that helps individuals understand which environments, team structures, and role characteristics best match their natural patterns, supporting sustainable career alignment. (Career Framework / Identity / Active)

Sepsis

A life-threatening condition caused by a dysregulated response to infection, leading to organ dysfunction; requires rapid recognition and treatment. (Clinical / Adrenaline Team / Active)

Sepsis Bundle

A time-sensitive set of coordinated interventions—labs, fluids, antibiotics—shown to improve outcomes in sepsis care. (Process / Adrenaline Team / Active)

Simulation Lab

A hands-on training environment using manikins or virtual reality to practice clinical scenarios safely. (Process / Education & Training / Active)

Sitting for Boards

The act of taking a national or state licensing exam required for professional certification. (Process / Education Pathways / Active)

SMART Goals

Objectives that are Specific, Measurable, Achievable, Relevant, and Time-bound, commonly used in professional development. (Process / Leadership League / Active)

Social Determinants of Health (SDOH)

Economic, social, and environmental factors that influence health outcomes beyond medical care. (Process / Prevention Pact / Active)

Soft-Robotic Micro-Actuators

Flexible robotic components inside equipment that move smoothly to support positioning, lifting, or comfort without rigid motion. (Device / Hopewell Hospital for Tomorrow / Active)

SpO$_2$ (Peripheral Oxygen Saturation)

The percentage of oxygen-saturated hemoglobin in the blood, measured noninvasively by pulse oximetry. (Clinical / Compassion Corps / Active)

Stark Law

A U.S. federal law that prohibits physicians from referring patients to certain healthcare services in which they or their immediate family members have a financial interest unless a specific exception applies. (Healthcare Regulation / Compliance / Active)

Sterile Field

A designated area maintained free of microorganisms during invasive procedures to prevent infection. (Clinical / Adrenaline Team / Active)

Structural Mismatch

A condition in which a clinician's identity or working style is fundamentally out of sync with their role, unit, or organization, leading to chronic strain or burnout. (Concept / Mason's Alignment Theory / Active)

Stryker OneFrame™ Bed

A next-generation hospital bed using sensors and soft robotics to redistribute pressure and reduce manual repositioning. (Device / Hopewell Hospital for Tomorrow / Active)

Suction Canister

A container that collects fluids removed during airway or surgical suctioning. (Device / Ginger Gauge / Active)

Surgical Count

A verification process ensuring instruments, sponges, and sharps are accounted for before and after surgery. (Process / Brad Bovie / Active)

Surgical Time-Out

A mandatory pause before incision to confirm correct patient, procedure, and site. (Process / Adrenaline Team / Active)

Sustainability Metrics

Measures tracking environmental impact, energy use, and waste reduction in healthcare operations. (Process / Leadership League / Active)

Suzette Soleil, RN

A **SCRUB*fit*™** character representing radiant empathy and teamwork within The Compassion Corps. (People / **SCRUB*fit*™** World / Active)

Synexis Command Hub

A centralized operations center monitoring real-time data across hospital and home-care settings to detect early warning signs and coordinate response. (Process / Hopewell Hospital for Tomorrow / Active)

T

Telemetry

Continuous electronic monitoring of a patient's heart rhythm. (Device / Adrenaline Team / Active)

Telepresence Window

A depth-aware video system that makes virtual clinician visits feel more immersive than standard video calls. (Device / Hopewell Hospital for Tomorrow / Active)

Theatre (Operating Room Theatre)

A term used in the UK and some international systems to refer to the operating room; emphasizes the coordinated, high-precision environment where surgical care is delivered. (Clinical / Surgical Settings / Active)

Therapeutic Communication

Intentional use of language, tone, and presence to promote trust, understanding, and healing. (Process / Compassion Corps / Active)

The Vital Link

A **SCRUB*fit*™** category representing information, data, and bridge-building roles connecting care and technology. (People / **SCRUB*fit*™** World / Active)

Time-Out Sacred

An OR phrase reinforcing that the surgical time-out is deliberate, protected, and non-negotiable. (Style / Brad Bovie / Active)

Tool of the Trade

Essential equipment or devices associated with a specific clinical role, highlighted in **SCRUB*fit*™** profiles. (Style /

SCRUB*fit*™ Templates / Active)

Transparency Atrium

Hopewell's glass-walled dashboard space displaying real-time financial, operational, and sustainability data. (Process / Hopewell Hospital for Tomorrow / Active)

Tranquil Path Candle

A sensory item used in forensic and trauma exam spaces to help restore calm and grounding. (Device & Style / Justice Jules / Active)

Trauma Surgeon

A physician specializing in rapid surgical management of critically injured patients. (People & Clinical Role / Adrenaline Team / Active)

Triage

The process of prioritizing patients based on urgency of need and available resources. (Clinical / Adrenaline Team / Active)

TrioPerf

A simplified infusion valve system designed to eliminate common human-factor failure points by reducing steps and reliance on memory during flow adjustments. (Medical Device / Human-Factors Engineering / Active)

Tubing Change Protocol

Scheduled replacement of IV or ventilator tubing to maintain infection control and patient safety. (Process / Compassion Corps / Active)

Turnover Shockwave

The ripple effect created when a key clinician leaves, impacting morale, workload, onboarding burden, and team alignment. (Concept / Workforce Strategy / Active)

U

Universal Precautions

An infection-control approach that treats all blood and bodily fluids as potentially infectious. (Process / Compassion Corps / Active)

Upcoding

Inaccurate billing of a higher level of service than was actually provided; considered fraudulent. (Process / The Vital Link / Active)

Urinalysis (UA)

A laboratory test of urine used to detect metabolic, infectious, or renal conditions. (Clinical / Diagnostic Division / Active)

User Interface (UI)

The visual layout and interaction design of digital systems affecting usability and workflow. (Device & Process / The Vital Link / Active)

V

Vera Vines, RN, MSN, MBA

A **SCRUB*fit*™** character representing the Hospital CEO—visionary, authentic leadership within The Leadership League. (People / **SCRUB*fit*™** World / Active)

Ventilator-Associated Pneumonia (VAP)

A lung infection that develops in intubated patients. (Clinical / Compassion Corps / Active)

Vital Signs

Core physiological measurements including temperature, pulse, respirations, blood pressure, and oxygen saturation. (Clinical / Throughout / Active)

Vyaire Avea Ventilator

An advanced neonatal and adult ventilator offering precise monitoring and lung-protective ventilation modes. (Device / Ginger Gauge / Active)

VTE Prophylaxis (Venous Thromboembolism)

Preventive measures such as compression devices or anticoagulants to reduce blood-clot risk. (Clinical / Brad Bovie / Active)

W

Wasserman Corridor

A passageway in Hopewell Hospital featuring the Wall of Voices—an interactive display of recorded staff and patient stories. (Style & Process / Hopewell Hospital for Tomorrow / Active)

Wasting with Witness

A required documentation step when discarding unused controlled substances to ensure accountability. (Process / Polly Pillcount / Active)

Wellness Rounds

A leadership practice focused on checking in with staff about workload, stress, and emotional well-being. (Process / Leadership League / Active)

Wheels In

OR shorthand signaling the patient's arrival and the transition from preparation to surgical time-out. (Style / Brad Bovie / Active)

Workflow

The sequence and organization of daily tasks within a healthcare role. (Work Environment / Operations / Active)

Workflow Optimization

The redesign of tasks and processes to improve efficiency, safety, and sustainability. (Process / The Vital Link / Active)

Workforce Gravity

The invisible force that keeps clinicians in roles where they feel valued and aligned. (Concept / Workforce Strategy / Active)

X

X-Ray Shielding

Protective lead barriers or garments used to reduce radiation exposure during imaging. (Device / Diagnostic Division / Active)

Y

Yellow Status (Feedback Flow Board)

Indicates an initiative is under review or pending approval before advancing. (Process / Hopewell Hospital for Tomorrow / Active)

Youth Volunteer Program

A Hopewell initiative introducing high-school students to healthcare careers. (People & Process / Prevention Pact / Active)

Z

Zero Harm

A safety philosophy aiming to eliminate preventable patient injuries through systems design and accountability. (Process / Leadership League / Active)

Zoom Interview

A virtual interview format used for healthcare hiring and residency selection. (Process / Education Themes / Active)

ZimmerStryker Nexus™ System

An integrated operating-room platform linking robotics, imaging, and instrument tracking to support safer surgeries. (Device / Hopewell Hospital for Tomorrow / Active)

100 Words Every Healthcare Professional Should Know

This section is a companion to the glossary — not a continuation of it.

These are not acronyms.

They are not protocols.

They are not tested on exams.

They are the words that quietly shape how care feels, how teams function, and how professionals stay human inside demanding systems. You'll hear them in hallways, sense them during hard shifts, and feel their absence when something is off.

Use these words not to *sound* like a clinician — but to **think** like one.

To notice what matters.

To find your rhythm in the world behind the scrubs.

A

Accountability — Owning your actions, even when no one is watching.

Adaptability — Shifting course without losing your center.

Advocacy — Using your voice to protect and uplift others.

Alignment — When your purpose and your practice move in the same direction.

Altruism — Helping without expecting credit.

Ambiguity — The gray space where judgment becomes skill.

Attunement — Sensing what someone needs without being told.

Authenticity — Being real in a world of roles.

Awareness — The first step toward meaningful change.

B

Balance — Not equal time, but intentional energy.

Belonging — The quiet confidence of knowing you fit where you stand.

Boundary — The invisible line that keeps compassion sustainable.

Bravery — Action in the presence of fear.

Burnout — A signal of misalignment, not weakness.

C

Calibration — Re-centering when your internal compass drifts.

Care — The universal language of healing.

Clarity — When confusion gives way to confidence.

Collaboration — What happens when every role matters.

Commitment — Staying steady through hard shifts.

Communication — The thread that holds care together.

Compassion — Seeing the person behind the symptom.

Competence — Skill paired with humility.

Composure — Grace under pressure.

Confidence — Earned through preparation, not ego.

Connection — The human spark in medicine.

Consistency — Reliability that builds trust.

Contemplation — Thinking deeply before acting quickly.

Courage — Showing up when outcomes are uncertain.

Curiosity — The engine of improvement.

D

Daring — Trying again when others stop.

Debrief — Turning experience into wisdom.

Dedication — The long game of showing up.

Dependability — Being someone others can count on.

Determination — Refusing to settle for "good enough."

Discernment — Knowing what truly matters in the moment.

Diversity — Many perspectives strengthening one system.

E

Empathy — Feeling *with*, not *for*.

Empowerment — Replacing hierarchy with humanity.

Endurance — Strength that outlasts exhaustion.

Engagement — Full presence in the task at hand.

Ethics — The moral compass of care.

Excellence — Doing ordinary things extraordinarily well.

F

Feedback — Information offered for growth, not criticism.

Flexibility — Bending without breaking.

Follow-Through — The final act of professionalism.

Forgiveness — Resetting teams — and yourself.

Fulfillment — Purpose that feels like peace.

G

Grace — Kindness without condition.

Gratitude — Seeing what's right, even on hard days.

Grounding — Returning to what steadies you.

Growth — The reward of reflection.

H

Healing — Restoring wholeness, not just fixing problems.

Honesty — The shortest path to trust.

Hope — The medicine that never runs out.

Humility — Letting the work matter more than the title.

I

Imagination — Innovation's first spark.

Improvement — The habit that builds excellence.

Inclusivity — Making space for every voice.

Initiative — Acting before being asked.

Integrity — Doing the right thing when it costs you something.

Intuition — Experience speaking in whispers.

J

Judgment — Choosing well under pressure.

Joy — Quiet satisfaction in purpose fulfilled.

Justice — Fairness applied to care.

K

Kindness — The universal protocol.

Knowledge — The foundation — never the finish line.

L

Leadership — Influence rooted in service.

Learning — The lifelong vital sign.

Listening — The skill that prevents the most mistakes.

Loyalty — Standing by your team when it's hard.

M

Mentorship — Passing the torch without dimming your own light.

Mindfulness — Presence without judgment.

Moral Courage — Doing right when silence feels safer.

Motivation — The internal pulse that keeps you moving.

N

Navigation — Finding direction in moving systems.

Negotiation — The diplomacy of teamwork.

Nurture — Feeding growth in others — and yourself.

O

Observation — Seeing what others miss.

Openness — Willingness to hear what's uncomfortable.

Optimism — Hope with sleeves rolled up.

Organization — Turning chaos into clarity.

P

Patience — The pause that prevents regret.

Perseverance — Staying the course.

Perspective — The lens that changes everything.

Precision — Caring enough to get it right.

Presence — The anchor of connection.

Professionalism — Respect in motion.

Purpose — Why you started — and why you stay.

Q

Quality — Doing it right the first time.

Questioning — The beginning of critical thinking.

R

Reflection — Learning before moving on.

Reliability — Showing up as promised.

Resilience — Strength that bends, not breaks.

Respect — The baseline vital sign of teamwork.

Responsibility — Turning awareness into action.

S

Safety — The sacred contract of healthcare.

Self-Awareness — The foundation of emotional intelligence.

Self-Care — Fuel for sustainable compassion.

Service — Purpose in action.

Simplicity — Clarity without excess.

Steadiness — Calm in the current.

Stewardship — Protecting trust, time, and truth.

Support — Holding space when words fall short.

Synergy — Collective purpose amplified.

T

Teamwork — The choreography of shared care.

Teaching — Passing wisdom forward.

Tenacity — Endurance rooted in belief.

Transparency — Truth told with grace.

Trust — The foundation of every healing act.

U

Understanding — Compassion translated into clarity.

Unity — Many hearts moving together.

V

Value — Knowing your worth — and your work's.

Vigilance — Watchfulness that keeps patients safe.

Vision — Seeing what could be, then building it.

Vitality — Energy aligned with purpose.

W

Well-Being — Balance of body, mind, and meaning.

Wisdom — Experience refined by empathy.

Worth — The reminder that you matter too.

X

X-Factor — The undefinable spark that elevates care.

Y

Yield — Knowing when to pause so others can lead.

Z

Zeal — Enthusiasm that fuels excellence.

Zen — Calm between crises.

Why These Words Matter

These words aren't a test.

They're a mirror.

When you find the ones that sound like you — or the ones you wish did — hold onto them. They are clues. They point toward alignment, toward sustainability, toward a version of healthcare that works *with* who you are, not against it.

Words shape care.

And care shapes people.

Chapter 1
Let Your Journey Begin...

Welcome to Your Guided Path to Finding Where You Truly Fit in Healthcare

The hallway is quiet now.

Not the kind of quiet that means "empty," but the kind that settles over a unit after the last call light has stopped blinking and the shift has finally exhaled. Monitors hum. A cart rolls in the distance. Someone laughs behind a closed door. The air is thick with stories — victories, losses, miracles, questions — the kind of stories that shape people in ways they only understand years later.

If you're holding this book, chances are you already feel the pull of those stories.

Maybe you're just starting to imagine a future in healthcare — curious, hopeful, a little nervous, wondering where you might belong.

Maybe you're already deep in the work — sleeves rolled, badge dangling, heart tired, purpose flickering but still alive under the surface.

Maybe you're searching — not for a job, but for your place: your people, your pace, your fit.

Wherever you're standing, this moment right here is your threshold.

You're not just opening a book.

You're opening a door.

On the other side is a different way of thinking about healthcare — one that doesn't start with credentials or salary tables or job postings, but with something far more powerful:

Who you are.

Where you belong.

And how you were wired to care.

Your healthcare career journey is personal.

It's practical.

It's visionary.

And yes — it's cinematic.

You're about to step into a world where alignment matters as much as ambition...

where your identity is your compass...

where your environment is your ecosystem...

and where your voice is your most essential instrument.

About the Journey We're About to Take Together

Before we dive into theories, frameworks, and career lists, let's get clear about where we're headed.

You're not just going to read this book.

You're going to travel through it.

We'll move in four big arcs:

First, we'll explore Mason's Alignment Theory™ (MAT) — why some roles feel like home while others feel like wearing someone else's scrubs two sizes too small.

Next, you'll walk through the Mini SCRUB*fits*™ Healthcare Career Assessment, using your responses to start zeroing in on one best-fit role as a starting point.

Then, you'll hear from healthcare leaders and legends in the Masters Series — people I consider to be some of the absolute best in the field today, including mentors who shaped my own journey.

Finally, you'll step into one of the most comprehensive healthcare career guides out there — a total of 345 careers in healthcare, including 185 of today's top roles, 25 standout careers, 85 careers of the future, and 50 side hustles or "dip-your-toe-in" healthcare paths.

By the end, you'll have something most people never get:

a full view of who you are, what you need, and where you can go in healthcare.

And right between "who you are" and "where you can go," there's a powerful little bridge I'm excited for you to walk across:

The Mini SCRUBfit™ Healthcare Career Assessment.

Your first glimpse into where you naturally fit in healthcare.

Before you wander into 345 career options and start circling roles with a pen, I want you to pause and do something most people skip:

Look in the mirror.

You already have clues about where you belong.

They're hiding in your preferences, your energy, your pace, your stress responses, your emotional wiring, and the way you instinctively show up for people.

The Mini SCRUBfit™ Healthcare Career Assessment is your first flashlight on those clues.

It's short.

It's simple.

It's fun.

And it gives you a snapshot of the kind of healthcare ecosystem that tends to bring out your best.

You'll begin to see whether:

• You thrive in urgency or steadiness

• You're drawn to diagnostics, procedures, coaching, tech, or coordination

• Your energy peaks with complexity, connection, structure, or autonomy

• You feel safer in high-intensity environments or slow, relational ones

• You're more fueled by puzzles, people, progress, or peace

This assessment will not say, "Here is your one perfect job forever."

It will say something much more useful:

"Here's the kind of ecosystem your nervous system understands.

Here's the lane where you're most likely to feel like yourself."

Many people think they're burned out because of workload, schedules, or staffing. Sometimes that's true.

But often, they're exhausted because they've been working against their wiring for too long.

This mini assessment is your first step back toward yourself.

Your results won't box you in.

They'll open doors.

They'll help you read the rest of this book with clarity instead of confusion, strategy instead of guessing, and alignment instead of accident.

So when you're ready, take the Mini SCRUBfit™ Healthcare Career Assessment.

Treat it like a conversation starter with yourself.

And remember — this is just the beginning.

The full SCRUBfit™ model — with all ten categories and deeper insights — is available online at:

www.masonmaison.pub

First Stop: The Alignment Theory

Once you've taken that first look in the mirror, we'll go deeper.

We'll talk about Mason's Alignment Theory™ (MAT) — the backbone of this entire journey.

You'll learn why some people come alive in the emergency department while others wilt there.

Why one person thrives in a quiet lab and another needs the buzz of a busy unit to feel engaged.

Why two people in the same job can have completely different experiences of it.

Mason's Alignment Theory™ (MAT) matters because:

If your career doesn't fit who you are, no amount of "self-care" can fix that.

But if it does fit who you are?

Then even hard days feel meaningful instead of pointless.

Next Stop: Leaders, Legends, and the Best of Healthcare

After we explore alignment, I'm going to introduce you to some of the brightest minds and biggest hearts in healthcare — people I consider leaders, legends, and in some cases, professional trouble-makers in the best possible way.

Some have been my mentors.

Some are people I've watched from a distance and thought, "They're changing healthcare just by being who they are."

You'll hear their take on:

• What alignment looks like in real life

• How they've protected their own alignment

• How they lead teams toward better fit, not just better metrics

• What they wish future clinicians, leaders, and students would understand now

Imagine sitting down for coffee with some of the best in the field and asking,

"How do I build a career worth staying for?"

That's what this section of the book is meant to feel like.

Final Stop: A Complete Healthcare Career Atlas

And then — once you understand alignment, know your wiring, and have heard from people living it at the highest levels — we'll zoom way out.

I'm handing you one of the largest, most comprehensive healthcare career guides you'll find between two covers:

• 185 of today's top healthcare careers

• 25 standout roles

• 85 healthcare careers of the future

- 50 side hustles or "dip-your-toe-in" healthcare paths

This isn't just a list.

It's a map — a way to see the scale of what's possible, not just the handful of roles people usually mention when they say "healthcare career."

Who's Taking You on This Trip?

You should probably know who's guiding you before we go any farther.

I've spent my life in healthcare — recruiting, developing, advising, innovating, building programs, and sitting in more conference rooms, nurse's stations, and physician lounges than I can count — and loving every minute of it.

I've served on boards and advisory groups.

I've judged national awards.

I've helped launch careers, fix pipelines, and repair teams.

I've watched amazing people walk away from healthcare — not because they didn't care, but because the fit was wrong and nobody showed them another way.

Somewhere along the way, one stubborn belief crystallized:

You are not here to contort yourself to fit healthcare.

Healthcare should be designed to fit you.

SCRUBfit™, Mason's Alignment Theory (MAT), PACES™, CARESET™, the career guides, and this entire book are my way of giving you language, tools, and options that didn't exist when I first started helping people find their path.

This is not just a book of careers.

It's a book of clarity.

How I Hope You'll Use This Book

Read this like:

• a map when you feel lost

• a mirror when you feel confused

• a compass when you're choosing next steps

• a conversation with someone who believes you're not "too much," "too sensitive," "too intense," or "too quiet" — you're just not aligned yet

You don't have to read it in one sitting.

You don't have to know the end of your story.

You don't have to have your life figured out.

You just have to stay curious... and keep choosing alignment, one step at a time.

Because when who you are matches what you do — and when where you work finally fits you — you don't just stay in healthcare.

You become one of the reasons it's worth staying.

Thank you for being here.

Thank you for choosing curiosity over resignation.

Thank you for believing that your career deserves alignment, not endurance.

I have a feeling we can find you a pair of scrubs that feels tailor-made for your wiring — and in a color that makes you absolutely glow.

Now take a breath, turn the page, and let's begin.

Your future is waiting.

Your healthcare journey starts now.

Chapter 2
Hopewell Hospital for Tomorrow

Hopewell Hospital for Tomorrow — Where the future is already on the floor

Throughout this book, you'll hear about a place called Hopewell Hospital for Tomorrow. It isn't a real hospital you can drive to, and it isn't a fantasy built from science fiction. It is a composite model—a near-future blueprint built from innovations already emerging and from human-centered redesigns that healthcare has needed for decades. Hopewell exists to show what healthcare can look like when systems finally evolve instead of collapse.

Some hospitals feel like they were built one policy at a time. Hopewell Hospital for Tomorrow feels like it was built from a single question: what would healthcare look like if it truly fit the people inside it?

You feel the answer the moment you step in.

The lobby opens into a sunlit atrium where adaptive smart glass filters daylight into soft gradients that change with the time of day rather than the demands of the clock. A living biowall breathes quietly along one side, pulling air through layers of botanical filtration. Beneath the main walkway, a shallow water channel absorbs sound and replaces the usual hospital cacophony with a steady, grounding flow. Seating curves into shapes that invite rest instead of resisting it. People move with intention, not urgency.

There is no front desk by design.

Hopewell learned early that desks create barriers, queues, and power dynamics that don't belong in a place built for care. Instead, trained Stewards—easily recognizable in their bright red blazers—move through the space with practiced attentiveness. They roam rather than wait, intercepting confusion before it becomes stress, translating the building into a story people can follow, and offering help before anyone has to ask.

What is less visible—but constantly felt—is how little anyone has to go searching.

Medications arrive without pages or runners. Supplies surface where they are needed and disappear just as quietly. **Autonomous service drones fly freely through the hospital's airspace—quiet, precise, and self-navigating— delivering medications, specimens, and supplies without runners, rails, shafts, or tubes.** Specimens leave patient rooms through sealed vertical shafts built into walls and columns, routed automatically to the appropriate labs without carts, labels waved in hallways, or staff pulled away from care. Overhead and underfoot, autonomous logistics systems move continuously, invisible by design, ensuring that clinicians never have to leave the moment to retrieve what the system already knows they will need.

At the heart of the atrium rises Reef Garland, a towering, zoo-scale living coral ecosystem that coils upward like a ribbon of color and light. Sun filters through open water columns and coral shelves, casting rippling reflections across the floor as patients, families, and clinicians pass beneath it. The reef is not decoration. It is part of Hopewell's nervous system—a living stabilizer designed to slow breathing, lower heart rates, and bring bodies back into rhythm.

Reef Garland carries a name chosen with intention. Garland was the founder's mother, a woman whose introductions always ended in laughter. "Yes, like Judy Garland," she would say with a grin, or, "Yes, like Christmas garland," when people hesitated over her name. In a hospital designed to remind people they are more than their diagnoses, it felt right that the building's emotional center would carry a name that made people smile.

Over time, the reef became something else entirely.

Schools of radiant blue fish thread through the coral like living punctuation, and every so often a dart of brilliant yellow flashes past the glass—Cousin Yvonne, the oversized Yellow Tang Garland insisted on naming at the dedication ceremony. Visitors learn to look for her. Children press their hands to the glass. Clinicians slow without meaning to. Stewards report hearing the same phrase echo through shifts, offered by toddlers, nurses, residents, and physicians alike: "There she is."

Hopewell understands that environments shape behavior long before policies ever do.

That philosophy extends far beyond the atrium. Patient rooms are built around healing rather than efficiency, with warm mineral tones, wide windows framing native courtyards, and lighting systems that restore circadian rhythm instead of flattening it. Beds quietly redistribute pressure and prevent injury before alarms are ever needed. Technology fades into the background, present and powerful without demanding attention.

Clinical intelligence at Hopewell works the same way.

Documentation no longer consumes clinicians because it no longer requires them to perform clerical work in the middle of care. Information is gathered ambiently, with transparency and consent, allowing clinicians to speak naturally, think clearly, and stay present. Safety systems operate as quiet backstops, catching mismatches and subtle changes long before they reach the bedside. When something goes wrong, support arrives early, informed, and calm.

Excellence here is not heroic. It is engineered.

Staffing is predictive and dynamic, designed around real-time acuity rather than averages. Learning time is protected. Specialty training is funded. Environmental services staff participate in safety huddles. Behavioral health is integrated everywhere, not siloed on another floor.

Care does not stop at the walls.

Virtual nursing functions as a staffed command center rather than a tablet on a stand, coordinating care so bedside clinicians can focus on presence and judgment. Hospital-at-home programs extend Hopewell's reach into living rooms and bedrooms without diluting safety, supported by continuous monitoring, automated medication delivery, and clinical oversight that travels with the patient rather than staying behind.

Throughout these spaces, you'll meet members of the **SCRUBfits™** world—some familiar, others newly emerging—moving through real systems, real teams, and real decisions. Hopewell is not built around superheroes. It is built around alignment: between people and roles, technology and judgment, care and the humans who provide it.

By the time you drift back toward the atrium, you understand why Hopewell Hospital for Tomorrow appears throughout this book. It is not a destination. It is a demonstration.

It shows what happens when healthcare stops forcing people to shrink to fit broken systems and instead stretches systems to fit the people inside them. It shows a future where care looks like care, support is built into the floor plan, and the work of healing—both giving it and surviving it—is finally allowed to be human.

The Russell and Bernice Preddy Library

None of this was meant to replace what already exists at Hopewell, please weave it all in. The Russell and Bernice Preddy Library expands the same human-centered redesign that runs through the atrium, the rooms, and the systems that quietly keep care moving.

The library absorbs weight so people do not have to.

It is open to the public to research their ailments. Every other Wednesday it is open to individuals interested in exploring a career in healthcare with recruiters onsite. Not just from Hopewell. Hopewell welcomes all neighboring hospitals, clinics, medical practices, the local fire & rescue use the space to its fullest recruiting and also conducting training and new hire orientation in the library. They all come and meet with potential candidates. Resume preparation, interviewing, etc. are all topics for Wednesdays.

Noise? No such thing with the Focus Nests for those those seeking a quiet space to study and learn.

No longer the shortage of space to host committee meetings, Hopewell features a bank of a dozen conference rooms. Small for committee meetings, medium for unit meetings and large for larger gatherings like the board of directors. Small, medium and large just like the Paris France themed open air barista bar. A unique pick up area allows clinicians and visitors to place orders for coffees, teas, sandwiches, etc.

The conference rooms are open to the community when not reserved for the hospital. Friends of Bill, Grief counseling, etc. all takes place.

Thursday evenings are especially fun with Karaoke on the Studer's Stage adjacent to Bistro Joie.

Midday — The Russell and Bernice Preddy Library

Late morning settles gently into the Russell and Bernice Preddy Library, the kind of hour that doesn't announce itself. Sunlight stretches across long tables, softening the edges of everything it touches. The pace here is unhurried by design.

Near the windows, a parent sits with a notebook open, reading slowly. Earlier, a diagnosis had been spoken aloud in a small exam room. Now the words live on paper, broken into manageable pieces. A Learning & Alignment Steward pauses nearby—not hovering, not interrupting—available without pressure. When the parent looks up, a question is answered plainly, without alarm or judgment.

Along the far wall, a Focus Nest seals closed with a quiet click. Inside, a student studies anatomy in complete stillness. Outside, the library continues at a different volume, silence and movement coexisting without friction.

At a conference table, a retired clinician turns the pages of a thin booklet on volunteering, lingering over possibilities without urgency. Nothing needs to be decided today. The library doesn't push. It waits.

Near Bistro Joie, cups clink softly. Someone laughs once, then instinctively lowers their voice—not because they are told to, but because the space teaches you how to be in it.

Nothing remarkable happens. No announcements are made. No conclusions are drawn.

And yet, when people stand to leave—the parent, the student, the retiree—each walks out carrying a little less than they brought in.

Wednesdays — The Healthcare Pathways Exchange

Every other Wednesday, the library shifts without fanfare.

Tables are arranged with intention, not urgency. Recruiters from Hopewell, neighboring hospitals, clinics, medical practices, and county fire and rescue services take their places—not to compete, but to explain.

Luke comes in on a Wednesday for the recruitment day. He's a local monorail operator who has become burned out with the monotony of the monorail. Luke signs up for Fire Fighting school after learning about the training provided by the local county fire and rescue.

Thursday Night — Studer's Stage

The singing doesn't start right away. Duck is emceeing. Duck, a nickname bestowed to him by his grandmother because he really liked Donald Duck orange juice.

A nurse from one of Hopewell's remote emergency departments is there.

Dr. Anna Remedy, one of the hospital hospitalists and her husband, a State Trooper come to enjoy themselves for "date night". He surprises her by serenading her, a surprise for their upcoming anniversary. He sings Can't Help Falling in Love by Elvis Presley.

Jessica, the Chief Nursing Officer jams to Madonna's Holiday & before you know it everyone is singing.

"If we took a holiday (Ooh, ooh-ooh-ooh)

Took some time to celebrate (Come on, let's celebrate)

Just one day out of life (Holiday)

It would be, it would be so nice........."

Duck nods toward Ray Beam from Radiology, a regular. Ray steps up and, with his baritone and unmistakable Southern accent, closes the evening with *The Calling*, sung in homage to the victims of COVID-19. Everyone stands. They always do. *The Calling* was written by healthcare thought leader Quint Studer and later arranged with Nashville artists.

Vera, the hospital CEO, stops by before heading home. Duck catches her eye and gives a small nod. Vera nods back, the kind of nod that says she knows exactly what this is doing for people.

By the end of the night, nothing headline-worthy has unfolded, and that is exactly the point. No one needed rescuing. No one needed fixing.

Chapter 3

Between Next and Now 2024-2026

THE LAST TWO YEARS: HOW HEALTHCARE RECALIBRATED (2024-2026)

Because this is the inaugural *What Color Are Your Scrubs?* — the Masters Series — this section looks back two years on purpose. Future editions will revisit this moment annually, capturing how healthcare continues to evolve year by year — what persists, what shifts, and what newly emerges — so career decisions are always made within a clearly understood context.

If Hopewell Hospital for Tomorrow shows what healthcare can become when systems are designed around humans, this chapter brings the reader back to where healthcare actually stood between 2024 and 2026 — not as a crisis snapshot, but as a system under pressure, actively recalibrating.

And recalibrating did not mean things suddenly became easier.

It meant the strain became visible.

What Actually Happened

Between 2024 and 2026, healthcare moved out of emergency mode and into something more complicated: structural correction. Systems were no longer just surviving — they were trying to decide what kind of future they were willing to build.

Health systems invested more heavily in retention instead of endless recruitment. Flexible scheduling expanded. Internal mobility programs grew. Career ladders became lattices. Some organizations began acknowledging what clinicians had known for years: sustainability matters — not just outcomes.

But none of this erased pressure.

Burnout did not vanish. Staffing shortages did not resolve. Administrative burden did not disappear. What changed was that misalignment became harder to hide. The conversation shifted from silent endurance to visible strain, and from denial to redesign.

Healthcare didn't stabilize — it clarified.

Public Sentiment: Strain Without Shutdown

What made this period distinctive wasn't only what systems were doing — it was how people were experiencing them.

National surveys showed growing dissatisfaction with cost, access, and system sustainability. Nearly one in four Americans described U.S. healthcare as being in crisis, while almost half said it had major problems. Affordability reached historic lows in public approval.

And yet, something subtle happened.

People didn't stop using healthcare. They didn't abandon their doctors. Many still trusted their own clinicians and local hospitals — even while losing faith in the system as a whole.

That tension mattered.

It created pressure without paralysis. Healthcare kept delivering care, training professionals, and innovating — but public tolerance for misalignment between cost, experience, and value thinned. That pressure became part of the recalibration.

Long-Term Care: Visibility, Not Resolution

One of the most politically charged healthcare flashpoints during this period was long-term care.

The federal government finalized a minimum staffing rule for nursing homes participating in **Medicare (gl)** and **Medicaid (gl)**, setting baseline expectations for nursing hours and **RN (gl)** coverage. The intent was clear: safer care required minimum standards.

What followed was not consensus.

Some states, nursing-home operators, and Republican lawmakers challenged the rule, arguing that workforce shortages made it unrealistic and financially destabilizing. Lawsuits, congressional resolutions, and administrative delays reshaped the rollout.

What remained true through all of it was this: staffing moved from an invisible burden to a visible national issue.

Frontline staff felt seen. Operators felt squeezed. Policymakers felt the tension between safety and feasibility.

The rule itself became less important than what it revealed: environments shape experience, and chronic understaffing is not a personal failure — it's a structural one.

Vaccinations, Immunity Gaps (gl), and the Next Decade

One of the most consequential shifts of this period wasn't just inside hospitals — it was in the public's relationship with prevention.

Between 2024 and 2026, vaccination behavior became more uneven. Not because science changed, but because confidence, access, and trust fractured. Some communities remained well-protected. Others developed widening immunity gaps (gl) large enough to allow outbreaks (gl) of measles (gl), pertussis (gl), and other vaccine-preventable diseases (gl) to return.

This didn't mean society rejected medicine. It meant healthcare became more reactive.

More testing.

More school closures.

More emergency visits.

More public-health strain.

For future clinicians, this matters. You will practice in a world where prevention is no longer assumed — it must be rebuilt through trust, communication, and access. Public health (gl) becomes part of bedside care. And alignment between science, policy, and community belief becomes just as important as the vaccine itself.

Prevention isn't just idealism.

It's a workload strategy (gl).

A safety strategy (gl).

A sustainability strategy (gl).

Technology Shifted From Flash to Relief

Between 2024 and 2026, technology stopped trying to impress and started trying to help.

Automated insulin systems like the **iLet Bionic Pancreas (gl)** reduced the daily cognitive burden of diabetes care. Robotic surgery platforms shifted toward modular, more flexible **OR (gl)** designs that acknowledged surgeon fatigue as a patient-safety issue. Remote monitoring, virtual nursing, and **AI (gl)**-assisted documentation began removing friction instead of adding it.

The common thread was relief.

Technology didn't replace clinicians.

It started carrying part of the load.

Second-Career Clinicians Changed the Culture

One of the quiet but powerful shifts of this period came from outside healthcare.

As layoffs swept through technology, media, corporate, and finance sectors, thousands of experienced professionals pivoted into healthcare. These second-career clinicians brought something rare: emotional maturity, communication skills, and a clear sense of purpose.

They didn't enter healthcare because it was easy.

They entered because it mattered.

In many hospitals, they became some of the strongest nurses, therapists, **informatics (gl)** specialists, and administrators — not despite their prior careers, but because of them. They reframed what "non-traditional" meant. They normalized starting over. And they brought new expectations about respect, boundaries, and sustainability.

Healthcare didn't just absorb them.

It evolved because of them.

A Healthier Cultural Conversation

Perhaps the most important change wasn't technological or **regulatory (gl)**.

It was cultural.

Between 2024 and 2026, healthcare stopped pretending that endurance alone was the goal. Conversations about fit, boundaries, environment, and longevity became legitimate. Choosing sustainability was no longer framed as weakness. Designing a career intentionally became a sign of professionalism.

People didn't stop caring.

They stopped self-erasing.

Why This Moment Matters

Healthcare did not emerge from this period "fixed."

But it emerged more honest.

More visible.

More open to redesign.

This chapter exists to ground you in the moment you are stepping into — not to warn you away from healthcare, and not to sugarcoat it either.

The system you are entering is strained, yes.

But it is also awake.

And in an awake system, alignment becomes power.

Chapter 4

A High-Schooler's Guide to This Book

Welcome, High School Explorers

If you're reading this as a high school student, you're already doing something most people don't do until years later: you're paying attention to who you're becoming. You don't need to have everything figured out right now. You just need curiosity, a sense of what matters to you, and a willingness to explore what's possible.

Healthcare is a world made up of hundreds of careers you've probably never heard of — roles in technology, science, leadership, imaging, therapy, public health, emergency care, and so much more. You don't have to know the "right" path today. This book will help you discover which roles fit your personality, interests, strengths, and the future you want to build.

As you move through the chapters, pay attention to what lights you up. Notice which **SCRUB*fit*™** characters feel relatable or exciting. Let this book become a way of trying on different futures without any pressure. And if you want to go deeper, the back of this book contains one of the largest healthcare career guides on the market, giving you more detail and direction than any resource you've ever held.

You're not choosing a job. You're discovering what kind of life you want — and where your talents can do the most good. You're not early, and you're not late. You're right on time.

Your On-Ramp Starts Here: You Don't Need It All Figured Out

You are not supposed to know your lifelong healthcare path at 16 or 17. What you *can* do right now is start noticing what energizes you, what overwhelms you, and what feels "just right." That's alignment in its earliest form — understanding your wiring before the world tells you who to be.

If you're curious, compassionate, unflappable, a hands-on helper, a tech kid, a science brain, or a creative problem-solver, there is a place for you in healthcare. This book will help you find it.

Chapter 5

Welcome, Second-Career Seekers

Welcome, Second-Career Seekers

If you're turning to this book while considering a new career, you're already demonstrating courage. Changing paths isn't a sign that your first career was wrong — it's a sign that you're listening to who you are now. People evolve. Values shift. Priorities sharpen. This book is here to help you honor that.

Many of the most successful people in healthcare didn't start here. They came from teaching, retail, the military, hospitality, corporate environments, parenting, caregiving, and jobs that shaped them in ways classrooms never could. Healthcare doesn't ask where you began. It asks what you can bring with you.

Inside these pages, you'll find clarity, direction, and tools to understand your strengths — and where they will feel most aligned. You'll meet the **SCRUB*fit*™** characters, explore real-world day-in-the-life narratives, and reflect on what feels like you. If you're worried about going back to school, balancing family, or navigating finances, this book will give you practical pathways and honest guidance — not pressure.

And if you want to explore the full range of opportunities waiting for you, the back of this book contains the largest healthcare career guide available anywhere on the market. Consider it your map, your menu, and your invitation to a future that fits.

You're not starting over. You're starting aligned.

Chapter 6
Welcome, Healthcare Insiders

Welcome, Healthcare Insiders

If you already work in healthcare, you bring a depth of insight that only experience provides. You know the pace, the weight, the joy, the frustration, and the stakes. You've seen what works and what doesn't. You've learned how to care for others even when the system makes it hard. That wisdom matters.

This book isn't here to reroute you. It's here to expand the map. Most people in healthcare only ever see a small corner of what's possible. They know their role well, but rarely get to explore the full landscape of careers that exist across the field. Whether you're seeking growth, better alignment, a new specialty, or a different kind of balance, you deserve a career that matches who you've become — not just the role you started in.

As you read through the **SCRUB*fit*™** characters, pay attention to the ones that feel familiar. Notice the patterns in your values, your strengths, and your frustrations. These clues will help you identify where your experience could flourish next, whether that means staying clinical, moving into leadership, exploring tech and informatics, or stepping into a role that finally gives you the alignment you've been craving.

And if you want a deeper look at every role available to you, the back of this book contains the largest healthcare career guide available on the market today. It's a resource designed for people like you — people with real experience who deserve real options.

You've given so much to healthcare already. Now it's time to find the place where healthcare gives something back to you.

Chapter 7

Mason's Alignment Theory (MAT)

The Real Crisis Isn't a Workforce Shortage — It's Misalignment.

"Get alignment right, and everything else improves. We protect our people and our patients. But it starts with awareness: leaders have to look honestly at whether the systems, expectations, and cultures they're creating are aligned with the values they promote. When alignment is missing at the top, it can't exist at the bedside."

— Ellen Menard, RN, BSN, MBA — Senior Vice President of Human Resources & Organization Development; Author of *The Not So Patient Advocate*

Mason's Alignment Theory (MAT)

Healthcare is full of people who care deeply about their work, yet feel exhausted, conflicted, or uncertain about whether they are in the right place. For decades, the industry has treated burnout as a personal failing—something to be fixed with resilience (gl) classes, stress-management (gl) handouts, or inspirational posters taped to break-room walls. But burnout is not a character flaw. It is a structural symptom of misalignment (gl). Mason's Alignment Theory (MAT) reframes the entire conversation, offering readers a clearer, more honest way to understand why some roles feel natural while others feel like constant friction.

MAT begins with a simple truth: people don't burn out because they care too much; they burn out because they're working in roles or environments that contradict who they are. Alignment is not about perfection, privilege, or luck. It is about fit—an everyday match between a person's identity (gl), the environment in which they practice, and the degree of agency (gl) they hold within that environment. When those three elements are in sync, the work feels sustainable, meaningful, and energizing. When even one is out of balance, fatigue accumulates, confidence erodes, and purpose becomes harder to access.

MAT is expressed through a straightforward formula:

Alignment = Identity × Environment × Agency.

Each variable strengthens or weakens the others. Each one determines whether a clinician thrives or merely endures. And each one can be shaped, developed, or redesigned over time. MAT gives you a way to understand yourself with more compassion and precision, while also naming the very real structural forces that shape your experience in healthcare.

Identity: Who You Are and What You Need to Thrive

Identity is the foundation of MAT. It captures your natural wiring (gl), your temperament (gl), your strengths, your stress responses, and the conditions in which you do your best work. Identity is not fixed, but it is deeply rooted. Some people thrive in motion and rapid decision-making. Some flourish through calm, steady, relationship-based work. Others find their power in complexity, data, pattern recognition (gl), mastery, precision, or advocacy (gl). Identity also encompasses what you need to feel grounded—predictability or variety, people or solitude, autonomy or structure, steady pace or controlled chaos.

When identity is honored, work feels intuitive and energizing. When identity is ignored, even the "right" job can feel wrong. Many healthcare professionals assume their dissatisfaction means they must leave the field entirely, when often the real issue is that they are practicing in a role that contradicts who they are at their core. MAT offers the language to identify those contradictions and the possibility of moving toward roles or environments that celebrate who you actually are.

Environment: The Conditions That Shape Your Experience

Environment is the external world you walk into every day—the culture, pace, leadership, expectations, staffing, team dynamics, and physical space. Two clinicians with identical credentials can have wildly different experiences simply because their environments differ. An Emergency Department (gl) rewards decisiveness and comfort with uncertainty; a dermatology (gl) practice rewards precision and patience; a research lab (gl) rewards curiosity and independence. The setting matters as much as the role.

Environment also encompasses access to resources, opportunities for growth, psychological safety (gl), mentorship (gl), teamwork, and clarity of expectations. When the environment supports and reflects the clinician's identity, work becomes sustainable. When it contradicts it, even the most passionate professionals struggle. MAT teaches readers to evaluate environments with honesty, naming what supports them and what strains them, rather than forcing themselves to adapt endlessly to conditions that cannot support long-term well-being.

Agency: The Freedom to Shape Your Work and Your Future

Agency is the often-overlooked dimension of alignment: the degree of influence, choice, and control a person holds within their career. Agency includes the ability to set boundaries (gl), make decisions, advocate for yourself, pursue opportunities, pivot roles, adjust schedules, advance your education, and design a pathway that matches your identity and aspirations. Agency is where possibility lives.

Some clinicians have abundant agency—they can transfer departments, negotiate flexibility, seek mentorship (gl), or shift into a new specialty. Others feel trapped by debt, policies (gl), culture, inflexible scheduling, or limited advancement. MAT recognizes these realities without judgment. Agency is not about willpower; it is about access. It expands with support, resources, and clarity. It grows when individuals understand their identity and environment and begin making intentional, small shifts toward alignment.

When agency is strong, clinicians feel empowered to shape their careers rather than merely endure them. When agency is weak, even the right job can feel constraining. MAT helps readers reclaim their agency not through unrealistic promises, but through practical pathways and long-view strategy (gl).

Why MAT Matters

MAT is not a motivational slogan. It is a structural explanation for real human experience. It validates what so many clinicians feel but seldom articulate: that sustainable, meaningful work requires more than grit. It requires alignment. MAT honors the truth that passion alone cannot compensate for a misaligned role or an unhealthy environment, and that resilience (gl) is not a replacement for proper staffing, fair policies (gl), or supportive leadership. At the same time, MAT empowers individuals by showing that alignment can be built, piece by piece, through self-understanding, intentional choices, and environments that support people rather than overwhelm them.

MAT does not promise perfection; it promises direction. It invites readers to assess their identity honestly, evaluate their environment courageously, and reclaim their agency strategically. It is a framework that meets people where they are and guides them toward where they can thrive.

Alignment Is for Everyone

Alignment is not reserved for those with unlimited resources, flexible schedules, or extraordinary privilege. It is also not reserved for hospitals and healthcare organizations with deep pockets.

Alignment belongs to the bedside nurse deciding whether to pursue certification (gl). It belongs to the medical assistant (gl) wondering if they should go back to school. It belongs to the respiratory therapist (gl) dreaming of leadership, the sonographer (gl) considering a specialty change, the pharmacist (gl) seeking a role with more connection, and the physician longing for a shift from volume to purpose. Alignment belongs to every person who contributes to healthcare.

And yet access to alignment is not equal. Not all environments offer the same level of agency (gl). Not all organizations provide the same culture, resources, or support. MAT acknowledges these structural inequities while still offering readers a pathway forward. Alignment is universal. The obstacles are structural. And the solutions require both individual clarity and system-level reform (gl).

Your Path Forward

Every chapter that follows—every framework, every **SCRUB***fit*™ category, every character story, every career exploration—builds on MAT. This theory is the compass for the entire book. It helps readers understand not just what they can do, but what they were meant to do, what they can sustain, and what will bring them back to life.

MAT is the starting point for reflection, the lens for choosing roles, and the roadmap for designing a healthcare career with intention. When identity, environment, and agency are aligned, people don't just work better—they feel better. They stay longer. They contribute more deeply. They thrive.

And that is the promise this book makes to every reader: alignment is possible, and your career can be redesigned around who you are—not the other way around.

Alignment in Practice: Who You'll Meet Along the Way

Healthcare is often taught as a system — protocols, pathways, credentials, ladders to climb. But no one actually *lives* it that way. Healthcare is lived through people: colleagues you lean on during impossible shifts, mentors who quietly change your trajectory, and professionals whose stories make you think, *Wait... maybe there's another way to do this.*

That's where the **SCRUB*fits*™** come in.

Throughout this book, you'll meet a group of healthcare professionals who act as guides, companions, and mirrors. They aren't mascots or caricatures. They're composites — grounded in real credentials, real career paths, real tensions, and real moments of alignment and misalignment. Each **SCRUB*fit*™** represents a way of being in healthcare, not just a job title.

Some of them thrive in high-adrenaline environments. Others find meaning in precision, prevention, systems, or long-term relationships with patients and teams. A few have pivoted more than once. All of them have learned, sometimes the hard way, that fulfillment in healthcare doesn't come from prestige alone — it comes from fit.

You don't need to memorize them. You don't need to follow them in order. Think of them the way you'd think of colleagues in a break room conversation or a late-night shift handoff: people whose stories help you see your own choices more clearly.

As you move through the Alignment framework, the Masters Series, and the 345 careers explored in this book, the **SCRUB*fits*™** will appear where they're most useful — offering context, perspective, and lived experience when the questions get complex or the decisions feel heavy.

You won't find one that's "right" for everyone. That's the point.

Healthcare doesn't need more identical professionals. It needs aligned ones. And sometimes, the fastest way to understand where you belong is to learn from a few guides who've already walked that path.

Chapter 8
PACES™ and CARESET™

Introduction to PACES™ and CARESET™

Choosing a healthcare career is rarely a straight line. Most people begin with a handful of job titles, a few assumptions about what they might enjoy, and a vague sense of whether they are "good with people" or "better behind the scenes." But the truth is deeper—and far more meaningful. Career alignment (gl) is not about guessing or hoping; it is about understanding the forces within you and around you that shape the lived experience (gl) of working in healthcare.

Before readers can evaluate a single role, they must first understand themselves and the conditions that either support or strain their ability to thrive. This is where the twin frameworks of PACES™ and CARESET™ come in.

These frameworks give structure to something most readers have felt for years but never had the words for: the invisible factors that make a job feel energizing, overwhelming, sustainable (gl), or impossible. Every clinician (gl) who has ever wondered why the same role feels wildly different from one department to the next—or why two people with identical credentials can have opposite experiences in the same job—will finally find clarity here. Healthcare careers don't succeed or fail in a vacuum; they rise or fall based on identity, environment, and the interaction between the two.

PACES™ captures the internal half of alignment (gl)—the wiring, strengths, needs, and realities each reader brings to the table. CARESET™ captures the external half—the cultural (gl), operational (gl), and team-based conditions that shape daily experience. Together, they form a complete map of why some people flourish in certain roles while others burn out in them, and why the same job can feel dramatically different depending on the setting.

What follows is more than a set of definitions. It is a translation key. It turns vague feelings into understandable factors, unspoken frustrations into identifiable patterns, and instinct into strategy. These frameworks give readers the language to describe their lived experience (gl), the clarity to see where they truly fit, and the confidence to pursue careers that match who they are and what they need. Alignment (gl) begins long before a job title. It begins with understanding yourself and the world you are stepping into.

PACES™: The Five Dimensions of You

Every healthcare career decision begins with you—who you are, how you're wired, and what you need in order to thrive. PACES™ is the five-part blueprint that helps readers understand their internal landscape (gl) before they look outward at job titles or salaries. These dimensions shape identity, influence satisfaction, and often determine whether someone feels energized or drained inside a role.

P — Personality (gl)

Personality describes the natural tendencies you bring into every room—your pace (gl), preferences, interpersonal (gl) style, and instinctive response to pressure. It shapes whether you feel more comfortable leading, supporting, analyzing, calming, fixing, teaching, or advocating (gl). In healthcare, personality is not about labels; it's about energy. Some roles reward rapid decision-making and confidence in uncertainty, while others flourish through patience, empathy, careful analysis, or nurturing. When readers understand the personality patterns that refill their energy rather than drain it, they can stop forcing themselves into roles that contradict who they are.

A — Aptitude (gl)

Aptitude reflects what you naturally do well—patterns of strength that appear without strain. Some readers excel in spatial reasoning (gl) or technical tasks; others have a quiet gift for comforting people or thinking in systems, patterns, or data. Aptitude is not intelligence; it is ease. When aptitude matches the work itself, confidence grows, performance improves, and stress decreases.

C — Constraints (gl)

Constraints are the real-world factors that shape what is possible today—time, money, geography, family responsibilities, scheduling limitations, prerequisite (gl) access, or competing obligations. Constraints are not barriers;

they are parameters (gl). The most sustainable (gl) careers are built by working with reality rather than fighting it.

E — Experience (gl)

Experience reflects what you bring with you—training, repetition, exposure, wins, setbacks, and the lived moments that have shaped your competence (gl) and confidence. It includes clinical hours, caregiving, leadership, customer service, volunteer work, military service, and the invisible skills learned through life. Alignment (gl) is influenced not only by what you want, but by what you have already built and what you can leverage today.

S — Situation (gl)

Situation captures the circumstances influencing decision-making in the present moment—life stage, career stage, financial goals, confidence, timing, and momentum. A decision that fits at 22 may not fit at 42. Understanding situation prevents impulsive (gl) decisions and supports strategic (gl) ones.

Together, these five dimensions form the internal half of alignment (gl). PACES™ helps readers understand the person making the decision—not just the decision itself.

CARESET™: The Seven Conditions That Shape Your Career Reality

If PACES™ explains the inner world, CARESET™ explains the world around you. These seven external conditions determine how well a role supports, stretches, or strains a healthcare professional. CARESET™ reveals why burnout is rarely caused by lack of passion, but by mismatches between people and systems.

C — Culture (gl)

Culture is the unwritten rulebook (gl) of a workplace—the tone, values, behaviors, and emotional climate that define how things are done. A healthy culture fuels belonging and stability. A toxic culture drains energy faster than any workload ever could.

A — Autonomy (gl)

Autonomy is the degree of control, voice, and decision-making power you have in your role. When autonomy is strong, professionals feel trusted and engaged. When it is stripped away, even meaningful work can feel unsustainable (gl).

R — Resources (gl)

Resources include staffing, supplies, equipment, time, technology, and support services. Many clinicians' stress stems not from the work itself, but from trying to do good work without the tools required to do it safely.

E — Expectations (gl)

Expectations are the spoken and unspoken standards that define success—productivity targets, documentation demands, responsiveness, schedules, and performance metrics. When expectations align with reality, work feels achievable. When they don't, burnout accelerates.

S — Structure (gl)

Structure includes workflows, policies, role clarity, reporting lines, scheduling norms, and career ladders. Clear structure creates stability. Poor structure creates friction that compounds (gl) over time.

E — Environment (gl)

Environment refers to physical and psychological (gl) workplace conditions—noise, layout, acuity (gl), risk exposure, and emotional intensity. Where you work shapes how you work.

T — Team (gl)

Team is the human ecosystem around you—trust, collaboration, mentorship (gl), communication, and mutual support. Strong teams buffer stress and make hard work sustainable (gl).

Together, these seven dimensions form the external half of alignment (gl). CARESET™ teaches readers how to evaluate whether a system can support the life they want to build.

Why PACES™ and CARESET™ Matter

Used together, PACES™ and CARESET™ provide a complete map of career alignment (gl). PACES™ reveals who the reader is. CARESET™ reveals what the world around them demands. The relationship between the two determines whether a role becomes a place of meaning and momentum—or a place of fatigue and friction.

This paired system sets the foundation for everything that follows in *What Color Are Your Scrubs?* (WCAYS), guiding you toward healthcare careers that fit—not just your credentials— but the person you truly are.

Chapter 9

Misalignment: Live from the Floor—The Shape of Misalignment in Real Life

Misalignment rarely announces itself. It doesn't walk into a manager's office and declare, "I'm overwhelmed," and it doesn't appear on an annual report (gl) as a neat little line item (gl) labeled emotional fatigue (gl). Instead, it arrives quietly—almost imperceptibly (gl)—and it shows up in people long before it shows up in numbers: a nurse who begins doubting the shift she once loved, a respiratory therapist who stops sharing ideas, a new graduate who seems smaller each week, or a seasoned physician who looks tired in a way that isn't purely physical. Misalignment lives in the pause between sentences, the sigh someone doesn't realize they made, and the slow narrowing of a clinician's world.

Across healthcare, we often wait until misalignment becomes burnout (gl) before we intervene (gl). By then, the damage is already in motion: recruitment (gl) begins, overtime (gl) rises, morale (gl) thins, culture destabilizes (gl), and patients feel the effects long before leadership sees the metrics (gl). But misalignment isn't a mystery. It has patterns, signatures (gl), and early warning signs that can be recognized—and addressed—before someone reaches a breaking point.

That is why these vignettes (gl) exist. The stories ahead offer a close, unfiltered (gl) look at misalignment as it actually unfolds inside Hopewell Hospital for Tomorrow: quiet at first, then disruptive (gl), and—when the system responds—transformative (gl). Each vignette centers on a person drifting out of alignment, sometimes for reasons they can't fully articulate (gl) yet. And in each case, Hopewell intervenes not by demanding more resilience (gl), but by restoring fit—between identity (gl) and environment (gl), between aptitude (gl) and role, between personality (gl) and the daily rhythm of the work.

You'll see PACES™ and CARESET™ woven throughout these scenarios—not as academic (gl) concepts, but as practical lenses that help name what we often sense intuitively (gl) but rarely define. These frameworks make the invisible visible. They help leaders understand why a high-performing nurse suddenly struggles on day shift, why a brilliant allied health (gl) professional withdraws (gl) after offering an idea, why a student hesitates before asking questions, why a physician loses joy in a specialty (gl) they once loved, or why an entire department begins to fray (gl) at its edges.

These vignettes are not meant to be dramatic. They are meant to be recognizable (gl). At some point, every healthcare professional has lived at least one of them—perhaps several. They are the stories behind resignations (gl) that looked surprising on paper but made perfect sense in hindsight (gl). They are the moments that quietly determine whether someone stays, grows, or begins writing a mental exit letter (gl).

What follows is the heart of Mason's Alignment Theory™ (MAT): alignment is not about changing the person. It is about understanding the person well enough to shape the environment to support them. When identity and environment meet, everything changes—performance steadies, emotional bandwidth (gl) expands, creativity returns, teamwork strengthens, communication improves, and retention (gl) becomes the natural byproduct (gl) rather than a desperate goal.

These vignettes represent the before. The alignment solutions that follow represent the after. And the financial impact that concludes this section reveals the cost of waiting too long to intervene.

Taken together, they form a mirror—one that reflects the real lives of clinicians and leaders, and the extraordinary organizational (gl) potential (gl) unlocked (gl) when alignment becomes a daily practice rather than a last resort.

Chapter 10
The Misalignment Epidemic

The Healthcare Misalignment Epidemic

The healthcare misalignment epidemic rarely arrives as one big dramatic moment. It usually begins in small, private spaces: a nurse sitting in the hospital parking lot with her hands still on the steering wheel long after the engine has stopped; a respiratory therapist staring at the ceiling at three in the morning, replaying the day in her mind; a student weaving through a crowded career fair, feeling overwhelmed by choices that all sound impressive but none of which feel like home; a physician walking out of a patient's room and realizing, with a jolt, that he no longer recognizes the person he has become in this work.

To everyone else, these scenes might look ordinary. To the person living them, something deep is shifting. There is a quiet ache, a hairline crack (gl) in the way the work used to feel, a sense that the person and the place no longer quite match. This is how misalignment spreads in healthcare. It does not arrive with alarms or announcements. It settles in slowly, almost silently (gl), as people who once felt certain about their calling begin to question where, and whether, they still belong.

Healthcare has never lacked heart. There is no shortage of people willing to comfort, to teach, to problem-solve, to heal. The crisis lives somewhere else entirely. It lives in the growing distance between who people are at their core and the environments they are asked to inhabit (gl) every day. Misalignment is not loud or theatrical (gl). It shows up in the long pause before a shift, in the heaviness someone feels walking down a hallway they used to love, in the private question that most healthcare workers hesitate to put into words: "Is this still me?" The answer is rarely that something is wrong with them. Much more often, something has changed around them.

When the Person and the Place Drift Apart

Misalignment becomes visible when the person and the place no longer move together. A technician wired for steadiness and predictability (gl) finds herself in an environment built on constant chaos. An analytical (gl) mind that thrives on careful thinking feels lost in a setting where everything is urgent and nothing ever feels finished. A relational (gl), high-empathy student is steered toward roles that reward speed rather than connection. A second-career professional with deep life experience and emotional maturity joins a unit that desperately needs those qualities, but where no one has time to mentor (gl) them. A leader who is skilled at bringing clarity and calm steps into a culture that is already running on confusion and overextension (gl).

Initially, people adapt. They stay late, pick up extra shifts, move faster, absorb more responsibility, and tell themselves this is just how healthcare feels. They compare themselves to coworkers who appear to be managing and assume the discomfort is a personal failing. But misalignment grows in these small compromises. Over time, the quiet realization emerges: "This does not fit me, no matter how hard I try." Misalignment is not about a lack of strength. It is about a mismatch (gl) between a person's wiring and the environment wrapped around them.

The Biology of Misalignment

Misalignment is not just an idea; it is a biological (gl) and physiological (gl) experience. The nervous system (gl) recognizes it long before someone is ready to say it out loud. When a person is consistently placed in environments that clash with their natural patterns of pace (gl), sensory load (gl), emotional intensity, and decision-making, the body sends early warnings. They may feel exhausted in a way that sleep no longer repairs, notice irritability (gl) that never used to be part of their personality, struggle to concentrate, or feel the flattening of compassion fatigue (gl) as they withdraw (gl) from patients and coworkers to protect what little is left of their reserves.

These are not signs of weakness. They are alarms. In healthcare, people are often taught to silence those alarms with phrases like "push through," "be tough," or "this is just how it is." But ignored alarms do not disappear; they accumulate (gl). Over time, misalignment pulls more and more energy out of the system until even the most dedicated, mission-driven people begin to feel hollowed out by work that once felt meaningful.

What Misalignment Steals

Misalignment gradually pulls at the threads of identity. It drains the color from a career that once felt bright. It turns a calling into a series of countdowns: counting hours left in the shift, days until the next day off, months until the end of a contract, years until retirement. It reshapes the way someone sees themselves, replacing "I am a helper" with "I am barely holding on." Misalignment also erodes (gl) confidence. Someone who once trusted their instincts now second-guesses every decision. The same person who used to volunteer to stay late for a struggling patient may find themselves quietly avoiding extra responsibilities because they simply cannot carry one more thing.

One of the earliest casualties is kindness. Not because people stop caring, but because caring from an empty well becomes physically painful. When misalignment is chronic (gl), the energy that once fueled patience and empathy is diverted (gl) to basic survival. People who entered healthcare ready to give their best find themselves simply trying to get through the day. The system looks at this and calls it burnout. Underneath, it is something even more fundamental: a profound (gl) misfit between person and environment.

Why the Crisis Feels Different Now

For decades, healthcare workers internalized (gl) one central message: be strong and push through. The work has always been demanding, but the landscape has changed. Patients are older and more complex. Documentation through the electronic health record (EHR) (gl) has multiplied. Families expect more communication. Regulations (gl) and quality reporting (gl) add new layers of work. Staffing ratios (gl) often stretch thin. Violence and incivility (gl) in emergency departments (gl), inpatient (gl) units, and behavioral health (gl) settings have increased. Breaks are shortened or skipped. Technology, which promised to make work easier, often adds more screens, more alerts, and more clicks.

Then came COVID-19 (gl), a mass-casualty (gl) event with no clear endpoint. For many clinicians, it intensified (gl) every existing pressure all at once. They worked through surges (gl), shortages, rapidly shifting protocols (gl), fear for their own safety, and the grief of witnessing large-scale (gl) loss. Some became the only person at a dying patient's bedside when families were not allowed to visit. Experiences like that leave marks that do not vanish when a pandemic (gl) emergency declaration (gl) ends. In that context, the quiet question many people had already been asking themselves—"Can I keep doing this?"—became much louder.

The Cycle That No One Can Outrun

Misalignment sits beneath much of what we label as a workforce crisis. When people are misaligned, they leave. Turnover (gl) creates vacancies. Vacancies lead to heavier workloads for the people who stay. Heavier workloads increase errors, missed care, and moral distress (gl). Those experiences become their own form of trauma (gl). Trauma increases the desire to leave, and the cycle repeats.

Organizations respond with sign-on bonuses, retention (gl) incentives, wellness programs, and resilience (gl) workshops. These can provide relief, but they cannot fix a fundamental mismatch. You cannot bribe a nervous system to stay in a misaligned environment forever. You cannot ask people to "be more resilient" when the real problem is that the work and the environment are fighting who they are. Misalignment has only one true remedy: bringing the person and the place back into fit.

How Misalignment Shows Up in People

For those who know how to look, misalignment becomes visible long before a formal resignation (gl) appears. A nurse who once greeted every patient by name and loved small talk now avoids eye contact in the hallway. A physician who used to teach students and residents (gl) at the bedside now rushes through encounters without looking up from the computer. A student who walked into their first clinical rotation (gl) feeling excited about their future leaves the semester asking whether they chose the wrong field. A second-career adult who entered healthcare with a deep sense of purpose begins quietly browsing other job postings late at night. A leader who once had energy for coaching and mentoring now answers emails at midnight and feels numb in staff meetings.

Individually, each of these may look like a bad week. Collectively (gl), they describe a workforce experiencing chronic (gl) misalignment. The danger is that when misalignment is unnamed, people assume it is a private problem and carry it alone.

Why It Begins Long Before the First Job

Misalignment does not start on someone's first day of work. It often begins in the decision-making process long before that. A high school student might be told that if they are "good at science," they should be a nurse or a doctor, even if their wiring might thrive in therapy (gl), imaging (gl), pharmacy (gl), public health (gl), or health information (gl). A college student might pick a major based on what is most visible or most praised, without ever exploring the quieter roles that might fit them better. A person may shadow (gl) only one unit or one role and assume the entire field looks and feels like that single experience.

When people make choices based on incomplete (gl) information, pressure, stereotypes (gl), or other people's expectations, they can end up in roles that never had a real chance of fitting. By the time the misalignment becomes clear, they have already invested years of study, tuition, and emotional energy. The fear of starting over keeps them stuck. The misalignment epidemic grows not because people do not care, but because the system has not given them the tools to understand where they belong from the beginning.

Why Naming the Epidemic Matters

When misalignment remains unnamed, people blame themselves. They may label themselves as not tough enough, not resilient (gl) enough, not focused enough, or not committed enough. They may wonder why their peers seem to be managing, without realizing those peers might be asking the same questions in private. This self-blame adds another layer of weight on top of an already heavy load.

Naming misalignment does not instantly fix it, but it changes the story. Instead of "I am failing," the story becomes "I am out of fit." That shift opens the door to new questions: What kind of environment matches my nervous system? Where do I feel more grounded and less drained? What tempo (gl) of work fits me best? Do I come alive in crisis, or in calm? Am I energized by constant interaction or by focused, detailed work?

The misalignment epidemic is not a story of people failing their roles. It is a story of roles and environments failing to match the people standing inside them. When we name that truth clearly, we can stop treating burnout as an individual flaw and start seeing misalignment as a system problem that can be redesigned.

The next chapter turns from diagnosis to blueprint—and begins the work of exploring what alignment really looks like when it is done on purpose.

Chapter 11

The Alignment Blueprint: Rebuilding Healthcare Through Alignment

The Alignment Blueprint: Rebuilding Healthcare Through Alignment

The solution to the healthcare workforce crisis is not mysterious, and it is not hidden behind layers of policy (gl) or impossible restructuring (gl). It does not begin with bigger bonuses (gl), bigger recruiting sprees (gl), or temporary agency contract (gl) fixes. The real solution begins at a deeper, more human level. It begins with the quiet truth that healthcare has always depended on alignment: the intricate (gl) fit between a person's wiring and the environment in which they practice.

Healthcare's greatest resource has never been technology or funding or infrastructure (gl).

It has always been people.

And people thrive when the work matches who they are.

For too long, healthcare roles have been designed around tasks, history, and habit. Many were shaped in an era when care moved slower, documentation (gl) was minimal, staffing models (gl) were predictable, and the emotional demands of the work were different. Over time, the work evolved, but the roles did not always evolve with it.

The future of healthcare requires something more intentional (gl) — a system built around human strengths, human nervous systems (gl), and human capacity. This chapter is a blueprint (gl) for that future.

Roles Built for Humans, Not Just Job Descriptions

A sustainable (gl) workforce begins with roles shaped around people, not people stretched to fit outdated roles. When clinical and support positions are designed with human wiring in mind, the entire system becomes more stable. The science behind this is simple and universal (gl):

People who thrive in fast, unpredictable (gl) environments belong in settings where rapid decision-making is essential.

Deep listeners find purpose in roles that allow sustained (gl) connection.

Those who love technology thrive in informatics (gl), imaging (gl), and systems work.

Analytical (gl) minds flourish in health information management (HIM) (gl), coding (gl), quality improvement (gl), and laboratory sciences (gl).

Problem-solvers come alive in triage (gl), trauma (gl), and acute care (gl).

A system that recognizes these natural patterns creates longevity (gl).

A system that ignores them creates turnover (gl).

When roles reflect human strengths, healthcare stops feeling like a test of endurance (gl) and instead becomes a place where people can grow into the best versions of themselves.

Advancement Without Abandoning the Work People Love

For decades, advancement (gl) in healthcare has followed a predictable path: climb upward, move away from the bedside, and accept leadership (gl) responsibilities whether or not they match your disposition (gl). This model unintentionally (gl) pulls experienced clinicians away from the work that gives them meaning.

In an alignment-based system, growth does not require giving up purpose. It allows experience to deepen instead of drift. This includes well-designed clinical ladders (gl), senior specialist roles (gl), advanced practice pathways (gl), preceptor (gl) and educator (gl) fellowships (gl), and leadership tiers that allow clinicians to influence (gl) practice without stepping completely out of patient care.

Cross-training (gl) should reward curiosity and strengths, not desperation to fill vacancies (gl). The more a clinician's expertise (gl) can grow roots instead of wings, the stronger and more stable the workforce becomes.

The Power of Second-Career Professionals

One of healthcare's greatest untapped (gl) strengths is the wave of second-career professionals entering the field. These individuals bring emotional maturity, real-world experience, steadiness under pressure, and communication skill that cannot be taught in textbooks. Many come to healthcare not by default but by choice, fueled by a sense of purpose that is deep and enduring (gl).

Supporting them through structured bridge programs (gl), flexible training options, thoughtful mentorship (gl), and tuition pathways (gl) creates a workforce enriched (gl) by life experience. These individuals often become anchors within teams because they arrive with clarity, motivation, and a strong understanding of who they are.

Alignment recognizes their value and invests in it.

Healthy Environments Create Healthy Workers

Burnout does not arise from lack of passion. It emerges when the demands of the work and the conditions of the environment are no longer in balance. Healing the environment is one of the most direct ways to heal the workforce. This means designing workplaces with safe assignments, emotionally intelligent (gl) leadership, technology that reduces burden instead of adding to it, flexibility in scheduling (gl), debriefing (gl) practices after trauma, mutual respect across disciplines (gl), and cultures where speaking up is interpreted as courage rather than inconvenience (gl).

When the environment supports human needs as intentionally (gl) as it supports operational (gl) needs, people reconnect with the reason they entered healthcare in the first place. Alignment between environment and person is not a luxury; it is the foundation of professional sustainability (gl).

Data-Driven Placement: The Precision Medicine of Workforce Design

Healthcare would never place a patient on a medication without checking for fit, contraindications (gl), and individualized (gl) needs. Yet the workforce — the very people responsible for patient care — is often placed in roles without the same level of precision (gl). Alignment changes this by bringing modern tools into workforce design.

Personality and strengths assessments (gl), realistic job previews (gl), simulation labs (gl), predictive analytics (gl), and structured decision-making can match individuals to environments where they will thrive. Instead of guessing where someone belongs, we begin to know.

SCRUB*fits*™ were built to do one thing well — never to filter people out, but to guide them toward environments that amplify (gl) their abilities and protect their well-being (gl). In healthcare, people don't struggle because they lack talent; they struggle because they're placed in systems that don't fit how they're wired, what they value, or how they do their best work. Alignment isn't about exclusion. It's about finally being seen — and finally being placed where you can thrive.

Alignment Begins Long Before the First Day on the Job

The seeds of burnout and misalignment are planted long before someone steps onto a unit. Students often choose majors based on limited exposure, outdated stereotypes (gl), or pressure. They might shadow (gl) only one lifestyle, one specialty (gl), or one unit, and assume that experience represents the entire field.

Alignment begins when students are taught to explore the full spectrum of healthcare worlds early — not as an afterthought. High school career exploration, transparent previews of specialties, mentorship (gl) with working professionals, and rotational internships (gl) help students make aligned decisions that will last.

Imagine a generation entering healthcare not by guesswork but with clarity about who they are and where they fit. The entire system would transform.

Restoring Purpose to the Center of Care

Healthcare is built on meaning. The quiet, powerful encounters between clinicians and patients — the teaching moments, the steady presence at the bedside, the safety someone provides during the hardest hour of another person's life — are the heartbeat of the profession.

When meaning is buried under documentation (gl), metrics (gl), and overwhelm, the workforce falters. Purpose must be intentionally (gl) protected and restored. This means celebrating impact, recognizing excellence across departments, protecting time for teaching and reflection, elevating stories of patient journeys, and encouraging innovation (gl) and contribution (gl).

Purpose is the renewable energy (gl) that powers healthcare. Alignment is what keeps that energy circulating.

A System That Sees People as Its Strength

A sustainable workforce is not built by replacing humans or demanding more from people who are already stretched. It is built by honoring them. The future of healthcare is a future where strengths guide placement, environments support well-being, advancement does not require abandoning purpose, second-career professionals are valued, technology lightens work instead of complicating it, and leaders understand humans as deeply as they understand operational data (gl).

Alignment reshapes the workforce from the inside out. It stabilizes teams, protects patient care, strengthens culture, and restores humanity to an industry that relies on it more than anything else.

Closing Note

The solution to the healthcare crisis will not be achieved by sheer numbers or by pushing people harder. It will be achieved by redesigning roles, environments, and pathways (gl) around the people who bring care to life. Somewhere in the vast world of healthcare, there is a role that matches each person's wiring — a place where their gifts are not stretched thin but strengthened, where purpose is sustainable, and where the work feels not only possible but right.

Alignment is not a trend or an idealistic (gl) hope.

It is the future.

And it is already within reach.

Chapter 12
The Alignment Revolution

How Healthcare Can Transform Itself in the Next Decade

The healthcare system of the next decade will not be saved by more recruiting (gl), more bonuses (gl), or more burnout workshops (gl). Those tools treat symptoms, not causes. The future will belong to organizations that understand a different truth: human alignment is the foundation of a stable, sustainable (gl) workforce.

The Alignment Revolution isn't abstract (gl) idealism. It is a practical blueprint (gl) for redesigning healthcare from the inside out—built around people, strengths, and the environments where they naturally thrive. Over the next ten years, alignment-based systems will outperform traditional systems in retention (gl), patient outcomes, safety, culture, and financial stability. This chapter lays out how.

1. The Next Decade Will Be Defined by Fit, Not Force

For decades, healthcare has relied on one core assumption:

If someone is trained, they can work anywhere.

But the research (gl) on burnout (gl), turnover (gl), and early-career exits (gl) shows otherwise. Whether someone stays in healthcare isn't determined by their training; it's determined by whether the environment matches their:

• nervous system (gl)

• communication style (gl)

• sensory tolerance (gl)

• decision-making pattern (gl)

• emotional processing (gl)

• cognitive wiring (gl)

• core values (gl)

• learning preferences (gl)

The next decade will pivot (gl) away from "staffing bodies" and toward placing humans—not randomly or out of desperation (gl), but intentionally (gl).

Systems that thrive will ask:

"Where will this person feel grounded, confident, and themselves?"

And then they'll match accordingly.

2. Alignment Will Become the New Standard for Workforce Planning

Currently, organizations workforce-plan (gl) by counting:

• how many nurses (gl) they have

- how many physicians (gl) they need

- how many techs (gl) they can recruit

- how many CNAs (gl) they can onboard

- how many travelers (gl) they can afford

The problem?

Numbers don't predict survival (gl).

What predicts survival is fit.

In an Alignment Revolution system:

- Units are staffed based on sensory load (gl) and cognitive demand (gl).

- Schedules are built around environmental tolerance (gl).

- Cross-training (gl) considers personality fit, not just skill.

- Roles are assigned based on **SCRUB*fit*™** Category (gl) alignment.

- Leaders know each staff member's alignment profile (gl).

- New hires are matched, not scattered.

This sounds futuristic (gl), but early adopters (gl) are already doing pieces of it—and their retention is outpacing national averages (gl).

3. Education Will Shift From a Pipeline (gl) Model to an Alignment Model

Right now, education is built on sorting:

- "Strong in science? Consider nursing."

- "Good with people? Become a social worker."

- "Technical? Try radiology."

This is surface-level (gl) thinking.

In the next decade, schools will embrace deeper alignment—helping students discover:

- Do they thrive in unpredictability (gl) or structure?

- Do they process emotion internally (gl) or externally (gl)?

- Do they think quickly or deeply?

- Do they enjoy constant interaction or focused independence (gl)?

- Do they prefer precision (gl), creativity (gl), or both?

Programs will begin with alignment assessments (gl), not end with burnout statistics (gl).

Imagine nursing schools that:

- guide high-intensity (gl) learners to emergency nursing (gl)

- guide steady, technical minds to perioperative (gl) environments

- guide emotionally intuitive (gl) students to behavioral health (gl)

- guide structured thinkers to health information (gl)

Education will no longer produce "generic clinicians."

It will produce aligned clinicians.

4. Systems Will Redesign Roles for Human Nervous Systems

For decades, healthcare has asked clinicians to conform (gl) to environments designed around:

- efficiency metrics (gl)

- legacy workflows (gl)

- historic staffing ratios (gl)

- old-school hierarchy (gl)

The Alignment Revolution will redesign from scratch:

- noise levels (gl)

- alarm loads (gl)

- sensory triggers (gl)

- documentation burden (gl)

- break structures (gl)

- team communication norms (gl)

- leadership presence (gl)

- safety expectations (gl)

Environments will be shaped around what humans can tolerate sustainably (gl)—not what spreadsheets demand.

This may include:

- quiet zones (gl)

- sensory-reduced medication rooms (gl)

- better alarm management (gl)

- protected deep-work time (gl) for documentation (gl)

- on-unit mental decompression (gl) spaces

- emotionally regulated (gl) huddles (gl)

- trauma-informed (gl) leadership (gl)

For the first time, human physiology (gl) will be part of workforce design.

5. Alignment Will Become the Root Strategy for Retention

Retention is currently reactive (gl):

- raise pay after people leave

- improve staffing after goodwill (gl) is lost

- offer wellness programs after burnout

- fix culture after it collapses

The Alignment Revolution flips this:

Retention becomes proactive (gl).

Retention starts at:

- hiring (gl)

- unit placement (gl)

- orientation (gl)

- mentorship (gl) matching

- scheduling (gl)

- leadership development (gl)

- career-pathing (gl)

Imagine retention beginning with:

"Where will this person thrive?"

Retention becomes a by-product (gl) of belonging (gl).

6. Technology Will Shift From Burden to Support

Technology has often increased burden through:

- constant alerts (gl)
- endless clicks (gl)
- rigid templates (gl)
- documentation bloat (gl)
- poor interoperability (gl)

The Alignment Revolution will leverage (gl) AI (gl) and automation (gl) to:

- reduce documentation time (gl)
- personalize (gl) workflows
- streamline (gl) communication
- anticipate (gl) burnout risk (gl)
- optimize (gl) staffing based on strengths
- pre-fill common EHR (gl) patterns
- protect clinicians' attention (gl)

SCRUB*fit***™** is part of this ecosystem—not replacing humans, but enhancing human fit.

]7. Leaders Will Be Measured by Alignment Metrics

Traditional metrics:

- turnover rate (gl)

- vacancy rate (gl)

- HCAHPS (gl)

- throughput (gl)• RVUs (gl)

Alignment metrics will emerge:

- alignment placement rate (gl)

- alignment-protected transitions (gl)

- misalignment risk score (gl)

- **SCRUB*fit*™** Category distribution (gl)

- time-to-stabilization (gl) for new hires

- alignment-informed scheduling (gl)

- reduction in sensory overload events (gl)

- alignment-driven psychological safety (gl)

Leaders will no longer manage "numbers."

They will manage human alignment ecosystems (gl).

8. The Next-Generation Workforce Will Demand Alignment

Gen Z (gl) and Gen Alpha (gl) are not driven by:

- hierarchy

- fear

- "pay your dues" culture

- suffering-is-part-of-the-job narratives (gl)

They want:

- mental health (gl)

- balance (gl)

- purpose

- belonging (gl)

- mentorship (gl)

- clarity

- psychological safety (gl)

- education that aligns with who they are

Systems that ignore these expectations will fall behind.

Systems that embrace alignment will become destinations (gl).

9. Alignment Will Save Healthcare More Money Than Any Bonus Ever Could

Misalignment is expensive. It drives:

- turnover (gl)

- absenteeism (gl)

- presenteeism (gl)

- errors (gl)

- extended length of stay (LOS) (gl)

- overtime (gl)

- travel-nurse dependency (gl)

- constant orientation cycles (gl)

Alignment:

- reduces turnover

- increases productivity (gl)

- stabilizes teamwork (gl)

- reduces harm events (gl)

- improves patient outcomes

- strengthens culture

- lowers total cost of care (gl)

Alignment is not "soft."

Alignment is financial strategy.

10. The Alignment Revolution Begins With Language

When people can name their environments—Adrenaline Team (gl), Compassion Corps (gl), Diagnostic Division (gl), and more —they begin to understand themselves differently.

They stop thinking:

"I'm not strong enough."

"I must not be cut out for this."

"Maybe I'm the problem."

And they start thinking:

"I simply wasn't in the right environment."

That shift changes lives.

It brings people back.

It keeps people in.

It restores dignity (gl) to the workforce.

It builds a future worth staying for.

The Next Decade Belongs to Alignment

Recruitment alone cannot fix what misalignment has broken.

But alignment can fix what recruitment never will.

Alignment is:

• the cure for burnout

• the solution to shortages (gl)

• the stabilizer of culture

• the key to safety

• the path to retention

• the foundation of future education

• the roadmap for redesign

• the bridge between human needs and healthcare demands

The Alignment Revolution is coming.

And it will transform healthcare not by adding pressure—but by honoring people.

Chapter 13
Alignment & Reflection

A Practical Look at How Your Healthcare "DNA" Shapes Your Fit

There is a moment—right before you step into a new chapter of your life—when everything feels both exciting and overwhelming. You may feel curious, hopeful, and a little unsure all at once, wondering:

How am I supposed to choose a healthcare path when I've never even been inside a hospital as anything other than a patient?

That question is exactly why this chapter exists.

You've already been introduced to Mason's Alignment Theory™ (MAT)—the lens that explains why burnout (gl), turnover (gl), and career dissatisfaction (gl) are not personal failures, but structural (gl) signals of misalignment. But alignment is not just something that happens inside healthcare systems. It begins inside you.

Long before anyone hands you a badge, schedules your shifts, or assigns you a unit, you already carry patterns—how you respond to pressure, how you relate to people, how you handle change, how you make decisions, and what kind of work gives you energy instead of draining it. Think of this as your personal healthcare "DNA." It is not a scientific (gl) code or a personality label. It is simply the collection of tendencies (gl), needs, and rhythms that make you who you are.

The sooner you understand those patterns, the easier it becomes to choose a path where you do not just survive—you thrive.

This chapter is your pause button.

Your deep breath.

Your moment to look inward before you start looking at job titles.

Because when you understand how you are wired, the rest of this book becomes much clearer.

The Alignment Promise

Alignment is for everyone — but access to alignment isn't equal. My theory isn't about overnight reinvention (gl); it's about reclaiming the right to do work that matches who you are. Every healthcare professional can move toward alignment through small day-to-day shifts, strategic (gl) pivots (gl) within their credential (gl), or long-term career redesign (gl). Some paths are immediate, some require planning, and some demand systemic (gl) reform (gl) — but the principle holds: people don't burn out from caring, they burn out from working in roles that contradict their identity (gl). Alignment is universal. The obstacles are structural. And the solution is a partnership between individuals, educators, and healthcare leaders who must begin removing the barriers that keep people stuck where they don't fit.

That promise is the heart of this entire book.

It is the lens through which everything else should be read.

Why Alignment Matters Before You Choose a Path

Here is the truth most people are never told when they are choosing a healthcare career:

Your job will not turn you into someone new.

It will turn you into more of who you already are.

You do not need clinical (gl) experience to begin understanding yourself. Even now, you likely already know:

• whether you prefer steady days or fast-moving ones

• whether people energize you or exhaust you

• whether you like structure or flexibility

• whether surprises feel exciting or stressful

• whether you are drawn to details, stories, puzzles, hands-on work, or systems

These are not skills. They are clues. They are how your nervous system (gl), mind, and personality naturally interact with the world.

Those same patterns show up inside every healthcare role. When your work environment matches them, the job feels sustainable (gl) and even joyful. When it does not, even a "good" job can feel unbearable (gl) over time.

That is why alignment cannot wait until after your first job. It has to begin now—before you spend years of time, tuition (gl), and emotional energy on something that was never going to fit.

Noticing Your Patterns, Before You Ever Wear Scrubs

People do not become different when they step into healthcare. They bring themselves with them.

Look at your own life so far:

Do you prefer steady, predictable (gl) rhythms—or do you light up when things move fast?

Do you recharge by connecting with people—or by focusing quietly on tasks and information?

Do you naturally zoom in on details, or zoom out to see the bigger picture?

Do you stay calm in uncertainty (gl), or do you do your best work when things are clearly defined?

These patterns show up in classrooms, friendships, hobbies, part-time jobs, and family life long before they ever show up in hospitals. They will show up again in whatever healthcare role you choose.

Alignment simply takes those patterns seriously.

Why This Chapter Comes Right Before the Mini SCRUB*fit*™ Assessment

The Mini **SCRUB*fit*™** Healthcare Career Assessment gives you a pattern.

This chapter gives you the meaning behind that pattern.

Without this reflection (gl), the assessment can feel like a quiz.

With it, the results become a map.

They begin to explain:

• why certain environments feel natural to you

• why others quietly drain you

• why some roles feel exciting while others feel heavy

• why your reactions to stress, pace, and people matter

That understanding will help you read every career profile in this book with clarity instead of confusion—and with strategy instead of guesswork.

Your Next Step

Turn the page.

You are now ready to take the Mini **SCRUB*fit*™** Healthcare Career Assessment—grounded in who you are, aware of your own patterns, and prepared to see how different healthcare worlds might fit you.

This is where clarity begins.

And where misalignment starts to lose its hold.

Chapter 14
Out of Alignment: The Human Cost

THE HEARTBREAK OF MISALIGNMENT

Most people choose a healthcare career the old-fashioned way: they follow a family tradition, chase a paycheck, or pick something that simply sounds good.

And then there are the Dr. Sunshines of the world.

Years ago, I placed a young orthopedic (gl) surgeon at a prestigious (gl) New York City practice — the kind of job people write LinkedIn (gl) victory posts about. Tall, bright, charismatic (gl), always polished. A guy who looked like he had been manufactured in a lab called Future Attending.

One of the first things he ever told me was:

"I look great in a white lab coat."

I laughed, assuming he was joking.

He wasn't.

(Yes, it went into my notes. I keep meticulous (gl) records —
the kind that surprise people years later.)

At the time, he carried every external marker of success:
prestige, paycheck, perception, presence. He was the walking,
talking prototype (gl) of I made it.

"I can do it," he told me.

And he was right. Technically, he could.

But alignment isn't about whether you can do something.

It's about whether the role fits the way your nervous system
was built to work.

Years later, when we reconnected, something had changed.

The operating room that once energized him now filled him
with dread. His knees ached. His patience frayed. The spark —
the thing that makes a clinician feel alive — had quietly
slipped out the door.

"Don't most of your cases run close to two hours?" I asked.

"Yeah," he said softly. "I can't stand it — literally."

Thirteen years of training.

Roughly $430,000 in education.

Thousands of patients.

And suddenly the path he had built no longer fit the body and
mind standing inside it.

He wasn't lazy.

He wasn't ungrateful.

He wasn't weak.

He was misaligned.

Here's the truth no one likes to say out loud:

A person can perform beautifully in a role while slowly disappearing inside it.

It's like wearing a suit tailored for someone else. From the outside it looks flawless. From the inside it pinches, constricts, and slowly makes it hard to breathe.

And eventually, even the best tailoring can't hide the fact that the body inside no longer fits the cut of the cloth.

Before we ended our call, he said something almost casually:

"I've been sketching a redesign for an orthopedic (gl) knee implant (gl)."

And just like that, the air changed.

The heaviness lifted.

The spark returned.

The light behind his voice flickered back on.

He didn't hate medicine.

He hated being trapped in the wrong expression of medicine.

Months later, he wrote to me: he had investors (gl), an engineer, and early-stage testing underway.

He hadn't left healthcare.

He had shifted lanes inside it — from endurance to innovation, from standing for hours to building something that moved the field forward.

That is alignment.

Not quitting.

Not escaping.

But finally standing in the part of the work that fits how you are built.

And that is the real heartbreak of misalignment:

You can be wildly successful...

and still be in the wrong place for who you truly are.

Chapter 15
Why Alignment Matters

Why Alignment Matters

Choosing a healthcare career isn't just about picking a job —
it's about choosing the conditions you will spend your life in.
Healthcare is demanding, fast-moving, emotionally complex
(gl), and deeply human. When someone enters a role that
doesn't align with who they are, the disconnect shows quickly.
Misalignment becomes exhaustion, frustration, burnout, and
eventually walking away from a career that once felt
meaningful.

Alignment changes everything.

Aligned caregivers (gl) feel energized instead of drained. They
communicate more clearly, connect more deeply, and make
safer decisions. They are more confident, more resilient (gl),
and more satisfied in their work. They stay longer, grow faster,
and create better patient experiences. When someone's
natural strengths match the rhythm of their work environment
— whether it's high-intensity emergency care, steady recovery

work, behind-the-scenes data precision, or supportive patient guidance — healthcare becomes sustainable instead of overwhelming.

Alignment is not about talent.

It is about fit.

It is about whether the environment supports your instincts.

Whether the pace matches your nervous system.

Whether the work feels meaningful to you at your core.

The **SCRUB*fit*™** Healthcare Career Assessment was created to help people discover that fit before they invest years of time, energy, training, and money. It identifies the environments where someone's strengths become advantages rather than obstacles, and where their natural tendencies — whether calm under pressure, attentive to detail, empathetic (gl), technical, structured, or collaborative (gl) — turn into sustainable career paths.

When people choose aligned roles, they aren't just better employees — they are healthier humans.

They feel more purpose, more clarity, and more confidence.

They grow rather than struggle.

They contribute rather than collapse.

And they stay in the field, strengthening a system that depends on them.

Alignment is the difference between a job that wears you down and a calling that lifts you up. It is the foundation of long-term success — for individuals, for healthcare systems, and for the future of care.

This is why alignment matters.

This is why **SCRUB*fit*™** exists.

And this is why every student, adult, and career-changer (gl) deserves to know where they truly belong in healthcare — before they ever step into the scrubs.

Chapter 16
Mini SCRUBfit Healthcare Career Assessment

THE MINI SCRUB*fit*™ HEALTHCARE CAREER ASSESSMENT

Every movement in healthcare has its method — and every method begins with a model.

SCRUB*fit*™ was built on one central truth:

Happiness, retention, and purpose in healthcare rise or fall on alignment — the match between who you are and where you work.

While that word alignment sounds personal, its roots are scientific.

Behavioral Science reveals how motivation and emotion shape performance under pressure.

Industrial–Organizational Psychology measures the fit between people and their professional environments.

Healthcare Workforce Research shows how that fit predicts burnout, turnover, and satisfaction.

Together, these disciplines form the foundation of the **SCRUB*fit*™** Framework — five domains that consistently forecast fulfillment and longevity in healthcare:

1 Pace & Energy — how you respond when urgency meets responsibility.

2 Compassion & Connection — how you build trust under pressure.

3 Precision & Process — how you create order, structure, and safety.

4 Innovation & Technology — how you adapt, troubleshoot, and improve.

5 Leadership & Growth — how you influence others and shape culture.

Each domain holds two unique callings — the 10 **SCRUB*fit*™** Categories, represented by the 21 characters you'll meet throughout this book:

The Adrenaline Team, Compassion Corps, Diagnostic Division, Med Heads, Recovery Regimen, Vital Link, Power Panel, Prevention Pact, Leadership League, and Care Crew.

Together, they form the **SCRUB*fit*™ Alignment Map** — healthcare's professional DNA.

THE SCIENCE OF SELF-DISCOVERY

This quick, 15-question assessment is designed to help you locate yourself on that map.

It's not a test — it's a mirror.

Each question represents a moment you've already lived: an emergency, a choice, a rhythm of your workday.

Your answers reflect the instincts that drive you when no one's watching.

When you're done, your responses will point to one of the ten **SCRUB*fit*™** categories — your natural alignment zone.

It's the color that fits not just your scrubs, but your spirit.

HOW TO TAKE THE ASSESSMENT

Answer instinctively — don't overthink it.

Circle the letter that sounds most like you on your best day at work.

When you're finished, here's how your results come to life:

• If you're taking the **online SCRUB*fit*™ Assessment**, you won't see a cheesy "mostly A's" answer key.

Behind the scenes, your responses are quietly weighted across the five domains and ten categories.

The system looks at your overall pattern — how you handle pressure, connection, precision, innovation, and leadership — and then reveals your **Primary SCRUB*fit*™ Category** and **Secondary Alignment**, along with the character who wears your color.

• If you're using this **mini assessment in the book**, you can still get a powerful snapshot.

As you review your answers, notice which letters repeat and which descriptions feel like home.

Then turn to the **SCRUB*fit*™ Alignment Guide** and read the categories that match those letters.

Don't treat them as a rigid label — treat them as the "chapters" of healthcare where your story is most likely to unfold.

The Questions

1. When everything starts happening at once, I...

A. Take command until calm returns.

B. Keep everyone grounded with reassurance.

C. Search for the pattern beneath the problem.

D. Recheck the data to see what we missed.

E. Encourage others to stay steady and keep moving.

F. Restore order by getting the workflow right.

G. Use it later as a lesson to prevent a repeat.

H. Bring the group together and focus on solutions.

I. Check the equipment or tech first — that's usually the culprit.

J. Keep the mood calm and cooperative.

2. My favorite part of a workday is...

A. The high-speed teamwork when things get intense.

B. A heartfelt thank-you from someone I helped.

C. Solving a puzzle that finally makes sense.

D. Seeing accuracy turn into safety.

E. Watching a patient take a new step toward recovery.

F. When the whole system clicks perfectly.

G. Knowing we stopped a problem before it started.

H. Helping people see their purpose again.

I. Getting a new device or idea to work flawlessly.

J. Ending the day with everyone smiling.

3. Under pressure, I...

A. Move faster and think clearer.

B. Focus harder on compassion.

C. Step back to see the whole picture.

D. Slow down enough to be precise.

E. Encourage progress, not panic.

F. Tighten the process so nothing slips.

G. Look for teachable moments.

H. Keep the group steady and confident.

I. Troubleshoot until the system hums again.

J. Crack a quick joke to keep the energy light.

4. When something goes wrong, I'm the one who...

A. Grabs the reins and steers it back on course.

B. Checks on how people are coping.

C. Runs the numbers or evidence.

D. Tracks the root cause line by line.

E. Helps everyone reset and try again.

F. Documents and clarifies what needs changing.

G. Designs education to prevent it next time.

H. Opens a huddle and guides the discussion.

I. Fixes what's broken — hardware, software, or process.

J. Communicates across the team so no one feels left out.

5. My coworkers rely on me to...

A. Stay cool when things heat up.

B. Listen when emotions run high.

C. Interpret results and find the truth.

D. Catch small errors before they matter.

E. Be patient and persistent.

F. Keep information flowing cleanly.

G. Educate and advocate for better health.

H. Model leadership that feels human.

I. Keep the tools and systems working.

J. Keep spirits high and people connected.

6. The environment where I thrive most is...

A. High-stakes, high-energy, and unpredictable.

B. Warm, personal, and full of empathy.

C. Data-driven and fact-based.

D. Structured, stable, and detail-oriented.

E. Encouraging, goal-focused, and positive.

F. Streamlined and organized.

G. Out in the community, solving problems upstream.

H. Purpose-filled, collaborative, and mission-driven.

I. Innovative, technical, and evolving.

J. Cooperative, supportive, and steady.

7. When a system isn't working, I...

A. Adapt immediately — we'll fix it later.

B. Protect the people affected.

C. Analyze until I see the cause.

D. Redesign the procedure.

E. Motivate others to stay calm and hopeful.

F. Clarify the workflow.

G. Turn it into training.

H. Rally leaders to align.

I. Repair the malfunction.

J. Keep communication flowing.

8. I'm happiest when I'm...

A. In motion — doing something that matters fast.

B. Bringing comfort to someone in pain.

C. Discovering something no one else saw.

D. Completing something flawlessly.

E. Helping someone rebuild strength.

F. Creating order from chaos.

G. Preventing harm before it happens.

H. Guiding a team to their best day.

I. Building or improving technology that helps care.

J. Making the workplace feel like family.

9. People often say I'm...

A. Fearless and decisive.

B. Kind and understanding.

C. Smart and curious.

D. Careful and consistent.

E. Optimistic and encouraging.

F. Dependable and systematic.

G. Insightful and proactive.

H. Wise and fair.

I. Clever and inventive.

J. Friendly and dependable.

10. My greatest satisfaction comes from...

A. Managing crisis with precision.

B. Turning fear into relief.

C. Solving the case no one else could.

D. Knowing my accuracy saved time or lives.

E. Watching progress unfold.

F. Seeing systems finally run right.

G. Inspiring healthier choices.

H. Watching leadership decisions lift morale.

I. Getting a complex setup to perform perfectly.

J. Seeing the team leave proud of the work we did.

11. When I notice a problem, I...

A. Act fast.

B. Listen first.

C. Investigate thoroughly.

D. Verify the data.

E. Support the people involved.

F. Document everything.

G. Educate and prevent recurrence.

H. Lead a conversation to fix it.

I. Test and tweak until it's right.

J. Communicate so everyone knows.

12. I define success as...

A. Staying sharp when the stakes are high.

B. Making others feel safe and cared for.

C. Finding truth through evidence.

D. Delivering exact, reliable outcomes.

E. Helping someone find their strength.

F. Running operations that never miss a beat.

G. Improving community health at scale.

H. Building teams that trust each other.

I. Creating solutions that last.

J. Uniting people around purpose.

13. When stress builds up, I...

A. Channel it — it sharpens my edge.

B. Slow down and reconnect with empathy.

C. Study it until I understand it.

D. Organize until it's under control.

E. Turn it into motivation.

F. Reassess processes for efficiency.

G. Learn from it and adjust prevention.

H. Lead others calmly through it.

I. Fix what's broken.

J. Bring humor or warmth to reset the mood.

14. If I weren't in healthcare, I'd probably be...

A. A firefighter or pilot.

B. A counselor or teacher.

C. A scientist or detective.

D. An engineer or accountant.

E. A coach or mentor.

F. An information manager.

G. A public-health advocate.

H. An executive or strategist.

I. An inventor or tech lead.

J. A team coordinator.

15. At the end of a long shift, I feel best when...

A. I know I made the critical difference.

B. Someone left comforted.

C. The data tells a clear story.

D. Every number checks out.

E. A patient smiled at their own progress.

F. The system ran seamlessly.

G. The community left safer.

H. The staff left inspired.

I. The machines hummed perfectly.

J. We all left proud of one another.

Scoring Your Results

Now that you've finished, take a breath.

The goal here isn't to "win" the test — it's to recognize your rhythm.

In the **full SCRUB*fit*™ system**, your responses feed into a behind-the-scenes model:

• Each answer is linked to one or more of the five **SCRUB*fit*™** domains.

• Those domains connect to the ten **SCRUB*fit*™** Categories.

• Your overall pattern — not any single question — shapes your **Primary Category** and **Secondary Alignment**.

In the **online assessment**, all of that scoring happens quietly in the background. You simply answer honestly, and your result appears: your color, your category, your character, and your alignment story.

In this **mini book version**, think less about tally marks and more about patterns:

• Notice which letters and descriptions showed up again and again.

• Pay attention to the phrases that made you think, *"That's me."*

165

• Use those patterns to guide you into the **SCRUB*fit*™ Alignment Guide** on the next pages.

The letter you gravitate toward most often will usually point to your primary **SCRUB*fit*™** category — the color and calling that best match your professional DNA.

Your next-strongest pattern represents your secondary alignment — the strength that supports how you work, lead, and grow.

Use your results as a compass, not a box.

They point you toward the environments, roles, and rhythms of care where you'll thrive.

Your SCRUB*fit*™ Alignment Guide

A — The Adrenaline Team

You come alive where time matters most. Swift, skilled, and steady under pressure, you turn urgency into mastery.

From the trauma bay to the OR suite, your world runs on instinct and focus. Jen-Jen Codedale races the clock in the emergency department. Brad Bovie keeps the surgical field safe through every "time-out" and turn. Krashlyn Riggs lifts off in a flight suit, calm even when chaos swirls below. Suzette Soleil helps new life enter the world under the bright lights of Labor & Delivery.

You thrive when minutes matter and teamwork feels electric — when calm hands save lives.

B — The Compassion Corps

You lead with heart. Empathy isn't a drain — it's your drive. You make patients and peers feel safe, seen, and human.

Ginger Gauge steadies a ventilator and a family's fears at once. Justice Jules walks survivors through the hardest hours with courage and care. In your world, compassion is clinical skill — measured not in tasks completed but in trust restored.

You thrive wherever care means connection and kindness becomes courage.

C — The Diagnostic Division

Curiosity is your compass. You see what others miss, transforming data into insight and evidence into action.

Ray Beam translates X-rays into life-saving decisions; Darcy Heplock decodes the mysteries of the lab bench. You think in patterns, probabilities, and possibilities — the quiet detective of healthcare.

You thrive where answers hide in pixels and petri dishes, and truth is the treatment.

D — The Med Heads

Precision is your superpower. You find peace in process, and your consistency keeps care safe and clear.

Polly Pillcount manages a pharmacy like an orchestra, every medication in harmony. Anna Remedy guards the fine line between safety and error, checking, charting, and recalibrating.

You thrive where accuracy saves lives and the math of medicine meets the art of care.

E — The Recovery Regimen

You believe progress is sacred. Step by step, you rebuild hope, strength, and confidence — in others and yourself.

Lilac Lift guides patients through rehab with steady encouragement. Hope Fulle helps them rediscover movement, independence, and joy. Your pace is steady, your optimism contagious.

You thrive where resilience is measured not in speed but in spirit — one milestone at a time.

F — The Vital Link

You keep information flowing and integrity intact. Behind every accurate record is your quiet excellence.

Clara Chartcheck knows that precision on paper means safety at the bedside. You translate the language of care into the logic of systems — converting every story into structured truth.

You thrive behind the scenes, where clarity and compliance protect every patient and empower every clinician.

G — The Prevention Pact

You think upstream — preventing harm before it starts. You educate, advocate, and protect the public's health.

Crimson Quest brings clinical insight to communities. Liv Well turns education into empowerment. Minty Mary reminds the youngest patients — and their parents — that prevention is the first prescription.

You thrive where outreach meets impact, where awareness saves more lives than intervention.

H — The Leadership League

You inspire alignment. Calm, strategic, and visionary, you see the whole system and move it toward better care.

Vera Vines writes notes of gratitude that ripple through an entire hospital. Sage Engage leads teams with both courage and kindness, transforming burnout into belonging.

You thrive where direction and empathy meet — where leadership isn't about power, but purpose.

I — The Power Panel

Innovation charges you. You make technology human and systems safe — the bridge between care and code.

Epic Circuit builds platforms that keep clinicians connected; Max Volt ensures every biomedical heartbeat stays strong. You're part engineer, part visionary — the spark behind seamless care.

You thrive in the hum of machines and the glow of screens, turning complexity into connection.

J — The Care Crew

You're the heartbeat of teamwork. Steady, adaptable, and kind, you make every shift feel possible and every day feel worth it.

Harper Helpwell greets patients with warmth and keeps clinicians grounded in grace. You lead from the middle — through kindness, reliability, and joy.

You thrive in the in-between moments that define great care: a smile, a handoff, a helping hand that keeps everything moving.

. . .

THE SCRUB*fit*™ ALIGNMENT PRINCIPLE

This isn't about who's "best."

It's about where you fit best.

Every color represents a rhythm of care — and together, those rhythms form the pulse of healthcare itself.

When you finish this assessment and turn the page, you'll meet the character who wears your color.

Their story will feel familiar, because in many ways, it's already yours.

That's the promise of **SCRUB*fit*™** —

The right person. In the right place. With the right purpose.

Chapter 17
Scrubbed In and Ready:

You've seen what alignment looks like — and why it matters. Now, meet the twenty-one professionals who live it every day.

The **SCRUB*fit*™** Squad is organized into ten categories — ten lanes of healthcare, each with its own rhythm, values, and way of showing up. Some roles thrive on urgency; others on precision. Some heal through speed; others through patience. None is "better." They're different — and that difference is the point.

Each category has its own heartbeat:

• The Adrenaline Team pulses with urgency — where seconds decide outcomes and calm under fire is the core skill.

• The Compassion Corps moves at the pace of connection — proving healing is relational (gl) as much as it is procedural (gl).

• The Diagnostic Division speaks in data and images —

turning chaos into clarity through precision and investigation (gl).

• The Med Heads live between knowledge and action — the cognitive (gl) command center that converts uncertainty into strategy.

• The Recovery Regimen advances by inches — rebuilding independence and dignity, one hard-won step at a time.

• The Prevention Pact works upstream (gl) — architects (gl) of wellness who build health before crisis arrives.

• The Leadership League sees the whole system — designing conditions where others can thrive, through connection and clarity.

• The Power Panel keeps the current steady — machines, systems, and data running so every signal is reliable.

• The Vital Link connects the dots — translators of trust who safeguard integrity (gl) across the record and the workflow.

• The Care Crew is the everyday glue — versatile, adaptable, and essential to making the day actually work.

Different on purpose. Together, in alignment, they create something larger than any single role: a system where care feels human again.

What's next: twenty-one stories. Ten categories. One shared mission — to show alignment lived, practiced, and perfected under pressure.

As you read, notice the clinical confessions, the small choices, the daily rhythms that shape a life in scrubs. Ask yourself:

Where do I fit? What pace feels right? Which environment brings out my best?

The answer might surprise you.

Scrub in? Let's begin.

Chapter 18
Obstacles, Nuances & Realities

Because alignment is real... but so are the roadblocks.

Healthcare professionals are some of the most committed people on earth. They don't wake up wanting to abandon patients or walk away from the work they trained for. What they want — what they deserve — is alignment: a role that matches their personality, emotional wiring, interests, values, and energy patterns.

But here's the nuance that often gets missed:

1. Alignment Is Universal — Access to It Is Not

Anyone can experience misalignment. Anyone can benefit from fixing it. But not everyone can pivot immediately. Finances, geography, childcare, licensing, limited program slots, or immigration (gl) constraints create real limits.

Acknowledging this doesn't weaken the message — it strengthens trust.

2. Alignment Happens in Three Levels

This is how alignment becomes viable for everyone:

Level 1 — Micro-Alignment (Today)

Small shifts inside the current job:

– changing units

– adjusting schedules

– shifting patient populations (gl)

– modifying responsibilities (gl)

These changes alone can reduce burnout dramatically.

Level 2 — Meso-Alignment (This Year)

Strategic pivots within the same credential (gl):

– ED RN → PACU

– CNA → monitor tech

– NP → new specialty

– PA → new practice model

These moves are realistic and achievable for most professionals.

Level 3 — Macro-Alignment (Long-Term)

Larger shifts requiring education, relocation, or major retraining. Not instant... but not impossible. And often life-changing.

3. The Individual Isn't the Problem — the System Is

This is where the narrative shifts:

Misalignment isn't a personal failure — it's a structural failure. When someone feels stuck or burned out, the question shouldn't be, "What's wrong with them?" but "What barriers are blocking their true fit?"

That single reframing invites leaders to the table instead of shaming the workforce.

4. Alignment Is a Journey — Not a Leap

This framing protects the message from critics and empowers readers:

- Some can start today.

- Some need a plan.

- Some need system changes.

But everyone deserves the right to pursue their true fit.

5. Systems Must Evolve Too

Leaders have a responsibility to:

- expand access to education

- create flexible pathways

- remove financial barriers

- redesign staffing models

- protect the workforce before they break

Without structural support, even the most determined clinician hits a ceiling.

Chapter 19
Bravo Zulu

When a System Tries to Protect Its Healers: What the VA Is Getting Right About Burnout

If you want to understand burnout in real life, don't just look at individual coping tips. Look at systems. Look at what happens when a large, complex healthcare enterprise decides —out loud—that clinician well-being is not a perk, not a poster, and not a "nice to have." It is a safety strategy. It is a retention strategy. It is a moral strategy. And if you ignore it, the bill always shows up—through turnover, errors, disengagement, and the slow disappearance of people who used to love the work.

That's why the U.S. Department of Veterans Affairs (VA) is worth paying attention to right now.

The VA is not a small organization experimenting on the margins. It is one of the largest integrated healthcare systems in the United States, serving millions of Veterans across a national network of hospitals and clinics. When an organization of that size makes measurable moves on burnout, it matters—not because it's perfect, but because it proves something important: burnout can be reduced when leaders treat it as a system problem, not a personality flaw.

And recently, the American Medical Association (AMA) did something that put a bright spotlight on that effort. Through its Joy in Medicine™ Health System Recognition Program, the AMA recognized multiple VA health care systems for their work to reduce burnout and support professional well-being—including VA Palo Alto Health Care System (CA), VA Boston Healthcare System (MA), and Minneapolis VA Health Care System (MN). That's not a participation ribbon. It's an external signal that real infrastructure is being built—policies, workflows, leadership expectations, measurement, and accountability—to protect the people doing the work.

So what is the VA doing that's working? What can the rest of healthcare learn from it? And what should we be honest about —because even strong systems can backslide when staffing, budgets, and politics squeeze the front line?

Let's walk through it.

Burnout Doesn't Mean You're Weak. It Means the System Is Asking for Too Much.

In healthcare, we've normalized a dangerous story: if you're exhausted, you need to be more resilient. If you're drowning, you need better time management. If you're emotionally numb, you need yoga.

But burnout is not a character issue. It's a mismatch issue. It's what happens when the job repeatedly demands a pace, emotional load, and administrative weight that a human body and mind cannot sustainably carry. It's what happens when work expands but resources don't. When documentation grows but staffing doesn't. When the environment punishes the very behaviors that keep patients safe—slowing down, double-checking, asking questions, taking a moment to think.

The VA's most important "win" is not a single program. It's the stance that burnout is measurable, preventable, and solvable through design—not just through individual grit.

That stance changes everything, because once you treat burnout like a system condition, you stop asking, "Why can't you handle it?" and start asking, "What are we doing to people that makes this feel unhandleable?"

What the AMA Recognition Actually Signals

The AMA's Joy in Medicine™ program recognizes health systems that demonstrate a commitment to reducing burnout and improving professional well-being. The key word there is systems. Not "a mindfulness day." Not "a pizza party." Systems.

When VA Palo Alto, VA Boston, and Minneapolis VA were recognized, it signaled that these organizations had built structures that go beyond good intentions. In plain terms, it suggests they have done things like:

Measure burnout and act on the findings (not hide them).

Create leadership roles and governance around well-being.

Reduce avoidable administrative friction.

Support team-based care so clinicians aren't isolated.

Treat well-being as part of quality and safety—not separate from it.

It also matters because the VA is a mission-driven environment. Many clinicians choose VA work because serving Veterans is not just meaningful—it's identity-deep meaningful. When purpose is strong, systems sometimes assume people will tolerate anything. The VA recognition pushes against that assumption. It implies: mission does not excuse harm to the workforce. Mission requires workforce protection.

A Quiet Power Move: Building Well-Being Into the Operating System

One of the VA's most important strategies is that it doesn't frame well-being as "soft." It ties it to operations, safety, retention, and performance.

Inside the VA, there are formal structures dedicated to employee well-being—often connected to organizational development and workforce support. The VA has described "Employee Whole Health" as an approach that supports employee well-being as part of broader Whole Health transformation. Whether you're in a direct care role or supporting the system behind the scenes, the message is that the organization is responsible for building conditions where humans can function well.

And that's the shift healthcare needs: from asking people to be superhuman to building systems that stop demanding superhuman performance as the baseline.

In many hospitals, burnout efforts are bolted on top of a broken workload. In the VA's best-performing sites, the aim is to redesign the workload itself—so that "well-being" isn't a separate lane. It's built into staffing decisions, workflow design, leadership expectations, and the way teams communicate.

What "Doing It Well" Looks Like on the Ground

When VA sites earn recognition for reducing burnout, you'll often see the same themes show up in different forms.

First, leaders treat burnout data as actionable intelligence, not a PR risk. They measure it, talk about it, and create specific interventions tied to what the data reveals. When a system actually closes the loop, it rebuilds trust.

Second, they prioritize team-based practice. Burnout grows faster when clinicians feel alone. Team design matters. A high-functioning team distributes cognitive load, creates real backup, and reduces the feeling that one person is holding the whole shift together with sheer willpower.

Third, they reduce friction where they can. Some stressors in healthcare are intrinsic—suffering, emergencies, uncertainty. But much stress is manufactured by duplicative forms, broken handoffs, unnecessary clicks, and unclear roles.

Fourth, they invest in psychological safety—the sense that you can speak up, ask questions, and admit uncertainty without being punished.

Why This Matters Beyond the VA

Even if you never work at the VA, the VA's progress matters because it demonstrates the direction healthcare has to go.

Healthcare is entering a long era where staffing will be tighter, patient complexity will be higher, and administrative demands will keep rising. You cannot meet that future with "try harder." You need alignment between humans and systems.

This is exactly why **SCRUB*fits*™** exists—not to shame people for struggling, but to help them choose environments where they can thrive and to push leaders toward building environments worth thriving in.

The Honest Part: Progress Can Be Fragile

A system can have excellent well-being infrastructure and still be threatened by staffing shortages, budget turbulence, and policy swings.

You cannot cut your way into a healthier workforce. You can cut your way into faster burnout.

What You Should Copy From the VA—Whether You're a Student, a Clinician, or a Leader

Students should choose environments, not just professions.

Clinicians should treat exhaustion as data, not shame.

Leaders must treat well-being as operational design, not an HR perk.

The VA is proving that clinician well-being can be engineered —at scale.

That's the future.

Not "be tougher."

Not "cope quietly."

Not "carry it alone."

A future where the system does some of the carrying too.

And when that happens, we don't just get happier clinicians.

We get safer care.

Better teams.

Better outcomes.

And careers that can actually last.

Chapter 20
SCRUBfit Squad: The Adrenaline Team

Where chaos meets control, and seconds decide outcomes.

The alarm sounds. A monitor beeps in the distance, a stretcher wheels across the floor, someone calls out a code — and in that instant, the room becomes a living organism. The air hums with tension, each step measured, each glance deliberate. This is where the Adrenaline Team thrives.

They are the professionals who move at the edge of urgency, balancing speed with precision, instinct with knowledge. They respond when others panic. They orchestrate when the room feels like a storm. They are nurses, paramedics, and operating room specialists who see emergencies not as chaos to avoid but as scenes to manage, lives to protect, decisions to make under pressure.

Alignment here is not theoretical. It's embedded in muscle memory, in the mental map of a trauma bay, in the anticipatory glance of a nurse monitoring six critical patients at once. It's in the way a paramedic stabilizes a broken body in the back of an ambulance while calculating hospital ETA, IV rates, and the likelihood of a decompensation (gl) before the patient even registers distress. It's in the way an OR RN anticipates a surgeon's next move, prepares the sterile field, and prevents a near-miss without a word spoken.

Every second is a decision, every decision a potential difference between life and death. Here, there is no pause button. Every patient, every call, every procedure demands attention, and the stakes are never theoretical. They deal in realities: the whine of the suction, the hiss of oxygen, the metallic ping of instruments, the rapid flutter of a heart monitor, the subtle color change of a patient's skin, the unspoken stress of colleagues pushed to the limit.

The Adrenaline Team doesn't work for accolades. They work for results, for the patient who will live another day because of their foresight, skill, and courage. They are the calm in the storm, the conductor of chaos, the heartbeat of the emergency room, the ambulance bay, and the operating room.

This chapter is their world. You will see what it takes to survive, thrive, and excel when every moment counts. You will witness the coordination, technical mastery, mental toughness, and emotional resilience that define these roles. You will feel the pulse of the work, the gravity of the responsibility, and the quiet victories that often go unseen.

Welcome to The Adrenaline Team. Here, clarity is forged in chaos, and alignment saves lives. The seconds don't wait. Neither do they.

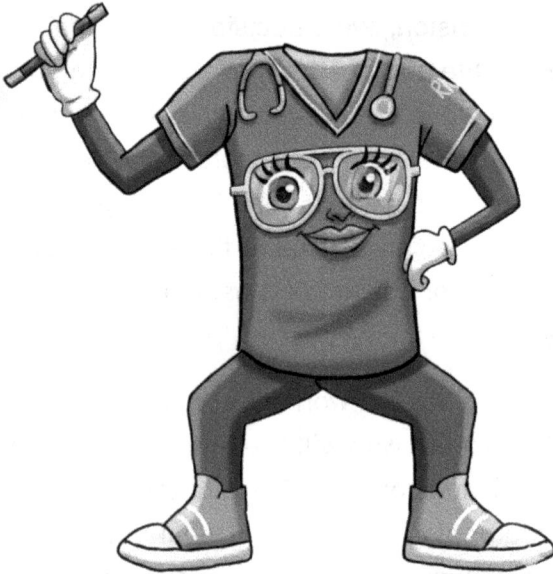

SCRUBfits™

Jen-Jen Codedale, BSN, RN

Jen-Jen Codedale, RN, BSN — Day in the Life — ER Charge Nurse (gl)

Shift: 07:00–19:00

Setting: Hopewell Hospital for Tomorrow (gl), Community

Hospital ED (gl), managing a pod with 180–200 patients per day

05:00 — Alarm & Pre-Shift Prep

The phone vibrates. Alarm hums faintly in the dark. Jen-Jen opens her eyes. The faint smell of coffee drifts from the kitchen. Her husband's bald head glistens in the soft morning sun as he hands her a piping hot coffee in her favorite aqua colored YETI travel mug emblazoned with the inscription, *"What Would Florence Do"* with an image of Florence Nightingale winking along with a Claritin. "Be careful today," he murmurs. Dolly Parton, their Boston Terrier, springs to her feet, tail wagging. The coffee warms her hands; Claritin swallowed. She scrolls overnight texts: "Short two nurses. Hallway psych hold. EMS chest pain pre-alert."

She pulls her navy scrubs on, badge clipped, hair in a tight bun, mentally triaging the day. As charge nurse (gl) today, she will orchestrate the pod, mentor staff, monitor patients for decompensation (gl), and jump in bedside whenever the situation demands.

06:45 — Commute & Mental Prep

Ten miles to go.

The familiar outline of Hopewell's Mini Hospital rises through the morning haze—once a failing community hospital that collapsed under financial pressure, like so many others. It sat empty for years until Hopewell stepped in, renovating it into a sleek 24-bed short-stay Mini Hospital as part of its plan to reach deeper into the community's backyard.

That's exactly what Hopewell does: *finds gaps and fills them.*

She takes a long sip of coffee and pulls up the Hopewell dashboard on her phone. Two chest pain workups pending, a possible stroke en route, a GI bleeder in triage, and a pneumonia patient who may qualify for Hopewell's hospital-at-home (gl) pathway.

Her heart rate rises—not fear, just readiness.

The Mini Hospital's façade glows softly with Hopewell's signature low-glare lighting as she mentally rehearses STEMI protocols (gl), sepsis bundles (gl), pediatric seizure interventions (gl), and rapid response (gl) steps. The future-forward part of Hopewell's system means she never walks in blind—she walks in prepared.

07:00 — Arrival & The Wall of Sound

Sliding doors hiss. The ED is alive: monitors beep, stretchers roll, phones ring incessantly. The ED board (gl) shows twenty stretchers full, six hallway beds occupied, two ambulances waiting. Jen-Jen scans the room, assessing acuity and staff availability.

Delegation begins immediately:

- "Taylor, take Rooms 7–8 — vitals every 15 min."

- "Alex, monitor Hallway D; watch for decompensation (gl)."

- "Emma, triage EMS chest pain — start IV (gl), EKG (gl) on arrival."

Already, she juggles six active patients, coordinating labs, imaging, meds, and constant patient reassessment while mentoring two new nurses. Every beep, groan, and call is data.

08:30 — Full Throttle

• EMS brings a 46-year-old male with chest pain. IV inserted, EKG leads placed; labs drawn. ST elevation — borderline STEMI (gl). Cardiology (gl) paged. Aspirin administered. Cath lab prep underway.

• Room 8 patient vomits violently — she adjusts IV fluids, administers antiemetic (gl), and reassures the patient.

• Room 6: 18-month-old with febrile seizure (gl) — acetaminophen drawn, parent coached, airway assessed, seizure activity monitored.

• Hallway D-1: agitated psychiatric patient — she calls security, implements verbal de-escalation, continuously monitors for decompensation (gl).

By 09:45, Jen-Jen is simultaneously:

• Overseeing six active patients in her pod

• Coordinating two new admits

• Mentoring a student nurse starting their first IV

• Assigning break coverage for short-staffed colleagues

Every second demands attention; a single missed sign could be catastrophic.

12:30 — The Non-Break Break

She squeezes down a protein shake between charts. Page: "New chest pain, triage level 2." Protein shake abandoned. Hand hygiene, back to chaos. Three discharges, two new admits, one Code Stroke (gl) later. Ambulance wheels in a drug overdose — naloxone (gl) administered, vitals monitored, team coordinated for safety.

15:30 — Afternoon Surge

• Room 11: fractured radius, awaiting orthopedic consult (gl)

• Hallway D-2: elderly hip fracture patient, in pain, waiting for Ortho

• Nursing home patient: signs of sepsis (gl), EMS pre-alerted

Vitals reassessed every 15–30 minutes. Oxygen titration precise. Pain meds timed exactly. Mentorship ongoing — student nurse whispers, "How do you keep up?"

Jen-Jen smiles wearily: "Because people need us. And I'm too stubborn to quit."

17:00 — Peak Chaos & Heavy Triage

Even with two hours left, she monitors new EMS arrivals, hallway holds, and rapid deterioration in frail patients. Scrubs stained, back aching, charting behind — she moves with purpose, orchestrating care like a conductor managing chaos.

19:10 — Overtime & Handoff

Clock-out irrelevant — COPD patient desatting. Oxygen titrated, Respiratory Therapy (gl) paged. Night shift handoff completed only when all patients stable.

20:15 — Decompression & Home

Ten miles home. Dolly greets her like she's returned from battle. Husband hugs silently — understanding without words. Salt air from the nearby beach. Her mind finally slows, replaying interventions, mentoring moments, and lives saved.

21:00 — Teaching & NP Studies

Thursday night she teaches at the Susan Dodd School of Nursing. Lesson: prioritization in high-acuity scenarios. Stories stripped of TV dramatics, lessons grounded in real ER experience. Simultaneously she is studying for her Nurse Practitioner (gl) degree — bedside care is her foundation.

22:30 — Quiet Resolve

The door swings open and Dolly could be mistaken for an incoming mini torpedo.

Twenty pounds of pure, squealing, tail-wagging velocity launches across the entryway and slams joyfully into Jen-Jen's shins. Dolly's tiny nails skitter on the hardwood as she tries to decide between jumping, spinning, and vibrating in place like a shaken soda can. Her whole body is one long exclamation mark.

Hubby reheats her dinner. Dolly is now snoring. Jen-Jen reflects: codes, decompensations (gl), hallway patients, teaching, successful interventions. Tomorrow, the cycle begins again.

"Every nurse was drawn here for a reason — your presence matters more than you know."

— Jennifer Mosedale, BSN, RN

A real-world nursing leader whose leadership spirit inspired Jen-Jen Codedale, BSN, RN

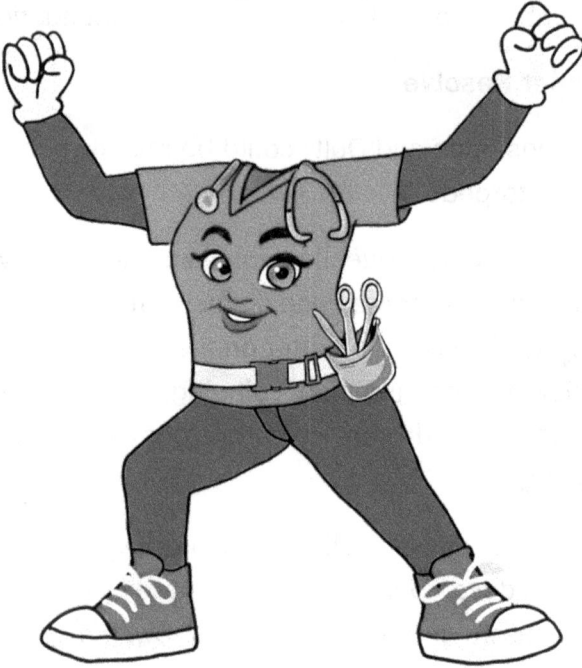

SCRUBfits™

Krashlyn Riggs, EMT-P

Krashlyn Riggs, EMT-P — "The Scene Stabilizer"

Scrub Color: Storm Gray

Primary Role: Paramedic (gl)

Also Aligns With: Flight Paramedic (gl); Critical Care Transport Specialist; EMS Field Training Officer

SCRUB*fit*™ Category: The Adrenaline Team

Personality Traits: Courageous, adaptable, resourceful, intuitive

Pros: Independence, community impact, hands-on critical care

Cons: Environmental unpredictability, physical strain, emotional fatigue

Clinical Tools: Cardiac monitor (gl); airway kit (gl); trauma pack; radio link

Clinical Confession: "I meet people on their worst day — and I give them a fighting chance."

Day in the Life — Paramedic (gl)

Shift: 06:30–18:30 / 18:30–06:30 (alternating rotation)

Setting: City EMS service, calls ranging from trauma to medical emergencies

05:40 — Sunrise Call Prep

The sun hasn't fully risen. Krashlyn sits on the tailgate of the rig, breakfast burrito in one hand, dented Stanley mug in the other. Radio check: clear. Patient care reports (gl) from last shift downloaded. LifePAK 15 (gl) tones, Hamilton-T1 ventilator (gl) passes, suction clear, QuikClot (gl) restocked. Video laryngoscope green. Power-LOAD rails smooth. She mutters a quick mantra: *"Check it before you need it."*

06:10 — Rig Check & Team Briefing

Partner nods. Radios synced. O2 tanks full. Trauma packs inventoried. Every strap, every line, every monitor double-checked. The street is quiet now — but within minutes, chaos can erupt.

07:05 — Multi-Vehicle Collision

She is still half-sunk into the massage chair in Wayne's Room, last bite of breakfast burrito in one hand, phone in the other, scrolling election results. The chair kneads a knot at the base of her spine while a blue Gatorade sweats in the side pocket of her cargo pants—her little insurance policy for whatever the day decides to throw at her.

She never really knows what the day will entail.

Dispatch hits like a slap through the quiet:

"Two-car collision. One trapped. Minor extrication."

She's up. Moving. Out the door. The massage chair is still vibrating as she allows the door to swing shut behind her.

Thirty seconds later, the rig screams away from Hopewell's main campus, cutting through the morning fog like a scalpel.

At the scene—wreckage, glass, chaos. One driver walking. The other pinned under a crushed dashboard.

Krashlyn moves fast, fluid, fearless:

• Manual cervical spine (gl) stabilization.

• Expose the thigh wound.

• Pack the bleed.

• Draw TXA (gl) — push.

- IV wide open (gl).

- Airway: intact.

- Breathing: shallow.

- Circulation: barely holding.

"Pre-alert Hopewell Trauma — ETA eight minutes."

The radio crackles back:

"Hopewell Trauma ready."

Of course they are.

It's Hopewell.

And it's only 7:05.

08:30 — STEMI Alert

12-lead ECG transmitted to ED. Nitro given, aspirin chewed, vitals monitored. Cath lab prepped remotely. Krashlyn rides the fine line: stabilize patient in-transit while anticipating ED needs, keeping oxygen (gl) titrated, ensuring IV flow rates correct.

09:40 — Midday Overdose

Drug overdose, unresponsive patient, pinpoint pupils. Naloxone (gl) administered, bag-valve-mask with PEEP applied. Heart rate returns. Eyes flutter. Partner secures scene, family calmed. Krashlyn documents minute-by-minute interventions. She leaves a Deterra pouch and a note: "If today's a pivot, here's your tool."

12:10 — Routine, Until It's Not

Call for suspected stroke. Patient slurred, face droop. FAST exam (gl) completed. Rapid transport. Pre-alert to ED. Careful communication, hands steady despite adrenaline. Notes on patient changes dictated over radio, vitals monitored every 2–3 minutes.

15:50 — Overdose Rescue #2

Adolescent patient, altered mental status, opioid suspected. Naloxone repeated, airway maintained, EMS partner observes for **decompensation** (gl). Family present — Krashlyn coaches them to remain calm while documenting interventions. Scene secure, patient stabilized, transported safely.

18:25 — Shift Swap / Night Transition

A structure fire standby interrupts the routine. Floodlights wash the helipad; rotor wash lifts the hem of her jacket. The rig is prepped for possible transport. Every tool checked again. She hands off patient care to incoming team with concise, critical information.

00:40 — Behavioral Health Call

Night shift. Bus-stop, distressed individual. De-escalation techniques applied — knees to curb height, hands visible, calm voice, verbs first. Transport agreed. Adrenaline high but measured.

03:30 — MCI Drill / Simulation

Multi-casualty incident drill. Triage tags placed. Radio redundancy tested. Routes mapped. Role assigned. Every second rehearsed — building muscle memory for real-life emergencies.

06:20 — Debrief & Home

Dawn smells like diesel and dew. Rig stocked, cleaned, prepped for next call. Cat greets her like she's been gone a week. Text to mentee: "Hydrate before next call." Mind decompresses slowly; body aches from multiple lifts, rapid movement, and adrenaline spikes.

Tools of the Trade (gl)

- LIFEPAK 15 (gl)

- Hamilton-T1 ventilator (gl)

- QuikClot (gl)

- Video laryngoscope (gl)

- Power-LOAD stretcher system (gl)

Quiet Superpowers

- Command presence without volume

- Scene choreography under pressure

- Mental whiteboard of next-best moves

- Rapid triage and stabilization

What Success Feels Like

- Perfect pre-alert called to ED

- Patient stabilized and delivered safely

- Team functioning seamlessly despite environmental chaos

Route to the Role

• EMT → Paramedic → CCP-C / FP-C (gl) → Tactical EMS (TEMS) integration

Myth vs. Reality

• Myth: "It's just driving to emergencies."

• Reality: Mobile critical care with life-or-death constraints, requiring split-second decisions, technical skill, and calm under extreme pressure.

SCRUB*fits*™

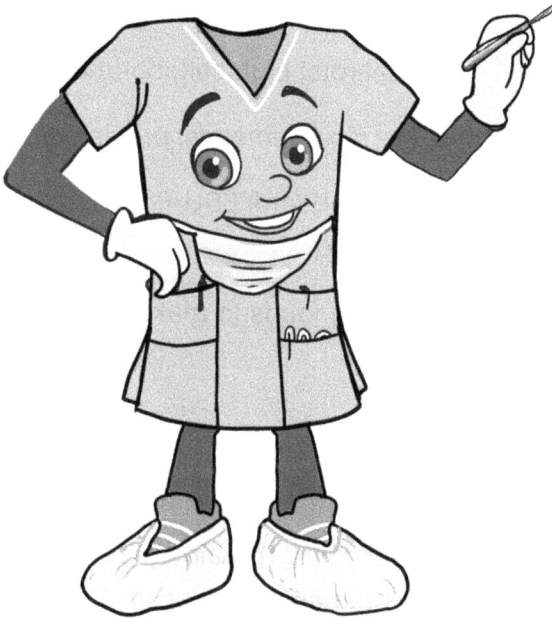

Brad Bovie, BSN, RN, CNOR

Brad Bovie, RN, BSN, CNOR — "The Surgical Sentinel"

Scrub Color: Teal

Primary Role: Operating Room Circulator

Also Aligns With: Perioperative Nurse; OR Clinical Coordinator; Surgical Services Educator

SCRUB*fit*™ Category: The Adrenaline Team

Personality Traits: Focused, meticulous, team-oriented, proactive

Pros: Critical technical role; high collaboration; clear flow

Cons: Long shifts; stamina demands; precise protocols

Clinical Tools: OR count board; ESU/ForceTriad (gl); surgical safety checklist; sterile gloves

Clinical Confession: "My job is to make sure every incision begins with trust."

A Day in the Life

18:45 — Arrival & Pre-Shift Ritual

Brad steps into the OR suite. The air smells faintly of antiseptic and warmed linens. He taps his badge on the scanner; the locker clicks shut behind him. On the counter, a perfectly lined tray awaits: sponges, instruments, surgical counts charted. Each item is in its place, but he inspects anyway — sterile gloves, RF-tagged sponges (gl), ForceTriad ESU (gl) ready, Bair Hugger (gl) warmers running. Every detail matters; every detail could prevent catastrophe.

19:05 — Team Huddle

The anesthesiologist, scrub tech, circulating nurse, and surgeon gather around the board. Brad leads the pre-op briefing: patient allergies, antibiotic timing, VTE prophylaxis, surgical positioning, instruments required, special implants.

He watches faces, gauging comprehension, detecting fatigue, adjusting instructions. He doesn't just communicate — he synchronizes. The team nods; tension eases slightly, trust begins to form.

19:25 — Surgical Time-Out

Lights flare above the OR table. Sterile drapes surround the patient. Brad calls the time-out: "Patient identity, surgical site, procedure, implants, counts confirmed." Each team member responds. The air is taut, every word carrying weight. Seconds feel heavier than minutes. Brad's eyes flick between the surgeon's hands, anesthesia lines, and scrub tech's setup — anticipating the first incision.

19:40 — First Incision & Orchestration

Scalpel touches skin. Brad coordinates silently: instruments passed in sequence, suction ready, cautery prepped, team fluidly moving as one. A slight tremor in the patient's pulse appears on the monitor — Brad calls for vitals check, oxygen adjusted, anesthesia confirms. All routine, yet critical.

20:10 — Mid-Case Complication

Unexpected bleeding. Surgeon's hands tense. Brad instantly communicates, "Suction up; count sponges; blood products ready." He signals the scrub tech to prep rapid infuser (gl). Instruments flow seamlessly. Sweat beads on his forehead, yet movements precise. Team trusts his calm decisiveness — adrenaline channeled, not chaotic.

21:00 — Teaching Moment

A student nurse observes. Brad guides subtly: "Notice how we anticipate, not react. Timing is everything; sequence is safety."

He doesn't slow the case, doesn't lecture — the teaching is in motion, woven into patient care.

21:45 — Equipment Alert

ForceTriad (gl) beeps irregularly. Brad pauses mid-pass, checks pad contact, confirms energy settings. No hesitation. A misfire avoided silently, without disruption.

22:30 — Complex Coordination

Surgeon requests a specialty instrument from storage mid-case. Brad visualizes tray layout, confirms sterile access, instructs tech without breaking focus. Blood pressure dips slightly. Brad signals anesthesia, positions fluid bolus — patient stabilized before complication escalates.

23:05 — End of First Case & Turnover

Incision closed, instruments counted, sponges verified. Brad documents meticulously, supervises sterile cleanup, hands off patient to PACU. Every step choreographed, executed with precision.

23:30 — Emergency Next Case

Trauma alert arrives: MVC victim, unstable pelvis. OR prepped instantly. Brad coordinates with scrub tech, anesthesia, ED nurse handoff — instruments staged, blood warmed, rapid infuser ready, Foley kit primed. Every movement rehearsed, every action critical.

00:15 — High-Stakes Trauma Case

The patient rolls in and the room snaps to attention. Vital signs are crashing, monitors climbing into a frantic chorus.

Above the field, **Hopewell's TraumaGrid display** auto-populates in real time: mechanism of injury, last recorded vitals, scanned blood type, labs streaming in as they're processed. An embedded **massive transfusion protocol** (gl) tile quietly updates the ideal ratio of packed cells to plasma with each unit Brad scans into the system.

Brad is the center of the storm.

He coordinates suction, clamps, instrument sequencing, and blood products with almost ridiculous precision. He's already handing the next instrument before the surgeon asks, reading posture and tone like a second language. The scrub tech mirrors him, responding instantly, filling in gaps before they appear.

Monitors beep, lines drip, alarms flirt with the edge of chaos.

Brad calls out changes in meds and fluids, and anesthesia adjusts before the numbers fully tank. The team trusts his orchestrations—and the way Hopewell's tech sharpens them.

In this room, **seconds aren't abstract.**

They're the line between "we lost him" and "he's going to make it."

02:00 — Stabilization Achieved

Patient stable, transferred to ICU (gl). Brad finally allows a brief breath. No downtime, only reset — next patient, next procedure. He logs interventions, updates surgical counts, coordinates cleanup.

04:00 — System Fixes & Documentation

A near-miss noted: wrong concentration medication nearly drawn. Brad updates protocol: barcode verification required, tall-man labeling implemented, huddle script revised. Safety improvements embedded.

06:00 — Final Case of Shift

Elective procedure for morning discharge. Routine yet must maintain vigilance. Brad ensures all instruments, medications, and counts are perfect. Procedure flows without interruption.

07:20 — SBAR (gl) Handoff & Exit

"All counts correct. Patient stable. Anesthesia aware. ICU notified." Handoff precise. Brad steps out. Lights dim. OR silent now. Success measured in safety, trust, and seamless execution.

Tools of the Trade (gl)

- Stryker OR bed (gl)

- ForceTriad ESU (gl)

- Bair Hugger (gl)

- RF-tagged sponges (gl)

- Sterile field maps (gl)

Quiet Superpowers

- Anticipatory setup & orchestration

- Situational awareness under extreme pressure

- Emotional triage through tone & presence

- Fluent scrub-circulator coordination

What Success Feels Like

- Every incision begins and ends safely

- Zero count discrepancies

- Team flows like choreography

- Surgeons trust his every decision

The Adrenaline Team — Alignment Under Pressure

When the alarms fade, the monitors quiet, and the stretchers roll empty, the work of **The Adrenaline Team** is far from over. They are the professionals who thrive where others falter — where seconds are lives, and every decision carries weight.

Jen-Jen Codedale moves through the chaos of the Emergency Department like a conductor guiding a symphony of crises. Her eyes read monitors and vitals as instinctively as a musician reads notes. A single second of hesitation could be the difference between **decompensation** (gl) and stabilization. Yet she moves with calm, teaching her team, mentoring students, and orchestrating a living system where chaos is inevitable and alignment is earned.

Krashlyn Riggs rides the sirens, every street a stage for life-or-death decisions. She stabilizes the unstable, anticipates threats before they arrive, and translates danger into action — all while keeping the patient, the family, and the EMS team grounded. Every pulse, every breath, every step is measured. Her hands may guide a needle, a bag-valve-mask, or an IV line, but her mind choreographs the entire scene, turning adrenaline into life-saving precision.

Brad Bovie inhabits the Operating Room like a sentinel. Lights glare, alarms hum, and every heartbeat echoes in the sterile theater. He orchestrates the team with invisible threads: instruments, monitors, anesthesia, surgeon. Every incision is a trust, every action a promise. Chaos is disciplined; risk is anticipated. His calm presence transforms tension into order, and the team moves in unison because he has created a rhythm that protects life with meticulous devotion.

Together, these professionals are **The Adrenaline Team (SCRUB*fit*™)** — healthcare's front line where precision, clarity, and courage meet. They don't chase excitement for thrill. They chase **alignment under pressure**, the razor-edge moment where skill, teamwork, and instinct intersect. They are the pulse of the hospital, the rhythm of the emergency, the invisible guardians who transform panic into purpose.

In their world, seconds matter. Every alarm, every call, every life — a chance to act decisively, to channel fear into focus, to turn crisis into survival. Their work is unsung but sacred, relentless but precise, high-stakes but humane. They are calm in the storm, leaders without titles, and in their hands, chaos becomes clarity.

This is The Adrenaline Team. Fast. Focused. Fearless.

Chapter 21

SCRUBfit Squad: The Compassion Corps

Where connection becomes clinical skill.

In healthcare, compassion isn't a soft skill — it's a precision instrument. It is the difference between a family that spirals and a family that steadies, between a patient who refuses care and a patient who finally exhales, between a room full of alarms and a room where someone feels safe enough to cooperate with healing. The Compassion Corps doesn't "add kindness" to clinical work. They operationalize it — translating fear into understanding, pain into partnership, and confusion into clear next steps.

These professionals work in the invisible spaces that determine outcomes: the moment a parent's face changes when they finally understand what a monitor is saying; the moment a survivor realizes they will be believed; the moment a patient with tight lungs stops fighting the mask because the person in front of them is calm enough to borrow. Their presence is not extra. It is an intervention — one that prevents panic, improves adherence, reduces escalation, and protects dignity when people are at their most vulnerable.

Alignment in the Compassion Corps lives at the intersection of empathy and expertise. They know when to speak, when to pause, when to advocate, and when to hold steady while someone else falls apart. Where others see tasks, they see people. Where others see symptoms, they see stories. And in their hands, connection becomes a clinical force that changes what happens next.

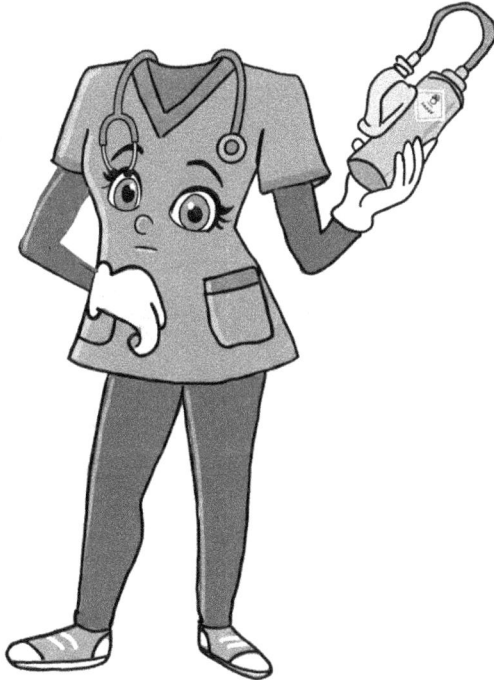

SCRUBfits™

Ginger Gauge, RRT

Ginger Gauge, RRT — "The Breath Bringer"

Scrub Color: Burnt Orange

Primary Role: Respiratory Therapist

Also Aligns With: Pulmonary Function Technologist; ECMO Specialist; Ventilation Safety Coordinator

SCRUB*fit*™ Category: The Compassion Corps

Personality Traits: Calm, attentive, thorough, quietly confident

Pros: Critical-care impact; strong team collaboration; clear patient outcomes

Cons: Emotionally intense cases; physically demanding; exposure to crisis events

Clinical Tools: Hamilton-G5 ventilator (gl); inline suction (gl); ABG kit (gl); pulse oximeter (gl)

Clinical Confession: "I breathe for people until they can breathe for themselves."

A Day in the Life

05:10 — Wake & Warm-Up

Alarm hums faintly in her bedroom — a rhythm she almost syncs to. She stretches, rolls out the tightness in her shoulders, and moves through a short run around her quiet neighborhood. Oats, banana, green tea. Mental checklist: vent census (gl) review — two patients weaning, one on high settings. She whispers to herself: "Let's get those lungs moving."

06:30 — Commute & Centering

Car ride soundtrack: Critical Care Scenarios podcast (gl). Cases of ventilator-associated pneumonia, spontaneous breathing trials (gl), ECMO troubleshooting. At the last light, she switches off the audio, inhales three deep breaths, visualizes the ICU, the patients, the monitors, the lines — preparing to meet urgency with calm.

06:50 — Pre-Shift Calibration

Hamilton-G5 ventilator (gl) and Dräger V500 calibrated. Inline suction (gl) checked. ABG kits stocked. She taps each line, listens to the hum of machines, feels the tubing under her fingers. The ICU is a symphony of breaths; she is the conductor.

07:10 — NICU Start

A 27-week preemie, fragile as porcelain. She adjusts FiO_2 (gl) 34% → 32%, whispers encouragement while checking chest rise. She positions the tiny patient, leaves a laminated breathing guide (gl) nearby. "Look at that chest rise — she's fighting with me," she murmurs, fingers steady on the ventilator.

08:30 — Family Check-In

Mom and dad peer anxiously over the isolette. Ginger bends, speaks softly, translates the numbers into human terms: "Her lungs are tiny but strong. Every breath she takes is a victory. She's doing this with us." The relief in their eyes is her quiet reward.

09:05 — Code Blue

Alarm screams. Neonate in respiratory distress. Ginger drops to protocol, bag-valve-mask in rhythm with heartbeats, coaching: "Slow the squeeze — match their effort." Tidal volume (gl) adjusted, O_2 saturations climb. Relief arrives, not as fanfare, but in steady numbers on the monitor.

10:40 — ICU Rounds

Sedation checked. Tidal volumes (gl) confirmed. Compliance (gl) measured. "Ready for a spontaneous breathing trial," she tells the team. Monitors beep in sync with hope. One minute in, patient breathing independently. She notes it with a smiley face — small victories, monumental in impact.

12:00 — Lunch & Laughter

Cafeteria, the smell of chili dogs. She laughs with a fellow RT about the morning's chaos. Humor is medicine too.

13:15 — Rapid Response (gl)

COPD exacerbation. Nebulizer started mid-sentence. Oxygen saturation climbs 86 → 95. She coaches: "In through the nose, out through the mouth. Feel the lungs expand." Patient exhales, relief palpable. "Best breath I've had all week," he whispers.

14:30 — Teaching Moment

Student RT shadows her. Ginger demonstrates inline suction technique (gl), ABG draws (gl), ventilator troubleshooting. She explains: "Every beep is a voice. Learn to listen, not just see." Presence is teaching; calm is mentorship; compassion is operationalized.

14:50 — Closing Checks & Reflection

All patients stable. Vent 12 secure. NICU twin A off phototherapy (gl). Notes complete. She checks machines one last time, straightens tubing, smooths blankets. Stepping outside, she inhales deeply. Another day spent breathing for those who cannot yet breathe for themselves.

Tools of the Trade (gl)

- Hamilton-G5 ventilator (gl)

- Inline suction (gl)

- ABG kit (gl)

- Pulse oximeter (gl)

Quiet Superpowers

- Translating numbers into patient-centered action

- Stabilizing ICU chaos with calm presence

- Teaching and mentoring through presence

- Operationalizing empathy into clinical precision

What Success Feels Like

- A patient weaning successfully from the vent

- Monitors steady, saturations stable

- Families reassured

- Quiet ICU, calm restored

SCRUBfits™

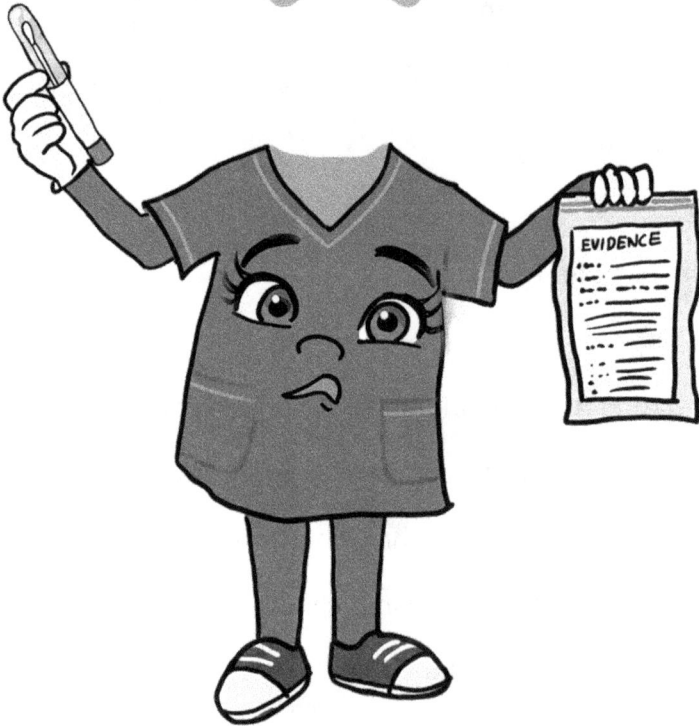

Justice Jules, RN, SANE-A

Justice Jules, RN, SANE-A — "The Trauma Witness"

Scrub Color: Ceramyst

Primary Role: Forensic Nurse Examiner

Also Aligns With: Sexual Assault Nurse Examiner; Forensic Program Coordinator; Evidence Collection Specialist

SCRUB*fit*™ Category: The Compassion Corps

Personality Traits: Empathetic, meticulous, unflappable, grounded

Pros: Deep purpose; trauma-informed care; cross-agency collaboration

Cons: Emotional weight; on-call intensity; legal pressure

Clinical Tools: Chain-of-custody kit (gl); Leica colposcope (gl); forensic light source (gl); documentation camera (gl)

Clinical Confession: "Compassion doesn't end when the chart closes — it testifies."

Day in the Life — Forensic Nurse Examiner (gl)**, Evening Shift 15:00–23:00**

13:40 — Ground & Gather

Justice begins with box breathing (gl), inhaling calm, exhaling tension. Ceramyst scrubs pressed, kit bag restocked, chain-of-custody (gl) forms double-checked. A hummus wrap and water, a quick scan of hospital policy updates — rituals that frame the evening. Every zip, click, and seal is a promise to patients she may never see again.

14:45 — Arrival & Calibration

Tranquil Path (gl) candle aroma softens the sterile hum of Hopewell's ED. She walks through the forensic suite, lights adjusted, Leica colposcope (gl) checked, documentation camera (gl) positioned. Her mind rehearses patient flow, privacy protocols, legal procedures. Alignment is clinical precision balanced with human care — every instrument ready, every step intentional.

15:20 — Case 1: Sexual Assault Survivor

Patient arrives, trembling. Justice kneels slightly, soft voice: "I'm Justice. You're safe here." Consent obtained, explanations repeated, every tool and touch measured. Leica colposcope (gl) captures forensic images; chain-of-custody (gl) documented meticulously. Artificial candles flicker softly in the private room — humanity in sterile surroundings. She coaches family to a quiet space, explains next steps gently, translating trauma into clarity.

17:10 — Evidence Transfer & Mentorship

Chain-of-custody (gl) verified with forensic coordinator (gl). Instruments cleaned, documentation logged. Justice pauses with resident nurses: "Label, log, lock. Respect the story, respect the process." She demonstrates proper handling, translating legal rigor into bedside care.

18:40 — Documentation & Decompression

Forensic EMR (gl) secured; critical details flagged. Justice reviews notes, checks photographs, reflects briefly. "We're learning to exhale," she whispers to manager — an acknowledgment of emotional labor.

19:45 — Staff Training Huddle

Justice leads a trauma-informed language session, pairing clinical expertise with patient advocacy. She models care:

"Awareness is where healing begins. Words are instruments; use them with intention." Students and staff take notes, learning empathy as procedure.

21:20 — Case 2: Domestic Violence Survivor

Patient presents with patterned bruising, abrasions. Justice examines with forensic scale (gl), alternate light source (gl), documenting precisely. Every word: calm. Every movement: deliberate. She validates: "I believe you. You're not alone." Medical care and legal documentation intertwine; alignment lives in compassion plus clinical rigor.

22:50 — Wrap & Reflection

Evidence secured, chain-of-custody (gl) double-checked, documentation finalized. Justice notes: "Light the candle after each case — the symbol matters." Emotional weight acknowledged, not ignored; professionalism maintained without sacrificing empathy.

23:20 — Drive Home

Soft jazz plays in the car. Streetlights reflect off courthouse windows. Badge hung on counter. Justice exhales: one truth documented, one soul honored. Each shift leaves marks on her mind, yet she carries the work forward with quiet steadiness.

Tools of the Trade (gl)

- Chain-of-custody kit (gl)

- Leica colposcope (gl)

- Forensic light source (gl)

- Documentation camera (gl)

Quiet Superpowers

- Balancing clinical precision with emotional support

- Translating trauma into actionable documentation

- Mentoring staff in forensic procedures

- Preserving dignity while navigating legal pressure

What Success Feels Like

- Patients leave feeling safe, validated, and cared for

- Evidence integrity maintained flawlessly

- Team aligned on trauma-informed care

- Emotional labor acknowledged, not forgotten

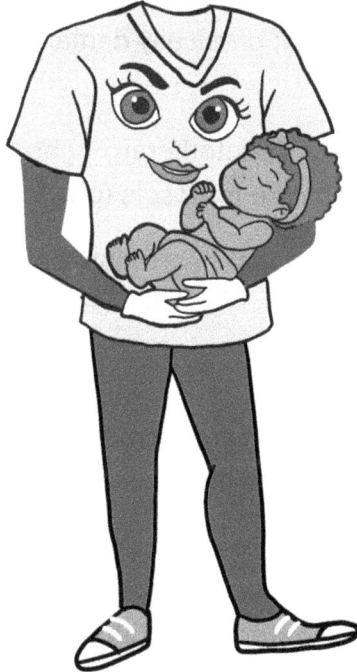

Hope Fulle, BSN, RN

Hope Fulle, RN, BSN — "The Tiny Guardian"

Scrub Color: Blush Pink

Primary Role: NICU Nurse

SCRUB*fit*™ Category: The Compassion Corps

Personality Traits: Tender, vigilant, nurturing, detail-oriented

Pros: Deep connection with families; life-saving precision; patient advocacy

Cons: Emotional intensity; physically demanding; high-stakes vigilance

Clinical Tools: CPAP (gl); phototherapy lights (gl); incubators (gl); EHR (gl); kangaroo care protocols (gl)

Clinical Confession: "I count heartbeats before I count steps."

Character Description

Hope Fulle didn't begin her career cradling preemies under the soft blue glow of isolette lights.

Her first degree — a BS in Developmental Psychology — led her into a decade of community outreach and early childhood programs. She loved the work, loved the families, loved being the steady voice in moments when parents didn't know what they needed.

But somewhere along the way, she realized she wasn't just fascinated by development — she was drawn to the very beginning of life itself.

Then came the turning point:

a grant program she'd managed was unexpectedly dissolved, and suddenly Hope was standing at a crossroads, her job gone but her desire to serve still blazing.

Instead of stepping back, she stepped forward.

Hope enrolled in a two-year BSN bridge program, stacking night classes on top of day jobs, clinical rotations on top of carpool duty, textbooks on top of faith. It wasn't easy — but she was finally headed toward the place her heart had been pointing all along.

When she graduated, she didn't just walk into Hopewell Hospital for Tomorrow... she ran, straight into their NICU Internship for second-career students.

The moment she entered that unit — the low hum of monitors, the tiny breaths, the fierce hope of families — she knew she'd found her alignment.

Today, Hope Fulle moves through the NICU like someone born for it.

Her pink blush scrubs glint softly under the phototherapy lamps as she charts with one hand and comforts with the other. She has the steady calm of someone who has lived whole chapters before this one — and the fresh fire of someone who refuses to waste the opportunity of a second career.

She hums to her babies.

She translates medical jargon into comfort for parents.

She can silence a room full of alarms with nothing but competence and kindness.

Hope's gift isn't just clinical skill — it's presence.

She brings a gentleness that settles the air, a confidence that steadies new residents, and a belief that no life is too small to fight for.

When families say, "Thank you for saving our baby,"

Hope just smiles and replies,

"I walk with them. They do the saving."

Her name fits her —

but her purpose defines her.

Hope Fulle didn't just change careers.

She found the place she was always meant to be.

A Day in the Life

19:30

Note: Hope's 12.5-hour shift is standard for NICU at Hopewell Hospital due to patient acuity, understaffing pressures, and critical continuity-of-care needs. Neonates on high-level support cannot be safely handed off every 8 hours without risking stability; continuity matters more than schedule convenience.

06:10 — Arrival & Mental Prep

The NICU hums with incubators and ventilators. Sanitizer scent mixes with anticipation and tension. Hope slips into blush pink scrubs, clips her badge, and scans the assignment board. Overnight notes: a 27-weeker on CPAP (gl), a post-op PDA ligation (gl), twins on phototherapy (gl). Every line, monitor, and alarm is a story that needs her eyes, hands, and judgment today.

07:15 — Handoff & First Assessments

Night shift provides a verbal handoff — details, subtle cues, potential alarms. Hope moves from isolette to isolette:

- Baby A: CPAP wean (gl).

- Baby B: post-op PDA ligation (gl), fragile vitals.

- Baby C: phototherapy day 2 (gl), jaundice trending.

She checks monitors, adjusts lines, listens with a stethoscope warm from her hands. Her alignment is in the steadiness between chaos and crisis, knowing tiny adjustments save lives.

08:30 — Early Surges

Two alarms: Baby B's BP trending low, Baby A showing bradycardia. Hope acts simultaneously: titrates fluids, calls for bedside echo, stimulates the neonate while maintaining monitoring of Baby A. Families in the room are guided through calm language, translating technical interventions into reassurance.

Why the long shift: Neonates' conditions fluctuate minute to minute. Handoffs mid-crisis risk errors. The 12.5-hour shift allows Hope to remain at the bedside, respond to instability, and see interventions through from start to stabilization.

09:45 — Family Teaching & Rounds

Interdisciplinary rounds: neonatologist, RT, dietitian, PT. Hope leads discussions, guides kangaroo care (gl), and models proper handling to parents. Tiny sighs, subtle chest movements, and tearful eyes are measured outcomes. Teaching isn't optional — it's life-saving.

11:15 — Critical Intervention

Baby B spikes a fever post-op. Blood cultures drawn. Antibiotics prepared. CPAP (gl) pressures adjusted. Every step documented in EHR (gl), every step measured to minimize stress. Hope coordinates staff and reassures parents — action under pressure, emotional labor intertwined with technical skill.

12:45 — Lunch & Charting

Salad in one hand, syringe feed in the other. EHR meticulous. Resident suggests a feeding plan adjustment; she evaluates vitals, lab trends, and tolerance. Feedback Flow Board (gl) shows Green — alignment maintained. Even lunch is a multitasking test of clinical precision.

14:30 — Afternoon Vigilance

Phototherapy lights (gl) adjusted. CPAP (gl) pressures monitored. Tiny oxygen desats corrected. Small victories: Baby C latches during kangaroo care, Baby A off brady monitor. Hope documents, celebrates, smiles at tiny progress, knowing every moment matters.

16:30 — Alarms & Rapid Response

Baby A's brady alarm escalates. Hope stimulates, repositions, titrates fluids, calls for backup. Baby stabilizes. Heartbeats normalized. Milestone cards printed; Polaroid photo taped to isolette. These small victories validate the long hours.

18:30 — Evening Handoff Prep

Evening shift arrives; Hope briefs them on each baby: ventilator settings, feeding tolerance, phototherapy schedules, parent teaching. She confirms continuity of care, ensuring high-acuity neonates remain stable through shift change.

19:15 — Closing & Reflection

Badge off, hands washed, monitor alarms silenced. She pauses to observe babies sleeping, breathing steadily. "See you tomorrow, little fighters." She exhales, allowing herself a moment of calm.

Reflection

"I count heartbeats before I count steps." The 12.5-hour shift isn't a burden — it's necessary vigilance, combining technical skill, emotional presence, and continuity-of-care precision to ensure the tiniest patients survive and thrive.

Tools of the Trade (gl)

- CPAP (gl)

- Phototherapy lights (gl)

- Incubators (gl)

- EHR (gl)

- Kangaroo care protocols (gl)

Quiet Superpowers

- Reading micro-changes in fragile patients

- Translating technical data into parental confidence

- Maintaining clarity and presence under extreme emotional intensity

- Delivering continuity-of-care across high-acuity neonates

What Success Feels Like

- Neonates stable and developing

- Families informed and empowered

- Every alarm, every breath, every heartbeat accounted for

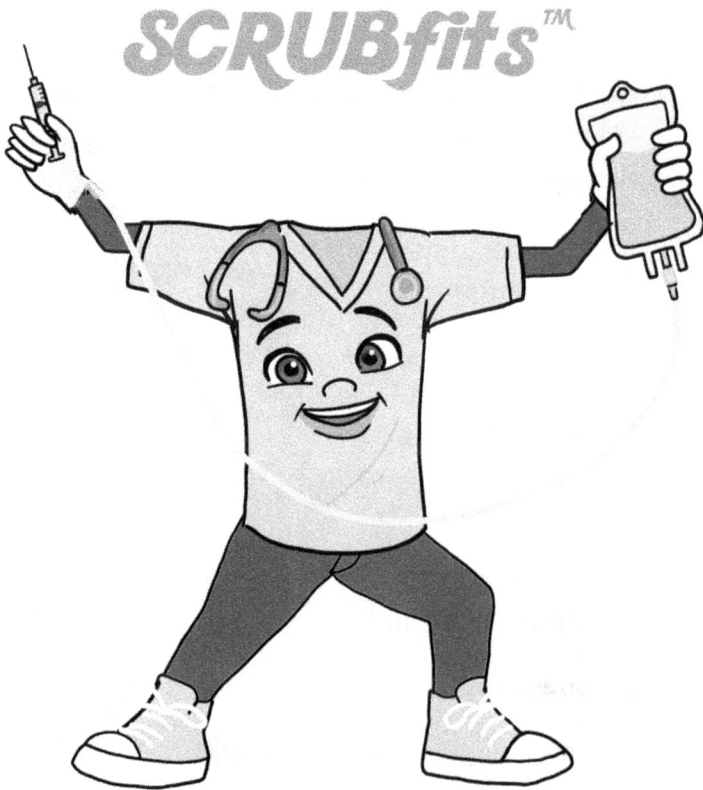

SCRUBfits™

Suzette Soleil, RN

Suzette Soleil, RN — "Med-Surg's North Star"

Scrub Color: Marigold Yellow

Primary Role: Medical-Surgical Nurse (Evening Shift)

SCRUB*fit*™ Category: The Compassion Corps

Personality Traits: Upbeat, intuitive, resilient, steady under stress

Pros: High variety; patient teaching; strong team culture; foundation for specialty growth

Cons: Heavy patient load; constant multitasking; emotional fatigue from repeat admissions

Clinical Tools: Stethoscope; dynamic acuity board (gl); IV pump (gl); barcode medication scanner (gl); comfort cart (gl)

Clinical Confession: "If I can brighten the room, I've already changed the outcome."

Character Description

Suzette Soleil has been caring for patients longer than most of her coworkers have been alive — and she wears that legacy like a well-pressed badge of honor.

Forty-five years ago, before Hopewell Hospital for Tomorrow existed, the land held a modest brick hospital with an onsite nursing school run by no-nonsense nuns in crisp habits. That's where Suzette learned to chart by hand, assess by instinct, and pray with her patients before she ever learned how to check an email.

Back then, she wore starched white uniforms and a cap you didn't dare tilt.

Now, in bright marigold yellow scrubs, she carries the same warmth, the same grit, the same unwavering devotion to people in their most vulnerable moments.

Ask her if she ever wished for a different career, and she'll give you the same answer she's given for decades:

"Not for a single day."

She has seen healthcare reinvent itself a dozen times — new technologies, new treatments, new philosophies. But nothing tested her quite like the transition to electronic health records. At first, Suzette approached the computers the way some people approach snakes: respectfully, but from a safe distance.

So Hopewell did what Hopewell does best when alignment matters — they paired her with someone whose strengths complemented her own. Her partner? A bright, very patient young Millennial nurse named Casey, who understood digital workflows like they were second nature.

Suzette taught Casey how to hear a patient's fear between sentences, how to catch the early signs of trouble before a monitor beeps, how to speak softly enough to calm a room but firmly enough to lead one.

And Casey taught Suzette where the "submit" button lived.

Together, they bridged two eras of nursing — one grounded in tradition, the other in transformation.

Now Casey serves as a Shift Team Leader on Hopewell's Med-Surg floor. He leads not by barking orders, but by setting a tone — one of steadiness, compassion, and pride in the work.

He's the person nurses instinctively look toward in a crisis, the one whose voice can quiet chaos.

Her walk is slower now, but her impact is stronger than ever.

She is Med-Surg's institutional memory, its mother hen, its compass.

Suzette jokes that she'll retire "the day Hopewell pries the badge reel from my hand," but even she admits the idea is starting to sound less like a joke and more like a well-deserved chapter break. She's not rushing it — just letting the possibility stretch and breathe, the way she teaches new grads to breathe before a tricky IV start. When she does go, she plans to exit with grace, gratitude, and absolutely no farewell sheet cake shaped like a stethoscope.

Day in the Life

Note: The evening Med-Surg shift demands vigilance across multiple high-acuity patients. While scheduled for 8.5 hours, intense multitasking, rapid-onset complications, and overlapping care needs can extend the cognitive and emotional demands far beyond the clock. Suzette's alignment thrives under this sustained pressure.

15:00 — Bed Assignments & Strategic Planning

Six patients on her pod, six stories, six sets of needs:

• Two fresh post-op surgical patients (lap chole (gl) and appendectomy)

• One new diabetic admission

• One COPD (gl) exacerbation

- One fall-risk patient

- One watcher flagged for early sepsis (gl)

The acuity board (gl) pulses like a live map of urgency. Suzette scans, plans, and prioritizes. Scanner beeps confirm med readiness. She inhales, centers, and hums softly — her mental calibration for the next high-stakes hours.

15:15 — Surgical Recovery: Room 612

Post-lap chole patient groaning. IV pump (gl) running analgesics. Suzette coaches deep breathing, instructs on incentive spirometry (IS, gl) ×10, and offers encouragement. "You'll thank me later," she smiles, hands steady, voice warm. Every breath, every cough monitored and logged in EHR (gl).

15:35 — Managing Nausea: Room 609

Antibiotics (gl) have triggered nausea. Comfort cart (gl) at the ready: ginger ale, dimmed lights, antiemetic. Suzette sits, gently rubs the patient's shoulder, monitors vitals. Alignment is not rushing — it's tuning into subtle cues, staying present, responding calmly.

15:50 — The Watcher: Room 606

Vitals whisper sepsis (gl). Suzette flags trends, pages the hospitalist, communicates clearly: "Lactate and cultures — let's catch this early." Every alarm, every lab, every glance at the dynamic acuity board (gl) reinforces urgency. This is preventive vigilance in action.

16:10 — Team Sync & Rapid Planning

A quick huddle at the nurses' station: "Yellow blinking — lactate trending up, cultures ordered." Suzette delegates tasks with clarity: one nurse draws cultures, another prepares antibiotics (gl), she monitors vitals and reassures the worried daughter. Alignment is team orchestration under pressure.

17:10 — Orders Land

Sepsis screen positive (gl). Fluids per MAP, cultures first, antibiotics second. Suzette directs choreography: two sites for cultures, allergies confirmed, IV pump (gl) calibrated. O_2 2 L NC (gl) started. Every step methodical, precise, and calmly communicated.

18:20 — Code Sepsis Activation (gl)

Lactate 3.4. Code Sepsis initiated. Suzette reports succinctly to rapid response team. She maintains composure, delegating while simultaneously mentoring a student: "See the trends? These whispers are our early warning." Critical interventions completed without panic.

19:12 — Stabilization & Family Reassurance

MAP rises to 66. Step-down bed pending. Daughter visibly relieved. Suzette explains: "We responded faster than most would catch it. You can breathe easier now." Emotional labor is part of the intervention — calming families is as vital as fluids and antibiotics.

20:30 — Multitasking Marathon

Syringe feeds, vitals, medication checks, rounding on post-op pain, restocking comfort cart (gl), charting EHR (gl). Each patient requires precision and attention. Suzette moves like sunlight across the floor — Marigold bright, steady, warming the environment while navigating high-acuity needs.

21:00 — Teaching Moment

Student whispers, "How did you know so early?" Suzette smiles: "Alignment is noticing whispers. Every trend, every subtle cue is a story." She models optimism as a clinical skill, mentoring by example.

22:30 — Wrapping Complex Care

Medications completed, vitals stable, EHR updated. Comfort cart (gl) restocked. Last patient teaching delivered. Alignment felt in the smooth flow of orders, calm presence, and stabilized patients.

23:30 — Badge Out & Reflection

Cool evening air. She exhales. "Good work, team." Each patient alive, comfortable, informed. Her optimism operationalized — a tangible effect on both patient outcomes and staff morale.

Tools of the Trade (gl)

• IV pump & barcode medication scanner (gl) — precision in motion

• Comfort cart (gl) — empathy on wheels

• Dynamic acuity board (gl) — teamwork in real time

• Pocket affirmations — for teammates who forget their own strength

Quiet Superpowers

• Emotional calibration — lowers a room's heart rate

• Mentorship by modeling — optimism as a clinical skill

- Remembers names, birthdays, small victories

What Success Feels Like

- Soft goodnights, pain finally eased

- Families reassured, students inspired

- Team saying, "You made this shift lighter"

Route to the Role

BSN → Med-Surg residency → mentorship under a calm, veteran charge nurse → Compassion Corps via Hopewell's Care with Character program

Myth vs. Reality

- Myth: Med-Surg is "basic floor" nursing

- Reality: Med-Surg is the backbone of acute care — coordinating disciplines, managing complexity, spotting decline before labs

Early Mistakes & How to Avoid Them

- Trying to fix everything at once → Prioritize, breathe, delegate. Alignment needs pacing, not perfection

Alignment Scan

- Thrives: Empaths with structure; multitaskers finding meaning in motion; optimists who ground emotion in skill

- Red Flags: Chronic cynicism; anti-team habits; avoidance of emotional labor

- Try-First Rotations: Med-Surg float pool; palliative consult shadow; patient-experience committee

- Non-Negotiables: Emotional maturity; clinical accuracy; collaborative spirit

- Readiness Signals: Energy in teamwork, clarity in chaos, purpose in people

Closing Note

If Hopewell runs on innovation, Suzette is the proof that wisdom — lived, weathered, and generously shared — is still the brightest form of caring.

The Compassion Corps — Alignment in Action

Where connection becomes clinical skill.

The Compassion Corps doesn't chase the siren — they steady the room after it arrives. They are the clinicians who lower a patient's heart rate with a voice before a medication ever hits the line, who explain the numbers until fear stops swallowing the air, who notice the subtle shift that says a patient is tiring out — physically or emotionally — before the monitor tells anyone else. Their work often happens quietly, but its impact is measurable: calmer rooms, safer care, stronger trust, better follow-through, fewer spirals.

Ginger Gauge, RRT turns breath into a bridge — reading alarms, ABGs (gl), and ventilator settings while translating the experience into language patients and families can hold. Justice Jules, RN, SANE-A carries both precision and tenderness, protecting dignity while honoring truth with documentation that must stand up long after the room goes quiet. Hope Fulle, RN, BSN fights for the smallest lives with vigilant steadiness, teaching parents how to touch their babies without fear and how to believe in progress measured in millimeters. Suzette Soleil, RN proves that Med-Surg is not "basic" — it is the backbone, where early decline is caught, families are taught, teams are steadied, and recovery begins long before discharge.

This is what the Compassion Corps shows the entire system: compassion is not decoration. It is strategy. It is skill. It is clinical.

Chapter 22

SCRUBfit Squad: The Diagnostic Division

Precision as a form of care.

Every diagnosis begins with clarity. The Diagnostic Division is healthcare's investigative core — the imaging professionals and laboratory scientists who turn uncertainty into direction. They work where the truth is fragile: in patient identifiers, calibration logs, specimen labels, positioning angles, tiny cellular details, and critical values that must be caught before the room even knows to worry.

Their alignment lives in the details because the details are the difference. A single mislabeled tube can rewrite a life. A single missed artifact can delay treatment. A single digit entered wrong can send care down the wrong road. So they build safety through discipline — verifying, cross-checking, rerunning, documenting, and defending accuracy like it's a promise.

They may work quietly, behind doors most patients never notice, but their impact echoes across every unit. When their systems are aligned, the fog lifts. Decisions sharpen. Treatment can begin with confidence. In the Diagnostic Division, precision isn't perfectionism — it's advocacy.

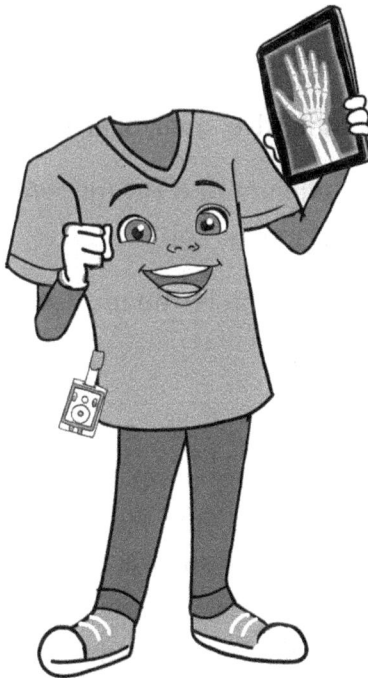

Ray Beam, RT(R) — "The Image Interpreter"

Scrub Color: Cobalt Mist

Primary Role: Radiologic Technologist

Also Aligns With: CT Technologist; MRI Technologist; Sonographer; Radiology Supervisor; Imaging Educator

SCRUB*fit*™ Category: The Diagnostic Division

Pros: High-tech environment; critical diagnostic role; meaningful patient interaction

Cons: Radiation-safety vigilance; long shifts; positioning strain

Personality Traits: Attentive, analytical, empathetic, precise

Clinical Tools: GE Definium 656 HD (gl); PACS (gl); lead apron (gl); positioning sponge (gl)

Clinical Confession: "I capture the unseen — and that changes everything."

Character Description

Ray steps into Imaging before dawn, Cobalt Mist scrubs glowing faintly under fluorescents. He calibrates the GE Definium 656 HD (gl), checks the PACS (gl) queue, and reviews orders. Each image is a puzzle piece — alignment between physics, anatomy, and empathy.

When trauma arrives, he moves fast but never hurried. He verifies identity, explains the scan, shields with care. Ray's alignment is precision married to compassion. To him, an X-ray isn't just a picture — it's a story told in grayscale.

Day in the Life

4:58 a.m. — When the City Is Still Dreaming, Ray Is Already Awake

Ray's alarm doesn't beep — it *glows*, a slow sunrise light that eases him awake like a radiograph developing in a darkroom.

His dog, Pixel (yes, named after the pixel matrix of a digital image), hops onto the bed and nudges his face as if to say:

Time to scan some skeletons, Dad.

Ray stretches, cracks his back (ironically satisfying for an X-ray tech), and heads to the kitchen. He drinks a protein shake that tastes like chalk and ambition. He eats half a banana, because he'll forget otherwise.

He checks his phone:

Morning Schedule:

- ER chest X-ray

- Pre-op knee series

- Trauma bay standby

- Portable rounds

- Outpatient ankle twist

He nods. *Light warm-up.*

5:37 a.m. — The Commute with a Purpose

Ray's drive is quiet except for the soft hum of his old Jeep and the subtle thrill of starting a day where every scan tells a story.

He pulls into the hospital lot as the sky starts to lighten.

Steel-blue scrubs. Lead apron folded in the backseat like a weighted cape.

He grabs his badge and steps inside with that Radiology stride — confident, steady, and a little faster than everyone else because imaging runs on urgency.

6:01 a.m. — Powering Up the Machines of Truth

The radiology department is still asleep, but Ray wakes it up.

He turns on the DR panel.

The monitors flicker alive.

The warm buzz of equipment fills the room.

He checks his radiation badge — zero overexposure.

He adjusts his collimator.

He runs his morning QC images.

The machine responds with a crisp, perfect test pattern.

Ray grins. *We're dialed in.*

6:22 a.m. — The ER Calls Before Even Saying Hello

A nurse rushes in:

"Ray, ER needs a STAT chest."

He grabs his portable like a knight grabbing a shield.

Room 12: A short-of-breath patient sits upright, scared, heart racing.

Ray's voice is calm, warm, grounding.

"Hey there, I'm Ray. I'm gonna take your picture, make sure your lungs look as handsome as you."

They chuckle — oxygen mask and all.

He positions the plate behind their back.

Shoulders forward.

Deep breath in.

Hold...

Click.

Ray reviews the image — sharp, centered, perfect exposure.

He sends it immediately.

The ER doc nods at him as he wheels out.

A silent exchange of respect.

7:04 a.m. — Pre-Op Knee Series: The Ballet of Positioning

Next up is a sweet older patient scheduled for knee replacement surgery.

They're nervous.

They apologize repeatedly for "not being flexible."

Ray kneels beside them, steadies their leg, and says with a wink:

"Don't worry. I've bent knees that haven't moved since the Carter administration."

They laugh — and relax instantly.

He positions them in a textbook AP, then lateral.

Comfortable. Precise. Quick.

It's not just imaging.

It's *care*.

9:18 a.m. — *Trauma Pager: BEEP BEEP BEEP***

Ray grabs his lead.

This is the part of radiology most people never see.

He positions himself at the foot of the trauma bay as the team floods the room.

He's ready before they call him.

"Ray, cross-table C-spine!"

He slides the plate under the backboard with the ease of someone who's done it a thousand times under impossible pressure.

No shaking.

No hesitation.

He becomes stillness in chaos.

Click.

A perfect cervical spine image appears.

Clean alignment.

Clear airway.

"Good job," the trauma doc says.

Ray nods — already prepping for the pelvic.

11:32 a.m. — Portable Rounds: The Radiology Olympics

Ray pushes the portable X-ray up and down halls like it's cardio day.

ICU, PACU, Med-Surg — everyone waves because everyone knows him.

He jokes with patients.

He warms cold hands.

He fixes pillows and untangles IV lines.

Every image he sends upstairs helps a provider make a decision.

He may not prescribe meds or perform procedures,

but he makes diagnosis (gl) possible.

12:41 p.m. — Lunch, the Radiologic Way

Lunch is 11 minutes long.

Maybe 12 if nobody calls a STAT.

Turkey sandwich.

Gatorade.

Half of a cookie someone left in the break room.

Ray sits with two CT techs as they debate contrast allergies and which scanner is "faster."

Portable X-ray calls him back mid-bite.

Every Radiologic Technologist knows the truth:

Lunch is a suggestion.

1:55 p.m. — Outpatient Ankle Twist

A teenager limps into his room, embarrassed, claiming he "didn't fall — just tripped in an epic way."

Ray nods.

"Say no more. Happens to the best of us."

He positions the ankle.

The kid winces.

"You know," Ray says, "I once sprained mine stepping off a curb trying to impress someone."

The kid laughs.

Shoulders drop.

Perfect positioning achieved.

He reviews the film:

Yep — clear fracture line.

He doesn't say anything — but he calls the provider immediately.

3:40 p.m. — The Surprise Add-On

Orthopedics calls wanting emergency images of a post-op patient.

Ray hustles.

He adjusts angles.

He gets perfect alignment despite a patient in pain.

The orthopedic surgeon reviews the films on the monitor and says:

"These are gorgeous."

Ray beams (pun intended).

4:57 p.m. — Shutdown Ritual

He cleans the room meticulously.

Wipes down equipment.

Shuts the machines down in sequence like a pilot powering off an aircraft.

His badge beeps as he clocks out — same calming beep as when he clocks in.

It's been a long day, but Ray feels proud.

Every image he took helped someone.

Every position he adjusted prevented misdiagnosis.

Every shot he captured served a purpose.

He steps outside and the sun is low, golden, cinematic — like it knows exactly who Ray Beam is.

6:10 p.m. — Home, Pixel, and Peace

Pixel nearly tackles him.

Ray laughs — tired but full.

Dinner with his partner is simple but warm: pasta, veggies, a glass of something cold.

They ask, "Anything interesting today?"

Ray shrugs and grins.

"Oh, you know... just captured the inside stories of half the hospital."

He showers, finds his softest T-shirt, and winds down on the couch.

10:03 p.m. — Ending the Day with Gratitude

Ray checks his badge dose log one last time (classic Radiologic Technologist move), then sets his phone to silent.

Pixel curls up beside him.

Ray whispers:

"Another day of pictures that matter."

He sleeps deeply — ready to do it all again tomorrow.

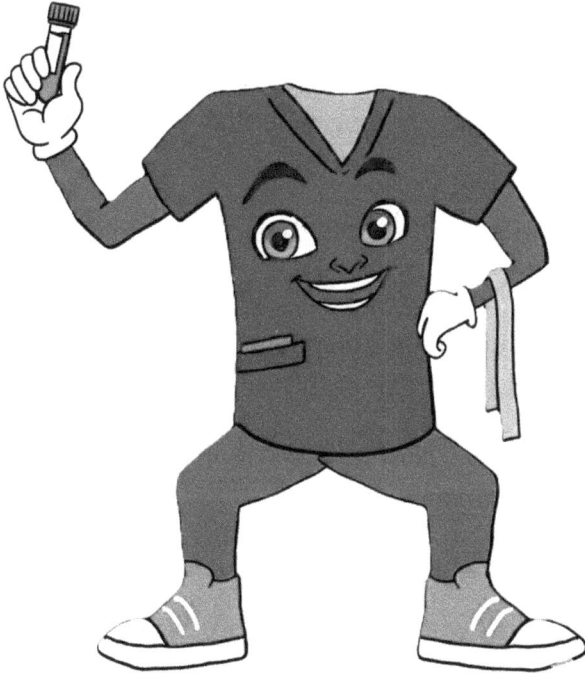

Darcy Heplock, MLS (ASCP)

Darcy Heplock, MLS (ASCP) — "The Silent Detective"

Scrub Color: Forest Green

Primary Role: Medical Laboratory Scientist

Also Aligns With: Clinical Microbiologist; Chemistry Technologist; Blood Bank Specialist; Lab Quality Coordinator

SCRUB*fit*™ Category: The Diagnostic Division

Pros: Essential to every diagnosis; clear accuracy metrics; strong scientific career path

Cons: Minimal patient contact; repetitive workflows; time-sensitive pressure

Personality Traits: Methodical, data-driven, detail-oriented, reliable

Clinical Tools: Centrifuge (gl); microscope (gl); hematology analyzer (gl); biosafety cabinet (gl)

Clinical Confession: "My patients live in test tubes — but their stories are human."

Character Description

Darcy's world hums with quiet precision. In Forest Green scrubs, she reviews samples, calibrates analyzers, and verifies results clinicians depend on. Every specimen is someone waiting for an answer — and she never forgets it.

Her alignment is repetition with reverence. If a result looks off, she doesn't guess — she investigates, reruns, documents. The lab isn't apart from patient care; it *is* patient care.

Day in the Life

4:46 a.m. — The World Sleeps, the Lab Prepares

Darcy wakes before her alarm.

Not because she's a morning person — she absolutely isn't — but because her brain is already sorting CBC values (gl) in her dreams.

Her cat, Hemmy (short for Hemoglobin), stretches across her chest like a warm, judgemental scarf.

Darcy whispers, "Shift change, little dude," and Hemmy slowly slides off with deep emotional resentment.

She makes coffee strong enough to power a generator.

She packs her lunch — yogurt, hummus, pretzels, and a cookie she absolutely deserves.

She checks her messages:

STAT troponin trending up

Two new COVID PCRs pending

Blood bank stock slightly low

She nods.

The lab never stops — and today, she won't either.

5:38 a.m. — Commute Under a Purple Dawn

Darcy drives through quiet streets with lo-fi beats playing.

Her car smells faintly of citrus and glove powder.

As she approaches the hospital, she feels the familiar shift — the moment when she transforms from regular-human Darcy into **Darcy Heplock, MLS**, guardian of the unseen, protector of the pipeline between samples and diagnosis.

She parks, swipes her badge, and walks through hallways that are still half-asleep.

But downstairs?

The lab is always awake.

6:01 a.m. — Enter the Lab: A World of Whirring and Wonder

Darcy steps into her kingdom:

• Analyzers rumble softly like dragons waking up

• Centrifuges whir with loyal urgency

• The faint smell of bleach hints at 10,000 lives saved

• Instruments blink in warm, soft, ready-for-battle light

She hangs her maroon scrub jacket, ties her hair back, and sanitizes her hands with ritualistic precision.

Then she speaks the words all MLS professionals whisper at the start of every shift:

"Let's save some lives indirectly."

6:18 a.m. — Morning QC: The Sacred Ritual

Darcy runs her quality control (QC) samples — the lab version of pre-flight checks.

She checks calibration curves.

She checks reagent volumes.

She makes sure each analyzer is giving results clean enough to tattoo on her arm.

Everything passes except *chemistry analyzer #2*, which today decides to be dramatic.

She gives it the Look™ — the one that says:

"We've been through worse. Don't start now."

It stabilizes.

Good choice.

6:55 a.m. — The STAT Storm Arrives

The pneumatic tube fires — *WHOOSH* — and a red-labeled bag drops into the station.

STAT blood samples.

Ray Beam in Radiology is probably already imaging the patient.

Darcy snaps into action:

• Spins the tube in the centrifuge

• Pipettes with flawless muscle memory

• Runs the chemistry panel

• Verifies the sodium, potassium, creatinine

• Checks the troponin — elevated

She releases the results to the EMR.

Somewhere upstairs, a provider changes a treatment plan because of her work.

Darcy doesn't see it.

But she *feels* it.

7:42 a.m. — Hematology: The Story Written in Cells

Darcy slides a blood smear under her microscope.

Pink and purple universes come to life.

RBCs floating like galaxies.

Neutrophils looking like tiny armored warriors.

Platelets — small, but ready to riot.

She spots something odd.

A cluster of blasts — abnormal cells.

Her voice goes quiet.

Her heart gets steady.

She reviews.

Confirms.

Alerts the pathologist.

Possible leukemia.

This is the moment most people will never know she caught —

yet everything hinges on her eyes.

9:10 a.m. — Microbiology: The Petri Dish Detective

Now comes micro — the part of the lab that feels like CSI but with more humidity.

Darcy checks yesterday's plates:

- One strep

- One staph

- Several cultures growing nothing (bless)

- One suspicious colony with a green hue

She performs a quick gram stain.

Purple cocci cluster like grapes.

She smiles.

Classic staph aureus.

She updates the chart, enters sensitivities, and lets the provider know what antibiotic will work best.

Invisible hero work: complete.

11:25 a.m. — Blood Bank Ballet

A trauma code hits.

Darcy rushes to Blood Bank.

She checks typing, crossmatches, and antibody screens — each step deliberate, careful, sacred.

The phone rings from the trauma bay:

"We need two units O-negative NOW."

Darcy grabs the cooler, double-checks every digit, and hands it to the runner with the words:

"Go. Safe transfusion."

In the right hands, her decision saves a life.

12:58 p.m. — Lunch, or Whatever's Left of It

Darcy sits in the break room, unscrewing her yogurt while answering questions from new grads:

"Why does hemolysis ruin potassium?"

"What color top do we use for coagulation?"

"Is it true someone once put urine in a chemistry tube?"

Darcy laughs.

"Yes. They absolutely did."

She gets six bites in before the tube system fires again.

She stands.

Sighs.

Returns to the bench.

Lunch: completed at 38%.

2:14 p.m. — The Mystery Sample

A mislabeled tube.

A wonky barcode.

A specimen that claims to be "arm: left?" but the word *left* is written like a suspicious ransom note.

Darcy channels her inner detective:

• Calls the floor nurse

• Tracks the phlebotomist

• Identifies the correct patient

• Stops a serious medical error

All because Darcy Heplock doesn't "just run samples" —

she protects the chain of truth.

4:03 p.m. — Final Verifications, Final Victories

Darcy signs off her last batch:

- 312 tests run

- 14 critical values reported

- 2 instrument calibrations

- 1 possible leukemia caught

- 1 trauma saved

- 0 mislabeled samples allowed to slip through her fingers

She hangs up her maroon coat and high-fives her coworker on the way out.

The lab doors close behind her, but the results she released today will ripple through the hospital all night long.

5:09 p.m. — Home, Hemmy, and Healing

Hemmy greets her like she's been gone for weeks.

She makes dinner, showers, slips into soft pajamas, and curls onto the couch with the comfort of knowing:

She didn't see a single patient today —

and yet she saved more lives than she can count.

She ends the night with tea, a crime show, and a sleepy cat on her chest.

Before bed, she murmurs:

"Good job today, Darcy."

And she's right.

10:18 p.m. — Lights Out, but the Lab Never Stops

The machines keep humming.

Samples keep coming.

Lives keep depending on people like Darcy Heplock.

And tomorrow, she'll wake up and do it all again —

quietly, brilliantly, heroically.

The Diagnostic Division — Accuracy as Advocacy

The Diagnostic Division proves alignment begins with truth. Care cannot move forward until facts do. Through images, slides, cultures, and critical values, they make certainty possible — one pixel, one smear, one specimen at a time. They are the guardians of the chain of truth, protecting patients from guesswork and teams from preventable error. And when they're in alignment, the entire system becomes safer — because the right answer arrives on time, every time it matters most.

Chapter 23
SCRUBfit Squad:
The Med Heads

Where intellect becomes intervention.

The Med Heads are healthcare's strategists (gl) — the clinicians who live where physiology (gl) meets precision. They decode symptoms into strategy, convert uncertainty into plan, and turn medication into meaning. In their world, thinking isn't a pause before action — it *is* the action. A well-timed order prevents a crisis. A clean differential (gl) saves hours. A corrected dose spares a kidney. A single clarifying question changes the entire trajectory (gl) of a patient's story.

They are the cognitive command center of care — physicians, nurse practitioners, and pharmacists who move fast *because* they think clearly, not because they guess quickly. Their alignment is both intellectual and ethical (gl): every directive balanced between benefit and risk, every decision shaped by evidence (gl), pattern recognition (gl), and humility. They don't chase certainty for comfort. They chase it because downstream lives depend on upstream clarity.

And when the Med Heads are in rhythm, the whole system breathes easier. Teams communicate cleanly. Plans hold. Patients feel steadier — not because medicine is suddenly simple, but because someone made it navigable (gl). They are thinkers who move with purpose: curiosity as fuel, collaboration as multiplier, and clarity as a form of care.

"The heart of pharmacy leadership is alignment: the right team, the right practices, the right purpose. Whether it's mentoring the next generation or guiding clinical decisions, a Director of Pharmacy ensures safety and stewardship (gl) across the entire system."

JoAnn Neufer, B.S. Pharm.

Former Director of Pharmacy, Sibley Memorial Hospital, Johns Hopkins Medicine

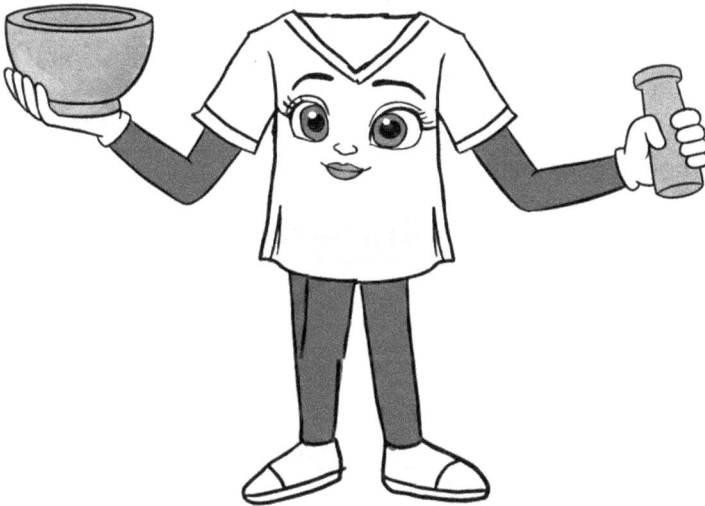

Polly Pillcount, PharmD

Polly Pillcount, PharmD — "The Dosing Detective"

Scrub Color: Violet Veil

Primary Role: Hospital Pharmacist (gl)

Also Aligns With: Clinical Pharmacist (gl), BCPS (gl); Medication Safety Officer (gl)

SCRUB*fit*™ Category: The Med Heads

Pros: Analytical; meticulous; systems-minded; trusted by clinicians

Cons: Can over-verify; slow to delegate

Personality Traits: Curious, steady, methodical, principled

Clinical Tools: Epic (gl); BD Pyxis (gl); smart pump (gl); Micromedex (gl); IV hood (gl)

Clinical Confession: "I still double-check saline bags like they're diamonds."

Character Description

Polly's world hums at the frequency of precision. Morning violet light spills across Central Pharmacy — measured calm inside controlled chaos. She doesn't just verify orders; she translates risk into reassurance. Every medication she releases is unseen protection, a quiet shield raised before anyone knows they were in danger.

Colleagues call her The Dosing Detective because she can trace a drug interaction (gl) like a forensic map (gl). A creatinine (gl) bump and her mind reconstructs the entire medication timeline before anyone reaches a calculator. Where others see numbers, she hears rhythm: dose → interval (gl) → effect → repeat. She trusts the math — but she trusts patterns more.

A residency near-miss made her a champion of safety culture, the kind that doesn't rely on "being careful," but on building guardrails (gl) strong enough to hold up on the worst day. Her whiteboard mantra is simple: **Clarity before speed.** Between verifications, she tapes medication puns to the laminar hood (gl) because humor keeps people awake, and awake people make fewer mistakes.

Catching a duplicate vancomycin (gl) order takes ten seconds and prevents a cascade (gl) that ends in renal failure (gl). Polly logs it on the Feedback Flow Board (gl):

Bright Spot — Caught Before Harm.

Polly measures success by absence: no codes triggered by errors, no frantic pages, no "How did this happen?" meetings. In her world, silence is proof.

A Day in the Life

Polly Pillcount, PharmD — The Dosing Detective

4:19 a.m. — Where Precision Wakes Before People Do

The hospital is dark, silent, and holding its breath. But down a long fluorescent hallway — tucked between sterile storage and the pneumatic tube station (gl) that coughs to life at inconvenient times — a violet glow hums awake.

It's the Central Pharmacy.

And it's where Polly begins her day.

Her scrubs are crisp. Her badge is straight. Her mind is already assembling drug interactions (gl) like puzzle pieces. Other clinicians wake up with coffee. Polly wakes up with pharmacokinetics (gl).

5:02 a.m. — The Calm Before the Orders Storm

The IV hood (gl) hums softly as she steps into the clean room. Her tools assemble like a ritual:

- BD Pyxis (gl) inventory report

- Epic (gl) queue blinking with overnight orders

- Smart pump (gl) safety logs

- Micromedex (gl) opened to a tab she never closes

A sticky note taped above her hood reads:

"Don't let your guardrails down."

Her own pun, of course.

Outside the hood: chaos waiting to happen.

Inside the hood: control.

6:14 a.m. — First Red Flag of the Day

A vancomycin (gl) order hits her queue. Then another. Two providers. Same patient. Two doses that could turn kidneys into confetti.

Polly scrolls the creatinine (gl) trend — up, creeping upward. She messages the resident:

"Duplicate vanco. Renal dosing (gl) concern. Recommend holding."

No drama. No ego. Just prevention.

She logs it under Bright Spot — Caught Before Harm.

Ten seconds of vigilance. A cascade avoided.

7:08 a.m. — Tube Station Roulette

The pneumatic tube (gl) wheezes, then launches a canister like a toddler who found caffeine. Polly cracks it open: electrolytes (gl), heparin (gl), and a note:

"Polly, pls check dose. I don't trust anyone else."

Trust is her currency.

She checks everything — dose, label, weight, renal function (gl). Assumptions are the enemy.

8:45 a.m. — Rounds: The Dosing Detective Goes Public

Pharmacists aren't always invited to rounds. But Polly is requested.

A sepsis (gl) case stalls the team.

"What's our dosing strategy?"

Polly answers without looking at a screen:

"Weight-based cefepime (gl), renal-adjusted (gl). Switch from q8h to q12h."

The attending (gl) nods. The nurses breathe again.

A new intern whispers, "She's the Hermione of dosing."

Polly pretends not to hear it — and grins.

10:32 a.m. — Behavioral Health Orders Arrive

Psych meds require a softer type of vigilance. A lithium (gl) level comes back high enough to make everyone sit up straighter.

Polly pivots: diet → diuretics (gl) → hydration (gl) → renal patterns (gl).

Her message lands clean:

"Holding lithium. Hydrate. Recheck at 1500."

Pharmacy isn't a basement job anymore. It's the brain trust.

12:11 p.m. — Polly's Lunch (If You Can Call It That)

Half a sandwich. Two string cheeses. One bite.

Pyxis alarm.

Lunch is over.

She logs the bite as a win.

1:28 p.m. — The Quiet Heroism of Verifications

Med after med scrolls:

Levofloxacin (gl). TPN (gl). Antifungal (gl). Pediatric amoxicillin (gl). Insulin (gl). A new anticoagulant (gl). A revised pain plan (gl).

To Polly, every med is a moment of protection.

A pharmacist isn't a cog. A pharmacist is a firewall (gl).

3:04 p.m. — The System Depends on One Quiet Catch

A nurse messages:

"This heparin (gl) bag looks weird?"

Polly sprints — pharmacy-style sprinting: purposeful, fast, already calculating.

The concentration is wrong. Not catastrophic yet — but wrong enough to become catastrophic in the wrong hands. She pulls the batch (gl). Quarantines (gl). Alerts leadership. A near-miss becomes a clean catch.

4:57 p.m. — End of Shift, Beginning of Vigilance

Final log:

- Duplicate therapy prevented

- Renal dosing adjusted

- Drug interaction (gl) identified

- Smart pump settings corrected

- Heparin batch quarantined

- Six resident teaching moments

Polly measures her day by absence: no harm, no crashes, no "How did we miss this?"

Silence means safety.

SCRUBfits™

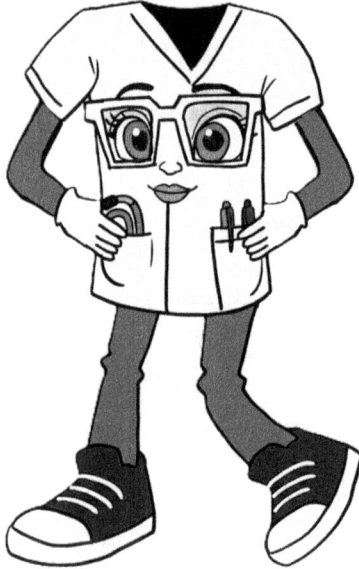

Anna Remedy, DNP, FNP-BC

Anna Remedy, DNP, FNP-BC, PMHNP — "The Therapeutic Translator"

Scrub Color: Navy Blue

Primary Role: Family Nurse Practitioner (gl)

Also Aligns With: Primary Care Physician (gl); Physician Assistant (gl)

SCRUB*fit*™ Category: The Med Heads

Pros: Empathetic; educator at heart; strong communicator

Cons: Absorbs patient stress; prone to over-explaining

Personality Traits: Grounded, approachable, observant, persistent

Clinical Tools: Stethoscope; EHR (gl); PHQ-9 (gl); SDOH (gl) screeners; BP cuff; telehealth kit (gl)

Clinical Confession: "I measure success by how calm the room feels when I leave."

Character Description

Anna sits at the intersection of medicine and meaning — where explanation becomes intervention and understanding becomes adherence (gl). She begins every visit with a question that makes space for truth:

"What's the hardest part of this for you?"

And she waits long enough for the real answer to surface.

She balances evidence (gl) and empathy with rare precision. She once color-coded a medication list for thirty minutes to prevent an ER readmission (gl) — not because she loves stationery, but because she understands something most people miss: confusion is a clinical risk (gl). Education, in her hands, is not a lecture. It's a safety measure.

Population dashboards (gl) don't intimidate her; they orient her. Patterns don't feel abstract. They feel like people she hasn't met yet. When she leaves a room, trust lingers — not because she promised perfection, but because she made the plan feel possible.

A Day in the Life

Anna Remedy, DNP, FNP-BC, PMHNP — The Therapeutic Translator

5:38 a.m. — The Remedy House Wakes Like a Small Town Coming Online

The day begins quietly, then all at once. Someone is arguing about yogurt downstairs. Cupboards open and close in the early light. And the English Bulldog grumble of Sig rises like a headline preparing to be read aloud.

Then comes the inevitable:

"Mom! SIG IS SMELLING MY CEREAL AGAIN!"

Anna smiles. There it is — the morning announcement.

She steps into the hallway flanked by her loyal escorts: Reba, the family Rottweiler — ninety pounds of devotion and questionable judgment about who counts as a threat — and Sig, her daughter's English Bulldog, forty-eight pounds of certainty that every human breakfast is actually his.

Downstairs, the chaos is perfectly alive. Her oldest daughter blends a smoothie with the intensity of a Food Network finalist. Her second daughter delivers a passionate case for being excused from school "for reasons too complex to explain right now." Her oldest son reads a cereal box like he's preparing to litigate one of its claims. And the youngest — the cereal victim — guards his bowl while Sig hovers, breathing heavily like a tiny steam engine.

"I can feel his breath on my milk," the youngest says without looking up. "It's warm. He's warming my cereal."

Anna slides her hands under Sig's barrel chest and lifts him — a move she's perfected with the muscle memory (gl) of someone who has rescued this dog from at least three trash cans, two laundry baskets, and once, a neighbor's open car.

"Buddy," she says, setting him gently on the floor, "that's what Bulldogs do."

Sig snorts, offended by the generalization (gl), and sits directly on her foot in protest. Reba sighs dramatically — the Rottweiler version of "enough with the drama."

Heavy boots tap across the tile. Her husband — crisp in his State Trooper uniform — steps into the kitchen holding a travel mug of coffee like it's classified evidence (gl). They met years ago in the Sheriff's Office, when Anna wore a different kind of badge. He stayed in law enforcement. She followed the pull toward medicine. The instinct is the same — protect, stabilize, translate danger into safety — just a new uniform, in her case scrubs.

"Long one?" he asks.

"Clinic all day," she says, taking a sip. "Hospital all night."

He kisses her temple. "Don't worry. I'll manage the evening chaos, canine scandals, and any cereal-related emergencies."

The kids groan in unison as Anna kisses him back, purely for sport.

By 7:13 a.m., the choreography is complete: shoes found, lunches packed, promises made, doors shut. Anna scratches Reba's ears, kisses Sig's wonderfully squishy forehead, grabs her stethoscope, and heads to the car.

Morning — The Beach-Adjacent Clinic

(Primary Care + Behavioral Health)

The clinic sits just a few minutes from the shoreline, and the building feels it — salt in the air, sun on the windows, a steady calm that makes even hard days feel a little less sharp.

Anna steps inside, and Michelle — guardian of the front desk, gatekeeper of sanity, unofficial mayor of the clinic — looks up already flipping through sticky notes, messages, and the day's schedule like a blackjack dealer with a supernatural gift.

"Morning," Michelle says, smiling brightly. "Two early birds are here. One's anxious. One's cheerful. You'll know which is which."

Behind her, Pat — Anna's nurse, former ICU clinical warrior — is already prepping charts, printing vitals sheets, and humming softly over an iPad. Pat is calm in the way only ICU veterans are calm: like weather has tried her and failed.

"Morning, boss," Pat says. "Your first three patients are roomed, I finally exorcised the cuff that's been possessed since Monday, and..." She produces a napkin-wrapped, comically oversized banana nut muffin and sets it in Anna's hand.

Anna raises a palm. "I'm being good today."

Then she forgets herself and takes a generous bite.

Pat smirks. "ICU training."

8:12 a.m. — First Patient: The Weight-of-the-World Teen

A teenage girl sits curled on the exam table, hoodie sleeves pulled over her hands. Anna pulls up a chair — not a stool, not a desk — a chair, eye level.

"What's the hardest part of this for you?" she asks.

The girl's face crumples. It's the kind of silent cry that only starts when trust arrives. Pat quietly hands Anna a tissue box without interrupting. Michelle adjusts the waiting room flow so no one feels rushed, because what's happening behind this door is real work.

10:27 a.m. — The Diabetes Tune-Up

A middle-aged man jokes his way through everything because he's afraid of disappointing people. Anna reviews glucose logs and says gently, "Let's take shame out of the room." Pat nods, taking notes, adjusting the care plan.

The patient leaves with a new strategy — and something harder to measure: the feeling that he can do this.

12:04 p.m. — Lunch (Aspirational)

Anna takes the first bite of a turkey wrap.

Michelle: "Your 12 is early, your 12:30 is already here, and someone wants to know if you can 'just take a quick look' at something."

Pat: "I screened the 12:30 — you're going to like her."

Anna: "Define 'like.'"

Pat: "She brought a list."

Anna: "How long?"

Pat: "Five items. Double-spaced. Bullet points. I'm proud of her."

Lunch is over. One bite counts as a victory.

2:41 p.m. — Behavioral Health Crossroads

A young man with anxiety sits stiffly on the edge of the chair.

"Tell me where in your body you feel the worry," Anna says softly.

He looks startled. Nobody has ever asked him that. Pat stands near the doorway — present, steady, not rushing.

By the time he leaves, his shoulders have lowered a fraction. That's how change starts: small, honest, possible.

4:52 p.m. — Closing Charts, Opening Another World

Michelle starts shutting down the front desk computer. Pat finishes cleaning rooms. The clinic hum fades.

"You're on nights?" Pat asks, knowing the answer but asking anyway.

Anna nods. "Yep. Round two."

Michelle hands Anna a small bag with two protein bars and a sticky note:

EAT SOMETHING. —M

Anna smiles as she walks to her car. The ocean is only a few minutes away, and she can smell salt in the breeze. Her second shift is waiting.

Evening — Hospitalist Mode Activated

5:31 p.m. The hospital doors open with a soft swoosh, and the air changes — cooler, sharper, charged. Her badge beeps. A nurse waves her over. Four admissions are waiting: COPD exacerbation (gl), complex post-op fever (gl), heart failure (gl) gasping between sentences, and an elderly woman waxing in and out of delirium (gl).

Anna washes her hands, adjusts her stethoscope, and steps fully into night-shift clarity.

7:18 p.m. — The Post-Op Fever

Handoff from the day team is muddy. Anna untangles it with calm precision. Labs ordered. Exam performed. Plan clarified. The spouse whispers as Anna leaves, "Thank you... I just needed someone who looked like they understood."

Anna does.

10:42 p.m. — The Delirium Patient

The elderly woman begins humming, disoriented, afraid. Anna sits beside her. Slow voice. Kind eyes. Hand on her wrist.

"You're safe. I'm right here."

She stays for five full minutes — the kind of five minutes that change outcomes.

1:03 a.m. — The Heart Failure Case

Respirations ease. Oxygen rises. The nurse exhales like she's been holding her breath for an hour.

"Good call," the nurse says.

Anna shakes her head gently. "Team call."

3:19 a.m. — A Quiet Moment

The hospital settles into that thin, late-night quiet that isn't peace exactly, but isn't chaos either. Anna finally opens one of Michelle's protein bars and thinks about the teen, the anxious young man, the post-op patient, and her own kids sleeping at home. Once, she wore a different badge — Deputy Sheriff — standing between danger and the people she served. Now her badge hangs from her scrub top, but the mission hasn't changed. She still shows up where the stakes are high and the outcomes matter.

6:07 a.m. — The Sunrise Drive Home

One more check. One more note. One more reassurance. Then badge-out. Outside, the sky begins to open — soft streaks of pink and gold at the horizon. The air holds that in-between feel, not quite night, not quite day.

Two worlds, one short drive apart. Clinic and hospital. Logic and heart. Binder tabs and intuition.

Anna is a steadiness people feel before they know her name.

"Mental health is not just about medication — those can be powerful tools, but healing begins with being truly heard. As a psychiatric nurse practitioner, my work is rooted in listening, empathy, and authentic human connection. Patients always know when care is genuine. Treatment is most effective when it is a collaboration — a partnership that honors not only emotional well-being, but physical health and the life circumstances each person is navigating. Mental health care is teamwork, built on trust, compassion, and understanding."

Dr. Joanna Robertson is the real-world clinical voice behind Anna Remedy, DNP, FNP-BC, PMHNP, the **SCRUB*fit*™** guide who walks readers through the emotional and psychological landscapes (gl) of healthcare. Her work as a psychiatric nurse practitioner brings deep listening, trauma-informed care, and genuine human connection into every page where Anna appears. In a world increasingly shaped by technology and speed, her perspective reminds us that healing still begins with something simple and powerful: being truly seen and heard.

[Image: Crimson Quest MD B&W.jpg]

Crimson Quest, MD — "The Crimson Blade"

Trauma Surgeon (gl) — High Velocity. High Stakes. High Vigilance.

SCRUB*fit*™ Category: The Med Heads

Scrub Color: Crimson Red (Trauma Bay) / Misty Sage (Academic Floors)

Primary Role: Trauma Surgeon (gl)

Also Aligns With: Surgical Intensivist (gl); Trauma Medical Director (gl); Quality & Safety Officer (gl)

Pros: Decisive; evidence-anchored; calm under pressure

Cons: Frustrated by delays; intolerant of sloppy handoffs

Personality Traits: Precise, inquisitive, protective

Clinical Tools: EHR (gl); trauma board (gl); telemetry (gl); resuscitation checklist (gl); massive transfusion protocol (gl)

Clinical Confession: "In trauma, hesitation is harm. Move, or move out of the way."

Character Description

Crimson Quest, MD moves like a blade through chaos — fast, quiet, precise. Her intuition is sharpened by thousands of seconds-matter decisions, each one etched into muscle memory (gl) and judgment.

Where others see confusion, she sees patterns:

• Seatbelt sign (gl) → occult bleeding (gl)

• Pale teen → internal hemorrhage (gl)

• Rising lactate (gl) → silent crash (gl)

Her mantra for trainees is blunt for a reason: "Trauma doesn't care about your feelings. But your intuition saves lives."

SCRUBfits™

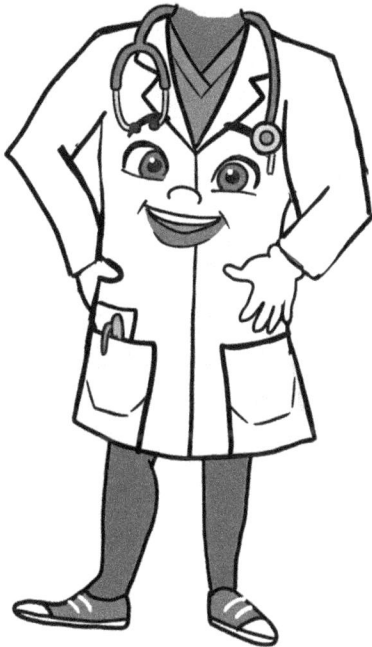

Crimson Quest, MD

A Day in the Life

Crimson Quest, MD — The Crimson Blade

05:15

The alarm cuts through the dark, but Crimson is already awake. Trauma surgeons learn to rise quickly, without bargaining with the morning. She drinks cold water, stretches her hands and shoulders, checks the pager, and scans the overnight list. Three laparotomies (gl). Two thoracotomies (gl). Multiple activations (gl). The city didn't sleep, and neither did the red phone.

06:30

Crimson steps into the hospital through the ED-side entrance — the one where paramedics half jog. Her Crimson Red scrubs catch the fluorescent light as she passes the trauma bay doors. The air smells like wipes, saline, and the unmistakable metallic note of adrenaline. The team is already moving: residents pre-charting, nurses warming irrigation fluids (gl), the trauma tech restocking chest tubes (gl). Crimson reviews the board, signs in, and runs a quiet ritual: scopes checked (gl), headlamp charged, loupes (gl) wiped, a fresh marker for incision notes.

07:00

Sign-out is brisk. The overnight attending gives a rundown: two post-op liver lacerations (gl) in the SICU (gl), one splenectomy (gl) recovering well, and a cyclist with an unstable pelvic fracture headed to IR (gl). Crimson listens, asks two pointed questions, and takes the baton. Trauma is a relay; each surgeon protects the next runner.

08:10

The first activation hits: rollover MVC (gl), unrestrained driver, prolonged extrication (gl). The room moves like choreography.

Crimson stations herself at the foot of the bed, scanning with seasoned eyes. Airway secure (gl). Breath sounds asymmetric (gl). Abdomen rigid. FAST exam (gl) positive.

"To the OR," she calls — decisive, clean.

The bed wheels toward the elevators at a jog, anesthesia already planning induction (gl). Crimson walks beside the gurney, one hand on the rail, voice steady, reassuring the patient who keeps whispering that she can't feel her legs.

08:27

Inside the OR, the lights flood the field. Crimson opens the abdomen in seconds, controlling hemorrhage (gl) with practiced precision. A splenic hilum (gl) bleed. A torn mesentery (gl). A lacerated diaphragm (gl). Instruments pass with wordless rhythm. Anesthesia calls out blood product numbers (gl). The scrub tech anticipates the next clamp before Crimson fully registers the need.

When the final suture cinches closed, a different kind of quiet settles. The patient is stable. Another life that shouldn't have made it now has a chance.

10:55

Back in the trauma bay, she drinks half a cup of cold coffee before the next page: fall from scaffolding (gl), multiple long-bone fractures (gl). Crimson kneels beside the patient and explains every exam maneuver before touching him. She coordinates with ortho (gl), orders imaging, and catches something the narrative doesn't explain — a breathing pattern that doesn't match the pain story.

A CT later confirms what she suspected: a subtle, dangerous splenic injury. Early detection saves a crash later. Crimson nods to herself. The little saves matter too.

12:40

Lunch doesn't arrive. Instead, she rounds again, reviews labs (gl), reassures families, and quietly steadies residents learning to carry the weight of decisions. A medical student shadows her, eyes wide at every page. Crimson lets the student close a laceration (gl) in the bay, guiding hands with respect, as if this were the only wound the patient would remember.

14:15

A stabbing arrives under police escort. The patient is hypotensive (gl), pale, drifting in and out. Crimson steps into command mode. Orders fly: massive transfusion protocol (gl), repeat FAST (gl), portable chest (gl). The team responds instantly. She recognizes the trajectory (gl) — angled beneath the rib cage, heading for trouble.

As they run the gurney down the hall, the patient reaches weakly toward a hallway light, disoriented and terrified. Crimson leans in and says, quiet but unbreakable:

"Stay with me. I've got you."

15:02

The operation is a blur of clamps, sponges, sutures, and rapid decisions. Trauma surgery is a conversation with the body — half science, half faith that hands will know what the clock won't forgive. Crimson moves fast but not frantic, the team in perfect sync. When the bleeding slows, shoulders drop a fraction. Victory by millimeters.

17:20

She steps into the hallway just as sunlight streaks through the windows. For a moment, she stands alone, letting the adrenaline drain. Then she's moving again — checking the earlier MVC patient in SICU (gl), reassuring a mother who keeps asking whether she said the right things before her son went to the OR. Crimson tells her she did. The mother believes her because Crimson says it like someone who has stood in that exact fear.

18:00

The pager erupts again: pedestrian struck. The bay fills with footsteps, monitors, urgency. Crimson steps back into the storm without hesitation. Trauma surgeons don't pace themselves — they pace the system. A resident beside her looks shaken.

Crimson offers one grounding line:

"We go one decision at a time."

19:30

Her shift ends, but she does one more walk-through — checking critical patients, speaking with night shift, reviewing notes, tying off loose ends that could become emergencies at 03:00. Trauma isn't a shift job. It's stewardship (gl).

20:05

Outside, the evening is quiet. The city hums under streetlights, unaware of the lives saved because a team and a surgeon refused to flinch. Crimson sits in her car for a moment before starting it, thinking about wins, losses avoided, and the faces of families who whispered thank you with trembling relief.

Then she exhales, starts the engine, and drives into the night. The red phone will ring again. It always does.

The Med Heads — Command and Clarity

The Med Heads define the cerebral core of healthcare — the clinicians who convert chaos into plan and uncertainty into action. Their alignment is intellectual, ethical (gl), and operational (gl): the ability to think clearly in motion, communicate cleanly under pressure, and protect patients through decisions that hold up at 2 a.m. and 2 p.m. alike.

Polly Pillcount, PharmD keeps the system safe through invisible catches — the duplicate therapy prevented, the concentration corrected, the near-miss turned into a clean save. Anna Remedy, DNP, FNP-BC, PMHNP translates fear into clarity and complexity into a plan people can follow — making education a safety tool and trust a clinical outcome. Crimson Quest, MD stands at the knife-edge where seconds matter, turning instinct into strategy and strategy into survival.

When the Med Heads are in rhythm, everything downstream moves with steadier breath: the right medication, the right intervention, the right timing, the right plan. In their hands, clarity becomes protection — and protection becomes healing.

Next up! **The Recovery Regimen**

Where the Med Heads provide precision, The Recovery Regimen provides endurance.

Here, healing becomes motion. Plans become persistence. Diagnoses become drive.

Every regained step echoes a Med Head's earlier decision.

Welcome to The Recovery Regimen — where healing learns to move again.

Chapter 24
SCRUBfit Squad: The Recovery Regimen

Rebuilding function with disciplined hope.

Healing doesn't end when the bleeding stops or the surgery is complete. The Recovery Regimen represents the clinicians who help patients rebuild strength, function, and independence after illness or injury. These professionals see possibility where others see limitation, and they measure success not just in vital signs, but in milestones like a first step, a regained skill, or the confidence to return home.

They are patient, persistent, and endlessly creative. They design treatment plans (gl) tailored to each person, adapting exercises, tools, and strategies to help bodies and minds recover. For patients, they are the encouragers who say "you can" when everything feels impossible. For the healthcare system, they are essential — reducing readmissions (gl), restoring independence, and reminding everyone that recovery is just as critical as treatment.

The Recovery Regimen reminds us that healthcare isn't only about survival. It's about restoration (gl), resilience (gl), and the dignity (gl) of reclaiming life after loss.

"As the Director of Physical Medicine and Rehabilitation (gl), I had the privilege (gl) of watching my team of physical, occupational, and speech therapists change lives every day. True alignment happens when highly educated professionals not only provide direct treatment, but also work with families and caregivers (gl) to extend care beyond the hospital. By developing comprehensive (gl), multidisciplinary (gl) treatment plans, they helped patients reclaim movement, communication, and independence — all while demonstrating compassion, patience, and devotion (gl). That is alignment in action."

— Catherine Christopher, M.Ed., CCC-SLP (Retired)

SCRUBfits™

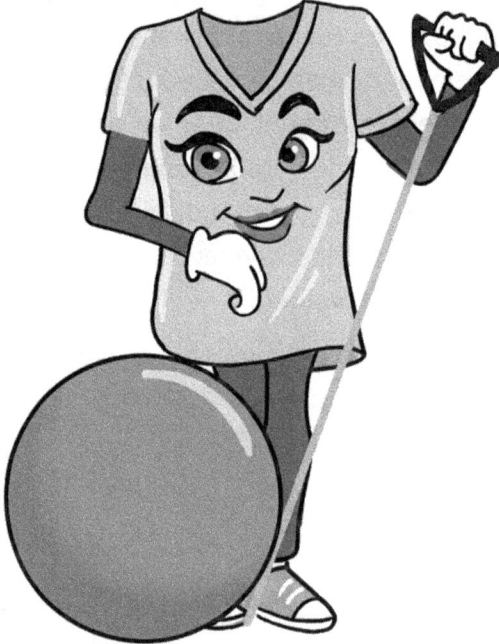

Lilac Lift, DPT

Lilac Lift, DPT — "The Mobility Mentor"

Scrub Color: Lavender

Primary Role: Physical Therapist (gl)

This Role Also Aligns With: Sports Medicine Specialist (gl); Neurological Rehabilitation (gl) PT; Home Health (gl) PT

SCRUB*fit*™ Category: The Recovery Regimen

Pros: Direct, visible impact on recovery; varied career paths; rewarding patient relationships

Cons: Physically demanding; progress can be slow; documentation (gl) heavy

Personality Traits: Energetic; determined; encouraging

Clinical Tools: gait belts (gl); resistance bands; therapy balls (gl); parallel bars (gl); transfer boards (gl)

Clinical Confession: "Nothing beats the sound of a patient taking their first steps again."

Character Description

Lilac Lift is the pulse of the rehab gym — a motivator wrapped in lavender scrubs and purpose. She helps people rediscover motion after loss: stroke (gl) survivors relearning gait (gl), athletes rebuilding confidence, elders reclaiming independence.

Equal parts coach and clinician, Lilac knows progress isn't linear. She reads fatigue in posture and hope in a trembling hand. "Push enough to stretch, never to snap," she tells her interns. Her laughter turns repetition into rhythm; her persistence turns minutes into milestones.

She anchors her day on the belief that recovery is collaboration. When a patient stalls, she re-tools the plan, never the person. She teaches caregivers side by side, turning therapy into teamwork that continues beyond the hospital.

By dusk, the gym quiets. Lilac reviews notes under the soft hum of disinfectant (gl) fans, her shoes flecked with chalk from parallel-bar practice. She looks up at the empty room, hearing echoes of first steps and the quiet chorus of belief returning. That's her favorite sound — progress you can feel.

Day in the Life

5:06 a.m. — When the World Is Still and the Body Remembers

Her alarm is a soft chime — intentional, gentle, nothing that startles a nervous system (gl) already tasked with healing others. Lilac Lift wakes slowly, stretching her arms overhead, feeling the small satisfying click of her own shoulder joint (gl).

It always reminds her:

Every body has a history.

The sky outside is just beginning to glow lavender — her color, her calm, her calling.

Her cat, Spindle, hops onto her stomach with the grace of a bowling ball dressed as a house pet. Lilac laughs, scratches behind Spindle's ears, and whispers, "Ready to help people move again?"

Spindle blinks like: You first.

Lilac rolls out of bed, plants her bare feet on the floor, and breathes in.

Movement is medicine.

Stillness is the first dose.

5:43 a.m. — Coffee, Journaling, and Prehab (gl) for the Therapist

Her morning ritual is simple:

- Hot mug of coffee

- Lavender candle flickering beside her notebook

- A five-minute reflection

Today's line she writes:

"Healing takes time. So does trust."

She repeats it twice. Some days, her patients need both. Some days, she does.

Then she does her own warm-up — cat-cow stretches (gl), a long hamstring (gl) reach, glute activation (gl), thoracic (gl) mobility (gl). She treats her body the way she wishes the world treated itself: with intention.

6:58 a.m. — Entering the Clinic, Entering Her Element

Her clinic smells faintly of eucalyptus (gl), warm foam rollers (gl), and a whiteboard full of half-erased reminders.

The lights flicker on. The treatment tables look like calm islands before the day's waves.

Her equipment — her instruments of restoration — sits ready:

- Therabands (gl) coiled like colorful serpents

- gait belt (gl) draped over a chair

- BOSU ball (gl) waiting to challenge someone's balance

- electrical stim (gl) unit warming up

- ultrasound gel (gl) in its holster like a gunslinger's weapon

Lilac ties her lilac-colored scrub jacket around her waist.

Her world is about to move.

7:15 a.m. — Patient #1: The Firefighter with the Frozen Shoulder

He arrives early — firefighters always do — stoic, polite, insisting he's "fine."

Lilac lifts an eyebrow.

"Fine?" she repeats, gently pressing on his shoulder.

He flinches.

"Fine-ish," he corrects.

She smiles warmly. "Better."

She begins with gentle mobilizations (gl), watching his breathing, noting the way he tries to hide discomfort. She talks him through each glide, each stretch, each subtle release.

"Pain isn't weakness," she reminds him. "Pain is information."

When he leaves, he raises his arm a few degrees higher than yesterday.

That's victory.

8:04 a.m. — Patient #2: The Elderly Woman Learning to Walk Again

Mrs. Henderson arrives with a walker (gl) decorated with floral stickers — the kind a granddaughter probably applied with pride.

Lilac kneels beside her.

"Ready to dance a little?" she asks.

Mrs. Henderson laughs. "If you promise not to step on my toes."

They practice weight shifting (gl), step initiation (gl), and confidence — the most underrated muscle in geriatrics (gl). Lilac counts softly:

"One... good... two... good... you're stronger than you think..."

Mrs. Henderson stands taller by the end of the session.

And Lilac's heart stretches with gratitude.

9:26 a.m. — Documentation... The Necessary Evil

Lilac sits at her computer with a sigh, her fingers tapping like she's performing a reluctant concerto (gl).

SOAP notes (gl) are her villain. Movement is her hero.

The clinic printer jams aggressively like it has personal issues.

Lilac whispers to it, "I'm doing my best too, buddy."

The printer does not respond.

10:03 a.m. — Patient #3: The Teen Athlete with an ACL Reconstruction (gl)

He arrives with swagger, headphones, and a confidence level not appropriate for someone wearing a knee brace (gl).

Lilac grins.

"Okay superstar," she teases. "Let's see how your quad (gl) is firing."

He tries a straight leg raise (gl) and shakes like he's bench pressing a refrigerator.

She doesn't laugh. She doesn't shame. She simply says:

"This is day one. Not day done."

They work through neuromuscular reeducation (gl), balance training (gl), scar mobility (gl), and then the first real conversation he's had about fear.

"What if I don't get back to where I was?"

Lilac crouches to eye level.

"You won't," she says kindly. "You'll get better. Different. Strong. Smart. That's the real comeback."

His eyes soften.

That's the session's breakthrough — not the exercise. The belief.

11:42 a.m. — Lilac's Lunch (AKA Patient #3's Leftover Protein Bar)

She eats a protein bar while leaning against a treatment table. Her stomach growls. She glances at the clock.

Fourteen minutes until the next patient.

She calls that "a feast."

12:10 p.m. — Patient #4: The Office Worker with Back Pain from Sitting on a Couch Too Long During Remote Work

He walks in crooked, grimacing like he aged forty years overnight.

"What happened?" she asks gently.

"I worked from my couch."

She winces in solidarity.

"No judgment," she says. "Just consequences."

They work on lumbar (gl) mobility (gl), core activation (gl), proper ergonomics (gl), and breathing that relaxes his sympathetic nervous system (gl).

When he stands straighter, he whispers, "Oh my God... I feel human."

Lilac fist bumps him.

1:37 p.m. — The Surprise Walk-In: A Post-Op Hip Replacement (gl)

A patient arrives unexpectedly after slipping on a wet bathroom floor.

Lilac doesn't panic. She pivots.

She checks incision (gl) healing, gait pattern (gl), muscle guarding (gl), hip mobility (gl), and pain levels. She coordinates with the surgeon's office and adjusts the protocol (gl).

"You're okay," she reassures. "You're not back at square one. Just taking a scenic detour."

The patient laughs — shaky but relieved.

3:04 p.m. — The Pediatric (gl) Hour

A five-year-old with toe-walking (gl) bounds in with sparkly sneakers and a tutu.

Lilac kneels, smiling. "Let's race to the cones!"

The girl gasps. "I ALWAYS win."

Lilac pretends to be devastated.

They work on gait correction (gl), motor control (gl), balance (gl) — all wrapped in the disguise of play. But the child only remembers:

"I beat Miss Lilac!"

And that's okay. Confidence is therapy too.

4:20 p.m. — Final Patient: The Burned-Out Nurse With Chronic Neck Pain

Lilac knows that slump. She knows that sigh. She knows that face — a fellow clinician carrying more than muscles can hold.

Lilac dims the lights. Gentles her voice. Treats not just the tissue but the tension.

Manual therapy (gl). Trigger point release (gl). Postural reset (gl). Breathing that unlocks trapped emotion (gl).

Halfway through, the nurse whispers, "I didn't realize how much I needed this."

Lilac squeezes her hand.

"Caregivers need care too."

5:57 p.m. — Closing the Clinic, Opening the Heart

Lilac wipes down the last table, turns off the machines, and lets the silence wash over her.

Today she:

- Helped a firefighter lift his arm a little higher

- Walked an elderly woman toward independence

- Reassured a teen athlete's shattered confidence

- Untangled a remote worker's spine

- Adapted for a hip replacement setback

- Played tag with a tiny tutu warrior

- Gave a nurse a moment of rest

She did not change the world.

But she changed seven worlds.

And that's enough.

6:20 p.m. — Sunset, Stretching, Stillness

At home, she stretches on her living room floor while Spindle judges her form.

She breathes deeply.

Movement restored. Strength renewed. Stories honored.

Lilac Lift doesn't heal for the applause.

She heals because she believes movement is hope — and she wants every person she touches to feel it.

SCRUBfits™

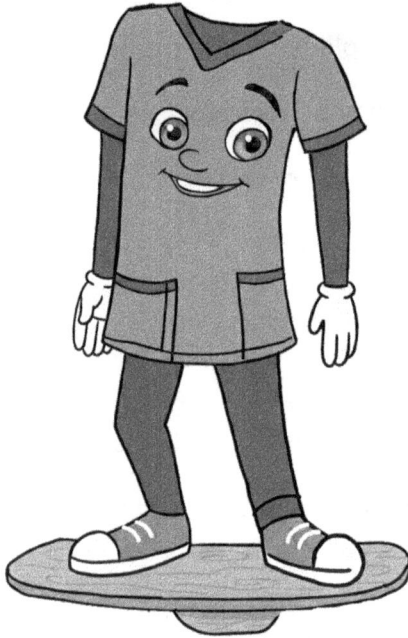

Liv Well, OTR/L

Liv Well, OTR/L — "The Restoration Specialist"

Scrub Color: Seafoam Green

Primary Role: Occupational Therapist (gl)

This Role Also Aligns With: Hand Therapist (gl); Rehabilitation (gl) Manager; Adaptive Equipment (gl) Designer

SCRUB*fit*™ Category: The Recovery Regimen

Pros: Creative problem-solving; deep patient relationships; visible functional outcomes (gl)

Cons: Progress plateaus (gl); emotional investment; complex discharge planning (gl)

Personality Traits: Inventive; compassionate; patient; resourceful

Clinical Tools: adaptive utensils (gl); splints (gl); putty (gl); fine-motor kits (gl); grab bars (gl)

Clinical Confession: "I fall in love with solutions nobody else sees."

Character Description

Liv Well brings artistry to rehabilitation. Her seafoam scrubs mirror the calm she cultivates in patients relearning the motions of daily life — buttoning shirts, writing notes, pouring coffee with trembling precision.

Her therapy station feels like a creative studio: colored putty (gl), adaptive silverware, and mock kitchens where success tastes like buttered toast. Independence, she says, is dignity in motion.

Liv's genius is adaptation. When tools fail, she invents new ones — a 3D-printed toothbrush grip (gl), a joystick for a paraplegic (gl) gamer, a color-coded med box for early dementia (gl). Innovation, born of empathy.

She's patient to the core. Where others see plateau, Liv sees preparation for the next leap. She celebrates tiny victories — a button fastened, a spoon lifted — as if they were miracles.

Evening finds her wiping splints and humming low. Above her desk, a card reads: "Because of you, I can cook breakfast again." She straightens it each night, a ritual of purpose.

A Day in the Life

5:18 a.m. — The Morning That Grounds Her

Liv Well wakes gently, not abruptly — her alarm is the soft sound of ocean waves. Deliberate choice. The nervous system (gl) can't help others regulate (gl) if her own starts in panic.

She stretches her fingers first — a ritual she teaches her patients. Then her wrists, then her shoulders, then the deep rib-space where breath gets stuck when life gets heavy.

At the foot of her bed, her terrier mix (gl), Button, yawns with a squeak and thumps her tail against the comforter.

Liv smiles. "Ready to go change some lives, Button?"

Button responds with a sneeze of enthusiasm.

Liv pads to the kitchen, makes warm lemon water, and writes in her five-minute OT reflection journal:

"Every task matters, because every task is someone's independence."

6:47 a.m. — The Clinic Before the World Arrives

She flips on the lights to her outpatient neuro-rehab (gl) clinic. The room wakes slowly: therapy putty (gl) on a tray, tactile (gl) bins arranged by texture, weighted utensils (gl) in a basket, reachers (gl) and sock-aids (gl) hanging like friendly tools on the wall, and a sensory integration (gl) swing swaying slightly in the corner.

She sets up her first treatment space: mat table (gl), grip-strength dynamometer (gl), visual scanning cards (gl), and functional tasks — zippers, buttons, pill organizers (gl), a practice stovetop dial.

This is not a gym.

This is a laboratory for rebuilding lives.

7:15 a.m. — Patient #1: The Stroke Survivor (gl) Learning to Use His Right Hand Again

Mr. Crane walks in with cautious steps, cane tapping rhythmically.

"Morning, Mr. C.," Liv says warmly. "Ready to show that hand who's boss today?"

He smiles shyly.

She kneels beside him, guiding finger flexion (gl), gentle wrist extension (gl), assisted reaching (gl). She watches his face more than his hand — OT is emotion as much as mechanics.

He grimaces at first. Then... a breakthrough. One knuckle bends smoothly.

Liv gasps. "You did that."

He looks at his hand like it just told him a secret.

This — right here — is why she loves her job.

8:09 a.m. — Patient #2: The Child With Sensory Processing (gl) Challenges

A little girl in glitter sneakers barrels into the room and dives onto the crash pad (gl) like she was launched from a cannon.

Her mom apologizes. Liv waves it off.

"Big energy is welcome here."

Liv guides her through sensory brushing (gl), deep pressure (gl) input, vestibular (gl) swing work, and fine motor (gl) puzzles — all wrapped in the disguise of play.

The girl giggles for the first time that week.

Mom wipes tears. Liv offers a tissue with a soft smile.

Sometimes OT isn't only about the child.

It's about healing the caregiver too.

9:38 a.m. — Documentation That Tries to Win, but Doesn't

Liv taps away at her SOAP notes (gl). She writes intentionally: improved functional reach (gl), increased grasp by ten percent, emotional regulation improved with deep pressure intervention (gl).

OT notes aren't boxes. They're stories wrapped in metrics (gl).

She sips lukewarm coffee and mutters, "You deserve better than this, darling."

She's talking to the coffee. But also... herself.

10:02 a.m. — Patient #3: The Car Accident Survivor Working on ADLs (gl)

A young man arrives, shoulders hunched, moving slowly, pain shadowing every expression.

They work at the ADL station (gl), practicing:

- tying shoes

- using a reacher

- carrying weight through the left arm

- getting in and out of a mock car

- brushing teeth with proper posture

He whispers, "I didn't think brushing my teeth would feel like climbing Everest."

Liv nods gently. "Everest is climbed one inch at a time."

His courage flickers back on.

11:34 a.m. — Patient #4: The Post-Op Hand Therapy Session

Sutures (gl) out. Scar tight. Movement guarded.

Liv warms the hand with paraffin (gl) wax, performs gentle scar mobilization (gl), then hands him a container of therapy putty (gl).

"Make spaghetti," she instructs.

He rolls the putty.

"Tighten the dough."

He squeezes.

"Now pinch the noodles."

He laughs. "It's working. And I'm hungry."

Liv grins. "Therapy goals: gain strength... and an appetite."

12:26 p.m. — Lunch That Is Mostly Not Lunch

She opens her salad. She stares at her salad. She closes her salad.

She answers two portal messages, updates two plans of care (gl), and writes three justifications (gl) for adaptive equipment (gl).

She takes one bite. Victory.

1:14 p.m. — Home Evaluation Visit (gl)

She drives to a patient's home — a retired teacher recovering from hip surgery.

Liv assesses:

• rug hazards (gl)

• bathroom layout

• grab bar needs

• bed height

• kitchen accessibility (gl)

• lighting for nighttime mobility (gl)

She walks through the home with the teacher's daughter.

"This is where your mom fell," the daughter whispers.

Liv kneels, touches the baseboard, and says softly, "We won't let that happen again."

She adjusts furniture, demonstrates safe transfers (gl), and recommends a shower chair (gl) and long-handled sponge (gl).

When she leaves, the daughter hugs her.

"You just gave me back my mom," she whispers.

Liv cries in her car — just for a moment.

2:50 p.m. — Pediatric Hour, Part II

A little boy with autism spectrum disorder (gl) tiptoes in, avoiding eye contact.

Liv meets him exactly where he is — sitting on the floor, quietly building blocks. Eventually, he joins.

They work on:

• bilateral coordination (gl)

• joint attention (gl)

• sensory exploration (gl)

• sequencing (gl) tasks

• emotional labeling (gl)

He places a block on top of hers.

Connection made.

OT magic.

4:07 p.m. — Final Patient: The Executive With Burnout

She arrives in dress slacks, perfect makeup, trembling hands.

"I can't keep up," she confesses.

Liv doesn't start with exercises. She starts with breathing.

Then:

• ergonomics (gl)

• joint protection (gl) strategies

• handwriting fatigue solutions

• mindfulness (gl) tools

• stress-reduction sensory inputs (gl)

Halfway through, the executive whispers, "I didn't know I was allowed to take care of myself."

Liv replies gently, "You're required."

5:55 p.m. — Closing the Clinic, Opening the Heart

She wipes down equipment, stacks sensory bins, logs her final notes. The lights hum softly.

Today she helped:

• A stroke survivor move his hand

• A child regulate her sensory world

• A young man rebuild daily life

• A teacher walk safely in her own home

• A child communicate through play

• A burned-out woman find her breath again

Lilac Lift restores movement.

Liv Well restores meaning.

Different magic. Equal power.

6:23 p.m. — Sunset Unwind

Back home, Liv sits on her porch while Button curls at her feet. The sky melts into shades of lilac, gold, and warm gray.

She exhales deeply.

Occupational therapy isn't only about muscles or joints.

It's about function. Identity. Choice. Independence. Dignity.

And Liv Well is a guardian of all five.

The Recovery Regimen — Resilience in Motion

The Recovery Regimen proves that healing doesn't end at discharge (gl). From physical and occupational therapists to dietitians (gl) and speech-language pathologists (gl), this category forms the bridge between illness and independence. Progress is measured in inches, but every inch reclaimed restores dignity.

Healing doesn't stop when strength returns — it transforms. And as recovery hands the baton forward, a new team steps in: the ones who keep every system alive and every signal flowing. While the Recovery Regimen restores the body, the next **SCRUB*fit*™** category powers the infrastructure that makes modern care possible.

Chapter 25
SCRUBfit Squad:
The Prevention Pact

Keep people well, upstream.

The best outcome is the one that never requires a hospital stay. The Prevention Pact is home to the clinicians and community builders who stop problems from becoming crises — the educators, epidemiology (gl) scouts, wellness coordinators, and oral-health (gl) guardians who shift care upstream.

They work where health actually happens: neighborhoods, schools, barbershops (gl), churches, job sites, and family kitchens. They turn data into action, barriers into bridges, and small daily choices into long-term wins. For patients and communities, they are the steady voice saying, "You can start here." For the healthcare system, they are the force that reduces risk, costs, and suffering before the first admission band is ever printed.

The Prevention Pact reminds us that prevention isn't passive — it's proactive care, policy (gl), and partnership (gl) in motion.

SCRUBfits™

Sage Engage, MPH

Sage Engage, MPH — "The Health Harbinger"

Scrub Color: Sage Green

Primary Role: Public Health Educator

Also Aligns With: Community Health Specialist (MPH, CHES) (gl); Population Health Manager (MPH, CPH) (gl); Health Promotion Coordinator (MPH) (gl); Epidemiology (gl) Field Officer (MPH, CSTE) (gl); Wellness Program Director (MPH, CHWC) (gl)

SCRUB*fit*™ Category: The Prevention Pact

Pros: High community impact; preventive-care (gl) focus; policy (gl) influence; cross-sector (gl) collaboration (gl); measurable outcomes

Cons: Patience needed for long-term results; limited direct patient care; funding challenges; political barriers; heavy data-analysis (gl) load

Personality Traits: Persuasive; resourceful; empathetic; strategic; culturally aware

Clinical Tools: Clipboards with survey data; mobile health van (gl) keys; health-fair banner; reusable water bottle covered in advocacy (gl) stickers; stack of bilingual (gl) brochures

Clinical Confession: "Prevention is the quiet revolution that saves more lives than any ER."

Character Description

Sage Engage is the steady current behind community health change. In sage-green scrubs and worn-in sneakers, he moves from school gyms to senior centers, meeting people where they already are. He's fluent in the language of trust — explaining screenings (gl) to hesitant parents in the morning and persuading city leaders to back a clean-water ordinance (gl) before sunset.

He doesn't measure success in applause, but in fewer emergency calls, more vaccinations (gl), and trends that bend toward well-being year after year. His work is part detective, part educator, part advocate (gl) — always focused on removing barriers before they become crises. Sage knows prevention can feel invisible, but it's the foundation of every healthy community.

Day in the Life

4:58 a.m. — When the World Is Quiet Enough to Hear Data Whisper

Sage Engage wakes before sunrise — not out of discipline, but because dawn is when patterns make the most sense.

He pushes open his curtains. The sky is a soft indigo (gl), just beginning to blush toward morning. His kettle clicks on automatically, filling the kitchen with the scent of chai.

His dog, Marble, a speckled Border Collie who believes public health is a sport, trots in with a hopeful tail wag.

"Morning, epidemiology (gl) assistant," Sage teases.

Marble sneezes, which Sage interprets as agreement.

He pours his tea, opens his tablet, and gazes at what he calls his sunrise ritual:

- Overnight COVID trend line (gl)

- Childhood vaccination (gl) rates

- Heat illness reports (gl)

- Emergency department utilization (gl)

- Local shelter capacity (gl)

This is his version of morning prayer — a communion (gl) with the population (gl) he serves.

He whispers his daily mantra:

"Protect the many. Teach the one. Listen for the pattern."

6:12 a.m. — Into the Field Office, Into the Fray

The Public Health Department building is waking up — copier warming, water cooler gurgling, fluorescent lights flickering reluctantly into consciousness.

Sage unlocks his office, a space filled with:

- Color-coded outbreak maps (gl)

- A towering stack of community health assessments (gl)

- A whiteboard scribbled with partnerships (gl), prevention goals, and half-erased equations

- Sticky notes that say things like "Equity (gl) or Nothing" and "Meet them where they are."

He pulls on his sage-green **SCRUB*fit*™** Prevention Pact jacket, adjusts his ID badge, and breathes in.

This is where medicine meets humanity.

6:48 a.m. — Community Health Briefing (gl)

His team gathers — epidemiologists (gl), health educators, outreach nurses, environmental health staff (gl), and one over-caffeinated intern.

Sage leads with calm command.

"Team, our asthma (gl) rates in the Riverside neighborhood just spiked. Could be seasonal... or environmental exposure (gl). We need eyes on it."

He circles an area on the map.

Then: "And let's finalize our heat safety campaign (gl). Daycares and senior centers first."

Finally, he smiles warmly.

"And someone please make sure the intern eats a breakfast burrito. I can feel his mitochondria (gl) crying."

The room laughs. The intern blushes.

Sage's superpower: delivering urgency without panic, delivering hope without denial.

7:32 a.m. — Home Visit (gl): A Mother, A Mold Problem, A New Plan

He drives to a home flagged by the case manager — two kids with asthma (gl), frequent ER visits (gl), suspected environmental triggers.

When the mother opens the door, she looks exhausted.

Sage softens his posture. "We're here to support, not judge."

He inspects the home:

• Mold around the bathroom vent

• Dust-heavy carpet

• Poor airflow in the kids' room

• Old humidifier (gl) with mineral buildup

He explains everything in kind, accessible language.

"We can fix this together. Small steps will make big changes."

He arranges:

- A free HEPA filter (gl)

- A landlord safety inspection (gl)

- An asthma action plan (gl)

- A follow-up from a community health worker (gl)

When he leaves, the mother's eyes shine with relief.

"You listened," she says quietly.

Sage touches her arm. "That's part of the treatment."

9:10 a.m. — School Coalition Meeting (gl)

Topic: Rising Teen Mental Health Concerns (gl)

The school's conference room smells like dry-erase markers and overstressed educators.

Sage guides the room with the patience of someone who has seen systems fail but still believes they can succeed.

"We're not just fighting statistics," he says. "We're fighting silence."

He coordinates:

- A peer counseling program (gl)

- Teacher mental health training (gl)

- Crisis hotline (gl) posters

• A trauma-informed (gl) classroom series

He advocates gently but fiercely.

One teacher whispers afterward, "We needed you."

Sage replies, "You needed resources. I'm just the delivery system."

10:58 a.m. — Outbreak Alert (gl): GI Illness Cluster at a Local Retirement Home

His phone buzzes with a message from the epidemiology (gl) team: "We're seeing a pattern."

Sage's pulse quickens — not fear, but readiness.

He heads immediately to the retirement home, Marble riding shotgun like an unofficial therapy dog (gl) who takes public health very seriously.

Inside, he meets with nursing staff, checks sanitation (gl) logs, reviews symptoms (gl), inspects food temperatures, and maps onset timelines.

His mind assembles the sequence like dominoes:

Day 1: nausea (gl)

Day 2: vomiting (gl)

Day 3: additional cases

Likely culprit: Norovirus (gl).

He implements:

• Isolation precautions (gl)

• Enhanced sanitation (gl) protocol (gl)

- Staff education

- A meal-handling audit (gl)

- Visitor restrictions (gl)

- Hydration (gl) strategy for residents

The nursing director squeezes his hand. "You came so fast."

Sage smiles. "Disease doesn't wait. Neither do we."

12:46 p.m. — Lunch: A Protein Bar and 42 Emails

He sits in his car under the shade of a tree. Marble rests her head in his lap.

He chews his protein bar and whispers, "Self-care (gl) is fuel, not fluff."

His inbox is a battlefield:

- Grant deadline reminders (gl)

- Heat index (gl) alerts

- Housing department replies

- Community event invitations

- A teenager asking for help launching an anti-vaping (gl) club

He replies to each one with warmth and clarity.

1:24 p.m. — Policy Meeting: The Invisible Side of Public Health

He enters a boardroom full of suits, spreadsheets, and budget anxieties.

Sage presents with calm conviction.

"Every dollar invested in prevention saves six in emergency care. Public health is not an expense. It's an insurance policy for the entire community."

Silence. Then slow nods.

Another small war won.

2:57 p.m. — Street Outreach (gl): Homelessness (gl) and Heat Risk

He joins the outreach team as they check on unhoused (gl) residents:

• Distribute water

• Offer cooling station maps (gl)

• Provide sunscreen (gl) and electrolyte (gl) packets

• Ask about medical needs

• Connect them with shelters

A man sitting under a bridge says, "No one ever asks if I'm okay."

Sage crouches to eye level. "I'm asking now."

The man smiles, toothless but sincere.

Human dignity (gl) is a public health intervention (gl).

4:36 p.m. — Back to the Department: Debrief (gl) and Data

He logs everything:

• Home visit improvements

• School coalition outcomes

- Outbreak containment (gl) progress

- Outreach encounters

- Heat-related vulnerabilities (gl)

He updates trend dashboards (gl) and high-risk population (gl) flags (gl).

The data sings to him — stories wrapped in numbers.

5:52 p.m. — Team Wind-Down

He thanks his team — individually, personally.

"Good work today." "Your instincts were right." "I appreciate your compassion." "Your analysis was sharp."

Public health is teamwork. Egos get in the way. Sage cuts around them like water.

6:31 p.m. — Sunset Drive Home

Marble rests her head on his thigh. The sky glows burnt orange against the silhouette (gl) of water towers.

Sage exhales. His day was long, messy, complex, heavy.

But his community is safer now than it was this morning.

That's the work — the sacred, invisible work.

7:14 p.m. — Evening Ritual: Release, Restore, Remember

He lights a lavender candle. Sits on his porch. Pets Marble's soft fur.

He whispers his closing mantra:

"Tomorrow, we protect again."

Public health isn't glamorous. It isn't loud. It isn't applauded.

It's the quiet, relentless defense of a community's future.

And Sage Engage stands at its front line — the watchtower, the compass, the heart.

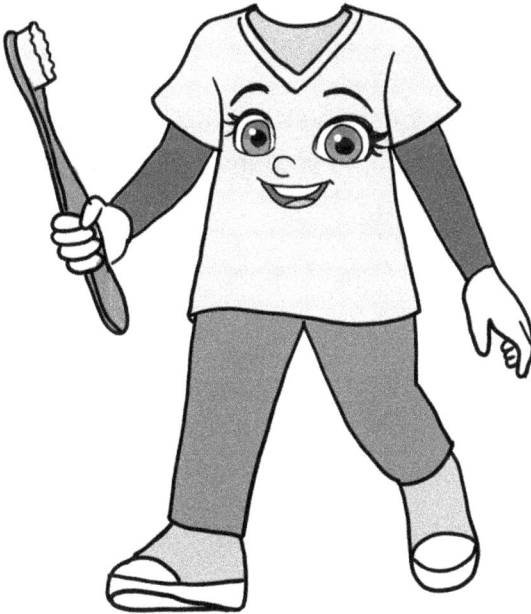

SCRUBfits™

Minty Mary, RDH

Minty Mary, RDH — "The Smile Saver"

Scrub Color: Mint Green

Primary Role: Dental Hygienist

Also Aligns With: Oral Health Educator (RDH, MPH) (gl); Pediatric Dental Hygienist (RDH, CPDHP) (gl); Community Dental Health Coordinator (RDH, CDHC) (gl); Dental Public Health Specialist (RDH, MPH) (gl); Preventive Dentistry (gl) Advocate (RDH) (gl)

SCRUB*fit***™** Category: The Prevention Pact

Pros: High patient interaction; direct prevention impact; strong job stability; flexible scheduling; hands-on skills

Cons: Repetitive tasks; posture strain; anxious patients; limited autonomy (gl) in some settings; insurance constraints (gl)

Personality Traits: Gentle; encouraging; detail-focused; approachable; consistent

Clinical Tools: Polishing tools; patient-education (gl) flipbook; floss samples in every pocket; peppermint lip balm; travel-size water flosser

Clinical Confession: "A healthy smile is a gateway to a healthy life — and I'm here to protect both."

Character Description

Minty Mary greets each patient with a reassuring grin and a subtle peppermint trail — her personal brand of calm. In mint-green scrubs, she turns anxious frowns into relaxed shoulders, blending technical precision with a soft, steady presence.

She's more than a clinician; she's an oral-health storyteller, weaving lessons about gum care, cavity defense, and the sugar traps hidden in daily habits. Her chairside skills are matched by her leadership — having grown practices, mentored new hygienists, and expanded prevention into underserved neighborhoods. To Mary, every smile is a preventive victory with ripple effects across a lifetime.

Day in the Life

5:11 a.m. — Mint Before Morning

Minty Mary wakes before her alarm — she always does. She says it's because morning is quieter before the world starts drinking coffee and chewing on granola bars that will become her problem later.

She sits up, stretches her jaw dramatically (a habit she picked up from Liv Well, OTR/L), and shuffles into the kitchen where her diffuser is already misting peppermint oil.

Her cat, Flossy, rubs against her leg with the grace of a marshmallow that has recently discovered affection.

"Good morning, cavity fighter," she whispers. It's unclear whether she means Flossy... or herself.

She makes green tea and writes a tiny affirmation (gl) on her sticky note pad:

"Gentle hands.

Kind words.

Fear melts when trust grows."

She tucks the sticky note into her scrub pocket like armor.

Today she will battle plaque (gl), fear, and tartar (gl).

Today she will win.

6:42 a.m. — Entering the Mint Zone

Her dental office hums awake with the soft buzz of overhead lights and the citrusy disinfectant (gl) wipe scent all hygienists know well.

She turns on her operatory (gl) light, lays out her tools with ritualistic calm:

• Cavitron ultrasonic scaler (gl)

• Mirror and explorer (gl)

• High-speed suction (gl)

• Fluoride varnish (gl)

• X-ray sensor (gl)

• Mint paste in three flavors: gentle mint, intense mint, and "I chew gum to feel alive" mint

She adjusts her lilac-and-mint mask, smooths her scrubs, and whispers to the room:

"Let's save some smiles."

7:02 a.m. — Patient #1: The Nervous Adult Who Hasn't Been in Six Years

He sits in the chair like he's bracing for turbulence (gl).

Minty Mary's voice softens to warm honey.

"You're safe. And you're here. That's what matters."

She walks him through every step:

- Bitewings (gl)

- Checking gum pockets (gl) with a periodontal (gl) probe (gl)

- Gentle ultrasonic scaling (gl)

- Hand scaling (gl) for sensitive areas

- Peppermint polish

He grips the armrest. She notices immediately.

"Deep breath in through your nose," she coaches. "Out through your mouth. I promise — I'm on your team."

By the end of the appointment, his shoulders have dropped an inch.

When he stands up, he smiles — really smiles — and she sees the spark of confidence reigniting.

"That wasn't so bad," he admits.

She winks. "That's the Minty Mary effect."

8:18 a.m. — Patient #2: The Eight-Year-Old with Rocket-Level Energy

He bursts into the room wearing dinosaur sneakers.

Minty Mary beams. "Ready to be a tooth explorer today?"

"YES!" he shouts.

She hands him sunglasses (blue, his choice) and lets him control the chair for a moment — the sacred pediatric ritual that grants trust.

She sings a silly brushing song while scaling, checks his erupting molars (gl), and shows him his plaque levels with disclosing solution (gl).

"It's not bad," she assures. "But your T-Rex teeth in the back need backup."

He salutes her with a superhero pose. Minty Mary fist bumps him.

She sends him out with a sticker, a tiny floss container, and the proudest grin a kid can have.

9:06 a.m. — X-Ray Sprint

The schedule compresses and suddenly she has two X-rays, one sealant prep (gl), and a chart review due — all in the same hour.

She slips into her focused mode:

- "Bite gently. Perfect."

- "Hold still — beautiful."

- "Sealant curing... and done."

She moves like choreography — precise, confident, soft-footed.

Her dentist mutters as he passes, "How do you stay so calm?"

She shrugs lightly. "Well... screaming doesn't sterilize instruments."

10:22 a.m. — Patient #3: The Teen With Braces (gl) and Attitude (gl)

He slumps in the chair, headphone in one ear, hoodie half up.

She smiles, unbothered.

"Scale of one to ten, how annoyed are you to be here?"

"...fifteen," he mumbles.

"Great. Then you'll love me in about twenty minutes."

She shows him how brackets are plaque magnets, demonstrates technique with a proxabrush (gl), and casually mentions that clean teeth make braces come off faster.

His eyes snap open. "Wait — seriously?!"

Minty Mary grins. Hook, line, sinker.

By the end he says, "Thanks... I guess."

That's teenager for: I trust you.

11:58 a.m. — Lunch: A Granola Bar and Charting Sprint

She sits in her operatory (gl), chewing quietly while typing notes:

• "Bleeding points: improving."

• "Patient tolerated scaling well."

• "Oral hygiene motivation excellent." (For some patients, "motivation present in spirit.")

She gets exactly six minutes. She uses five of them to chart and one to breathe.

12:47 p.m. — Patient #4: The Elderly Woman With a Soft Voice and Softer Bones

Mrs. Dawson speaks barely above a whisper. Minty Mary kneels beside her chair, eye level.

"We'll go slow," she promises.

She supports her neck gently, adjusts the chair angle to avoid vertigo (gl), and uses the softest polishing prophy cup (gl).

She learns about her garden, her grandson's graduation, and how her late husband used to bring her daisies.

By the time she finishes, Mrs. Dawson rests a hand on Mary's.

"You're very kind," she says quietly.

Minty Mary squeezes it. "You're very brave."

2:18 p.m. — Emergency Walk-In: The Cracked Filling Mystery

A woman rushes in, holding her cheek. "My tooth feels wrong!"

Minty Mary guides her into the chair.

She performs quick radiographs (gl), assesses the filling, checks for fracture lines, and uses cold testing (gl) to determine sensitivity.

"It's cracked," she confirms softly. "I'll get the dentist."

She stays with her until the dentist arrives — hand on her shoulder, anchoring (gl) her through fear.

Some days she cleans. Some days she comforts.

Both matter.

3:42 p.m. — Patient #5: The Man Who Calls Himself "Your Worst Nightmare"

He jokes his way through everything. She laughs at half of it and kindly steers him back into stillness for the other half.

When she finishes, he sits up and says, "Minty Mary... you're a magician."

She bows dramatically. "All in a day's plaque!"

He groans. She cackles.

4:57 p.m. — Closing Time, Deep Breath

She sterilizes instruments (gl), wipes down chairs, restocks her fluoride tray, and turns off her operatory (gl) light.

She stands in the doorway for a moment, taking in the quiet.

Today she:

• Eased dental fear

• Helped a kid feel brave

• Motivated a teen

• Comforted an elder

• Solved a cracked filling mystery

• Brought confidence back to a dozen smiles

Minty Mary doesn't just clean teeth.

She restores courage.

She builds trust.

She gives people back the confidence to smile without thinking twice.

5:33 p.m. — Sunset and Self-Care (gl)

She drives home with Floss waiting in the window, the peppermint aroma still lingering on her scrubs.

She lights another candle, stretches her neck, and breathes deeply.

Tomorrow, she'll save more smiles.

Tonight, she rests hers.

The Prevention Pact — Upstream Alignment

The Prevention Pact proves that the best care is the care you never need. Public-health educators, epidemiologists (gl), hygienists, wellness coordinators — they are the architects of healthier tomorrows.

For readers, the Pact opens pathways where advocacy (gl), education, and proactive care protect communities — and safeguard futures.

Chapter 26
SCRUBfit Squad: The Leadership League

Design the conditions where others thrive.

Leadership in healthcare isn't about stepping away from the bedside — it's about widening the circle of care. The Leadership League represents clinicians who have transformed skill into stewardship (gl), seeing leadership not as a title, but as a daily act of alignment.

These are the nurse managers, medical directors (gl), educators, and executives who build bridges between policy (gl) and practice — ensuring every decision still echoes the heartbeat of the bedside.

Members of the Leadership League create systems where people flourish — not through command, but through connection. They mentor emerging talent, stabilize teams, and bring calm to chaos. They understand that retention (gl), culture (gl), and safety rise or fall with the tone they set. To them, metrics (gl) aren't just numbers on a dashboard; they're stories of human care, clarity, and trust.

True leadership is less about power and more about presence. The Leadership League turns burnout into purpose by modeling alignment from the top down. When they lead well, patients heal faster, teams stay longer, and the entire organization breathes easier — because every person feels seen, supported, and inspired to give their best.

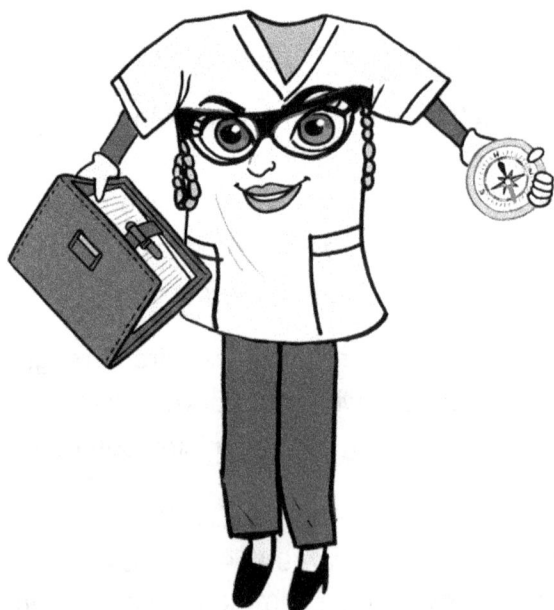

SCRUBfits™

Vera Vines,
MSN, MBA, MHA, FACHE

Vera Vines, FACHE, MBA, MHA, MSN — "The Steward of Alignment"

Scrub Color: Etoma Lavender Mist

Primary Role: Chief Executive Officer (CEO) (gl)

Also Aligns With: Chief Operating Officer (COO) (gl); Chief Nursing Executive (CNE) (gl); Chief Strategy Officer (CSO) (gl); Executive Director (gl); System President (gl)

Pros: Broad system-wide impact; visible influence; ability to shape culture and strategy

Cons: High-stakes decisions; emotional burden of accountability; limited personal downtime

Personality Traits: Visionary; composed; empathetic; strategic; grounded

Clinical Tools: Leadership dashboards; cultural playbooks (gl); strategic plans; handwritten recognition notes

Clinical Confession: "True growth is measured in people, not projects."

Character Description

Vera Vines brings a steady strength of service and experience into the halls of leadership. In her white scrubs with Etoma Lavender Mist accents, she stands as a symbol of renewal and growth — traits carried from her years as a nurse leader into her current leadership role.

Her passion lies in guiding her team. Vera believes leadership is about cultivating potential — building programs that outlast a single encounter. She thrives on watching new grads grow into confident clinicians and, eventually, leaders themselves.

Vera Vines spent years as a nurse leader and Chief Nursing Officer (CNO) (gl) before stepping into the CEO role, and she refuses to let that history fade. Though administration means less direct patient care, she never loses her grounding in practice; she still joins bedside rounds and unit huddles (gl) to stay connected, reminding herself — and her teams — that leadership is rooted in service. A scrub top remains part of her daily wardrobe, ready for her to jump in and assist when needed, while a navy blue suit jacket hangs on the back of her office door — a quiet reminder of the title she carries and the board meetings (gl) that come with it.

As CEO, Vera embodies alignment in action: she's found a way to stay true to her clinical calling while expanding her influence to shape entire systems of care. For her, leadership isn't stepping away from the bedside — it's stepping up so she can lift everyone she serves.

Day in the Life — Vera Vines, FACHE, MBA, MHA, MSN

Chief Executive Officer, Hopewell Hospital for Tomorrow

SCRUB*fit*™ Category: The Leadership League

Shift Type: Day Shift — 07:00–20:00 (gl)

07:00 — Command Bridge Calibration

Vera arrives early, coffee in hand, white scrubs with lavender mist trim beneath her blazer. From the Command Bridge (gl), she surveys live dashboards (gl): overnight trauma alerts, NICU (gl) census (gl), system readiness. Outside the glass wall, a helicopter skims into the dawn — another critical patient for Hopewell's Level I Trauma Center (gl) and Level IV NICU (gl), the highest neonatal care (gl) level in the region.

"Data is how we listen when people aren't in the room."

07:05 — The Call

Her executive assistant, Becky, calls with tension in her voice.

"Vera... The Joint Commission (gl) just walked into WellNow Hospital."

WellNow Hospital is the for-profit hospital down the road owned by CCA, Clinical Corporation of America. Always collegial, they are just as often in court against each other. Their state is a COPN (gl) — Certificate of Public Need (gl) — state, which means every time a hospital wants to expand, it has to go through a state review process to prove the community actually needs those beds, that new imaging suite (gl), or that shiny surgical robot (gl). No one can just throw up a new wing because the board is feeling ambitious; they have to submit thick applications, sit through public hearings (gl), justify the cost, and sometimes battle competitors who argue, "We already provide that service." CCA always meets them in court with every expansion attempt.

Not a surprise — unannounced surveys (gl) have been the norm since 2006. Every three years, managers brace, closets are scrubbed, and someone whispers, "Mr. Joint is in the building." The rituals begin.

08:15 — Budget and Vision Review

In a glass-walled room overlooking the entrance, the capital plan comes into view: helipad upgrades, expanded Bundle Room (gl) suites, NICU ventilator bays (gl).

Vera keeps asking:

"What's the return on reassurance?"

She anchors every budget line to Hopewell's core value: trust.

09:30 — Rounding for Outcomes

Vera walks the Trauma Center. A nurse kneels beside an elderly spouse, explaining every monitor with calm clarity. Vera writes a note to thank her.

Hopewell's tradition: every leader sends handwritten notes to team members' homes — stamped, mailed, never handed off.

It tells families: your person's work matters.

10:45 — Interview for Chief of Neonatology (gl)

Her questions probe integrity and alignment:

• "Tell me about an ethical dilemma (gl) in the NICU."

• "How do you lead through crisis?"

She listens for signs the candidate protects families as fiercely as ventilator settings.

Hopewell's Level IV NICU uses Mother–Baby Suites (gl) — a model Vera benchmarked after Inova Loudoun. She's looking for a chief who understands family presence is medicine.

11:30 — Orientation, but Everyone's Watching the Doors

Rumors of "Mr. Joint" swirl. Frames are polished. Closets rediscovered. A betting pool forms in the "Compliance Fund" mug.

Vera quietly predicts: early next week. She's almost always right.

12:00 — Leadership Lunch at Discovery Café

Her refrain:

"Thank you for turning data into dignity."

Managers discuss bright spots and barriers. The conversation spans HCAHPS (gl), falls (gl), turnover (gl), culture (gl). Vera keeps tying numbers to human stories — the heartbeat of Hopewell's pursuit of its sixth Magnet® milestone (gl).

13:30 — Magnet® Steering Committee

In the Transparency Atrium, surrounded by dashboards (gl), Vera centers the room:

"Excellence isn't achieved once — it's sustained through alignment."

Leaders review CLABSI (gl), falls (gl), turnover (gl), HCAHPS (gl). Overhead, a helicopter roars — a reminder of outcomes too large to fit on slides.

Hopewell is pursuing its sixth consecutive Magnet® designation — achieved by fewer than 0.4% of U.S. hospitals. (gl)

15:00 — The Bundle Room

Walking the wing with Cindy Leo, Vera watches parents practicing diaper changes and feedings — quiet rehearsals for real life.

"Parents are nervous," Cindy says.

"That's why we built this," Vera replies. "Confidence is part of care."

The Bundle Room is strategy, not décor.

16:30 — Strategic Debrief (gl)

In the Command Bridge (gl), leaders review staffing grids (gl) and surge plans (gl). A soft alert: ED (gl) to yellow status (gl).

Vera lets the tone hang:

"That sound is what these numbers are about."

Every spreadsheet cell is tied to a hallway, a handoff (gl), a human.

17:30 — Kinzie Gallery (gl) Event

She speaks at Sustaining Excellence Through Alignment:

"Hopewell isn't built on architecture or algorithms (gl). It's built on alignment — thousands of quiet decisions to do the right thing when no one's watching."

19:30 — Evening Exit

In the hospital diner, family bundles are boxed for staff and visitors. Outside, a nurse teaches car-seat safety (gl); the new father trembles slightly.

"You're already doing great," the nurse reassures him.

Vera writes the nurse's name for another handwritten note.

Leadership is presence, not spotlight.

20:00 — The Drive Home

Vera reflects as the city lights move past.

The Joint Commission (gl) doesn't shut hospitals down; it reveals who they already are.

Her yellow lab, Duke is waiting. So is tomorrow. So is the next chance to steady the pulse.

The Leadership League — System Alignment

The Leadership League shows that alignment isn't defined by where you work, but by how you lead. From nurse managers and executives to educators and quality directors (gl), these roles magnify impact by shaping systems, mentoring teams, and building environments where others can excel.

The Leadership League illuminates careers where influence extends far beyond the bedside — proving that leadership itself can be a powerful form of healing.

Chapter 27

SCRUBfit Squad:
The Power Panel

Choreography, sterility (gl), and shared timing.

Healthcare runs on energy — not just human energy, but the literal power that keeps technology alive. The Power Panel is made up of professionals who wire, safeguard, and synchronize the machines and systems modern care depends on.

These are the problem-solvers who make sure ventilators (gl) hum, monitors (gl) tell the truth, and IT systems don't blink in the middle of an emergency. They thrive where failure isn't an option and where readiness is measured in uptime (gl).

For patients, their work is unseen but lifesaving. For clinicians, they are the safety net that ensures every beep, scan, and spark is reliable. The Power Panel proves that alignment is about more than people — it's about the machines and systems that empower them

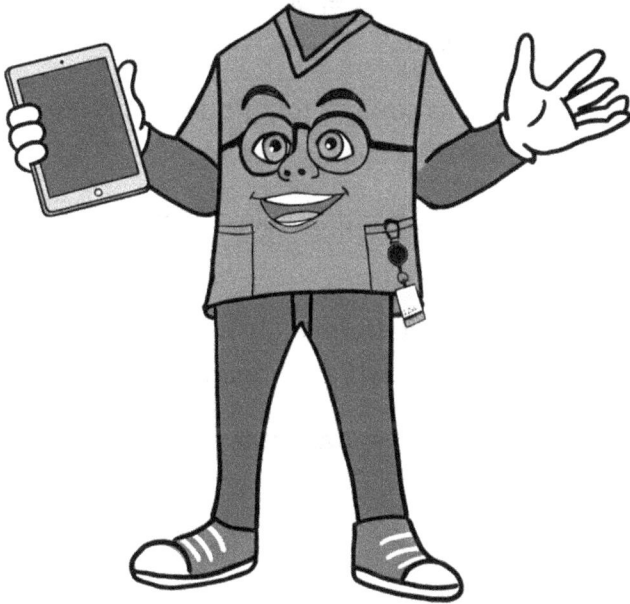

Epic Circuit, MS, CPHIMS

Epic Circuit, MS, CPHIMS — "The Systems Synchronizer"

Scrub Color: Steel Gray

Primary Role: Clinical Informaticist (gl)

Also Aligns With: EHR Optimization Specialist (gl); Clinical Systems Analyst (gl); Health IT Trainer (gl); Data Workflow Engineer (gl)

SCRUB*fit*™ Category: The Power Panel

Pros: Central to tech-driven care; bridge between clinicians and IT; strong growth field

Cons: Long hours during go-lives (gl); troubleshooting pressure; constant learning curve

Personality Traits: Analytical; adaptable; collaborative; systems-minded

Clinical Tools: EHR build platforms (gl); workflow charts (gl); interface-testing tools (gl); data dashboards (gl)

Clinical Confession: "The best system is the one you don't notice — because it works."

Character Description

Epic Circuit is the bridge between IT and ICU (gl) — a translator fluent in both code and clinical language. In Steel Gray scrubs, he embodies the precision of technology balanced with the empathy of care. His focus is making systems serve people — not the other way around.

He comes alive during go-lives and upgrades, when tension runs high and every second counts. Epic is the calm explainer, the midnight troubleshooter, the steady voice in a room full of alerts. Physicians trust him because he listens first, then fixes fast.

His alignment lives in the invisible: the clicks saved, the errors prevented, the workflows that suddenly make sense. He's proof that alignment isn't abstract — it's coded, tested, and taught into the systems that deliver care. And when everything runs flawlessly, no one notices him at all — which is exactly how he likes it.

Day in the Life — Clinical Informaticist (gl)

05:32 — The alarm glows before it sounds. Coffee brews while overnight dashboards load: uptime stable, ticket queue long, one critical medication-alert error flagged at 02:18. Breakfast is yogurt, granola, and the quiet foreboding only an informaticist understands — if the system hiccups, the hospital holds its breath.

06:25 — Commute through gray drizzle. The hospital looms ahead, a constellation of monitors behind every window. In this role, patients aren't seen but still felt — every keystroke in the EHR (gl) traces back to someone's care.

06:52 — Badge tap. The command center hums, walls lined with dashboards (gl). First task: verify the CPOE (gl) module's overnight update. New drug-allergy interaction (gl) logic deployed without a crash — small miracle.

07:30 — Morning huddle with pharmacy, nursing informatics (gl), and IT security (gl). Today's mission: finalize smart-pump integration (gl) for new Alaris smart pumps (gl). The discussion toggles between mL/hr and code syntax. "Safety is measured in seconds," someone says. Everyone nods.

08:46 — Testing in the sandbox (gl). Orders entered, meds verified, flowsheets (gl) checked. A mislabeled dropdown pops: "Heparin flush 1,000 units/mL" displayed as "10,000." Flagged immediately. One label can rewrite an outcome. Correction submitted.

10:02 — Clinical rounds with internal medicine. Tablet in hand, they watch how clinicians actually interact with the system. A resident grumbles, "It's still asking for a second cosign (gl) on PRNs (gl)." "On the fix list before lunch," comes the reply. The alliance between bedside and backend matters.

11:18 — The Epic (gl) dashboard blinks yellow — latency spike (gl). Logs triangulated: an errant interface (gl) between lab and pharmacy servers. A five-minute slowdown avoids a five-hour outage. Relief arrives as silence — everything running, as it should.

12:07 — Lunch at the desk: salad, cooling coffee, a sticky note — "deploy alert-override metrics (gl)." Scripting while eating. Like doses, code must be precise; one extra character and the order chain misfires.

13:15 — Nursing Education pilot: barcode scanning workflow (gl) to reduce med-admin errors (gl). "Will it flag expired meds?" Yes — red box, audible tone, auto-generated log. Guardrails (gl) that talk back.

14:47 — Afternoon downtime drill (gl). Systems drop to outage mode (gl). Paper orders, backup printers, downtime MARs (gl). Power returns; timestamps compared. "Seventeen minutes. Still safe." Collective exhale.

16:02 — Email from Quality: "Analyze alert-fatigue rates (gl)?" Dataset: 72,493 pop-ups in 30 days. A dashboard appears, highlighting which alerts are most bypassed. The goal isn't fewer alerts; it's smarter ones.

17:20 — Final review. The Feedback Flow Board (gl) glows green: alert-logic patch — approved; workflow redesign — approved; downtime test — completed. Laptop closes. Exhale.

18:10 — Drive home through dusk. The radio hums under the satisfaction of invisible victories. No one will thank them for catching that mislabeled order set — which is exactly the point.

19:03 — Dinner at home: soup reheated, cat on the counter. One last status check — all systems normal. Notebook entry: "Clinical informatics isn't about data. It's about trust translated into code."

SCRUBfits™

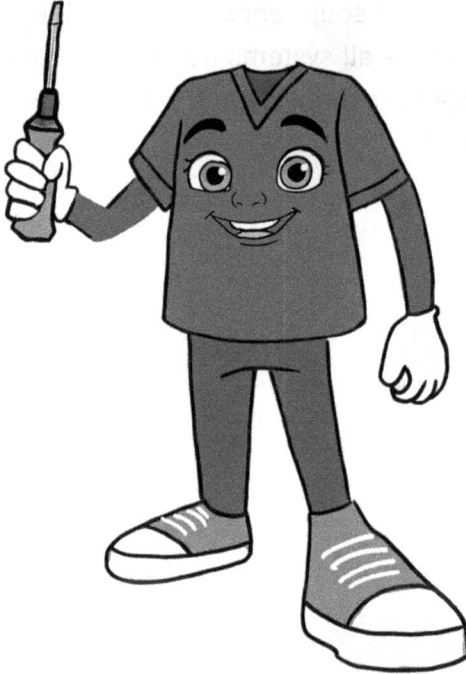

Max Volt, BMET

Max Volt, BMET — "The Power Protector"

Scrub Color: Electric Blue

Primary Role: Biomedical Equipment Technician (BMET) (gl)

Also Aligns With: Clinical Engineer (gl); Imaging Service Specialist (gl); Equipment Safety Officer (gl); Biomedical Systems Manager (gl)

SCRUB*fit*™ Category: The Power Panel

Pros: Hands-on technical role; vital to patient safety; varied career paths

Cons: Pressure of equipment failures; 24/7 call demands; safety-compliance burden (gl)

Personality Traits: Problem-solver; meticulous; dependable; practical

Clinical Tools: Multimeter (gl); calibration devices (gl); service manuals (gl); electrical-safety analyzers (gl); tagging software (gl)

Clinical Confession: "Every machine has a heartbeat — I just keep it steady."

Character Description

Max Volt is the guardian of machines. In Electric Blue scrubs, he's the unseen professional who ensures every monitor (gl), ventilator (gl), and infusion pump (gl) performs exactly as designed. To patients, he's invisible — to clinicians, indispensable.

He treats every device as if it holds a life in its circuitry — because it often does. Whether crawling beneath a bed to fix a faulty connection or racing to repair an MRI coil (gl) minutes before a scan, Max treats precision as protection.

He thrives on quiet pressure — the hum of diagnostics, the faint click of calibration, the moment a red error light turns green. His alignment comes from vigilance: reliability is safety, and every spark, switch, and sensor must earn a clinician's trust before it earns his signature.

Max lives by a simple belief: every machine has a heartbeat, and his job is to keep it steady.

Day in the Life — Biomedical Equipment Technician (BMET) (gl)

05:28 — The alarm vibrates before sunrise. Coffee brews while the ticket report loads: infusion pump calibration, ventilator alarm, defibrillator (gl) check, one high-priority OR (gl) call. Breakfast is a protein bar eaten one-handed over yesterday's PM logs (gl). The day starts not with patients, but with the machines that help save them.

06:10 — Commute through fog. The parking lot glows with security lights (gl) and the quiet pulse of generators (gl). Every hum matters — power means life.

06:42 — Badge tap. The Biomed shop smells of solder (gl), rubber tubing, and fresh coffee. Ritual: boot the CMMS (gl), scan work orders, verify alerts. One ventilator flagged for low pressure tolerance; one IV pump due for PM. Tools assembled: torque driver (gl), multimeter (gl), calibration syringe (gl), battered clipboard.

07:18 — ICU ventilator, tagged SERVICE REQUIRED (gl). Into the alcove, test lung (gl) connected, self-diagnostic run. Flow error confirmed — clogged expiratory filter (gl). Replace, recalibrate, log the result. Pass. A quick wipe of the control screen. "You're clear, partner," he whispers.

08:33 — Cath lab (gl) defibrillator calibration. Leads to analyzer (gl), 200-joule test shock. Numbers match spec. Green "INSPECTED" sticker applied. A cardiologist walks in: "You keep us alive more than you know." He grins. "I just make sure the heroes have working toys."

09:57 — Pager buzz: urgent OR call — "anesthesia gas module fault" (gl). System logs show a false O_2 sensor reading. A loose connector, easily missed. Reseat, recalibrate with gas analyzer (gl), error clears. Thumbs-up from anesthesia: "You saved us ten minutes — that's a lifetime in here."

11:12 — Back in the shop, quarterly infusion-pump (gl) round. Pressure tests, battery checks, leak inspections. Hissing air and clicking relays form their own soundtrack.

12:14 — Lunch: turkey sandwich, chips, banter about whose soldering station smells worse. "We're the hospital's pit crew," someone jokes. Nods all around — not glamorous, but vital.

13:03 — L&D (gl) install: new fetal monitors (gl). Network drops run, EHR (gl) interface (gl) synced, real-time data verified. "Will this actually work?" a nurse asks. "If it doesn't, you'll be the first to know — and so will I."

14:56 — Preventive maintenance (gl) on the defibrillator cart (gl). Pads replaced, battery swapped, charge cycle verified. Fresh green "INSPECTED" sticker — Hopewell's quiet signature of reliability.

16:08 — Med–Surg service call: "Infusion pump alarming — error 404." Silence, open casing, kinked pressure line (gl). Two minutes to resolve. Log the fix in CMMS (gl); barcode scanned (gl) for tracking. Another whisper: "Back in the fight."

17:30 — End-of-day summary. Tickets closed, PM certificates printed (gl), bench wiped clean. The soldering station winds down. Screen flashes: All systems nominal (gl). The phrase never gets old.

18:22 — Commute under a motherboard sunset. City lights shimmer like LEDs (gl). Every beep, pulse, and light depends on invisible hands keeping everything alive.

19:04 — Home. Dinner reheated, boots off, mind still tuned to circuits and safety. A message from the ICU charge nurse: "Ventilator's working perfectly. Patient stable." He smiles. Best readout of the day.

[Image: Max Volt B&W.png]

Max Volt, BMET

The Power Panel — Wiring Reliability

The Power Panel proves that healthcare alignment is powered by more than people — it's fueled by the systems and machines that never stop running. From biomedical engineers (gl) and imaging specialists (gl) to IT troubleshooters and safety officers (gl), this category highlights careers where technical expertise keeps care alive.

For readers, the Power Panel opens doors to roles where solving problems behind the scenes makes all the difference at the bedside. Technology hums; data flows. When the power is steady and the systems are stable, the next link in alignment activates — the one that turns energy into understanding.

That responsibility belongs to The Vital Link — the translators of data, the guardians of integrity, and the keepers of every patient's story.

→ Next Up: The Vital Link — Translating Chaos into Clarity.

Chapter 28
SCRUBfit Squad:
The Vital Link

Information as medicine; accuracy as compassion.

They are the quiet architects of order in a world built on complexity. When the Compassion Corps heals the body and the Adrenaline Team saves lives in motion, The Vital Link ensures the system itself can stand.

These professionals translate chaos into clarity — bridging the clinical and the operational, the data and the human story. They can trace every medication, lab, and signature to its rightful source, guarding privacy (gl) as fiercely as others guard airways. If healthcare is a body, they are its nervous system — carrying signals that keep every part in sync.

You'll find The Vital Link in offices that hum with printers (gl) and policy binders (gl), in command centers glowing with dashboards (gl), in meetings where silence falls when they speak. They see patterns others miss: an outlier lab value (gl), a missing document, a coding inconsistency that could cost the hospital thousands — or delay a patient's care. To them, information is medicine, and accuracy is compassion.

They don't wear capes; they wear badge reels (gl). They carry clipboards, compliance binders (gl), and an unshakable belief that every detail tells a story. Their work protects not only patients but the integrity of the profession itself. They are guardians of the record, stewards of systems, translators of trust.

At Hopewell Hospital for Tomorrow, The Vital Link connects departments that never used to speak the same language. From the HIM (gl) director safeguarding privacy to the informaticist refining Epic (gl) workflows, their alignment creates the invisible infrastructure that makes safe, equitable, efficient care possible.

Without The Vital Link, there is no continuity. With them, every patient's story becomes complete.

At Hopewell Hospital for Tomorrow

Hopewell doesn't run on power or policy alone — it runs on connection. Behind every beep, barcode (gl), and chart entry is a quiet network of minds keeping the mission alive. Across its glass corridors, real-time dashboards (gl) pulse with live data — patient flow, staffing, quality metrics — each color-coded to signal safety and progress.

Clinical teams and informatics labs test workflow prototypes (gl) in simulated environments before they touch a real chart. Across campus, every department feeds into The Command Bridge (gl) — Hopewell's real-time operations hub, where analysts, clinicians, and executives monitor system health like vital signs for the entire hospital.

At Hopewell, alignment isn't just discussed — it's built into the walls, the wiring, and the work. For those in The Vital Link, it's more than a workplace. It's a living, learning organism — one they translate, protect, and continually refine.

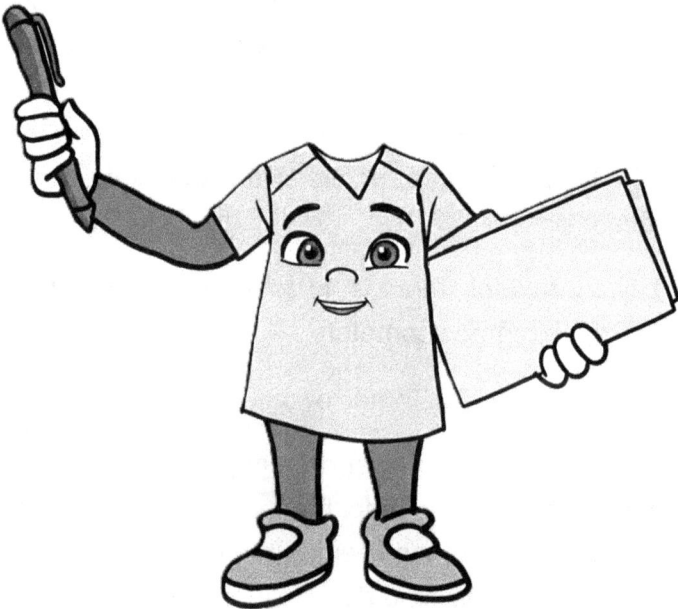

Clara Chartcheck, RHIA — "Second Career Trailblazer"

Scrub Color: Coral Spring

Primary Role: Health Information Management (HIM) Director (gl)

Also Aligns With: Coding Manager (CCS) (gl); Clinical Documentation Integrity Specialist (CDIP) (gl); Privacy Officer (CHPS) (gl); Data Governance Analyst (RHIA) (gl); Compliance Director (CHC) (gl)

SCRUB*fit*™ Category: The Vital Link

Pros: Mission-critical to data integrity; cross-department collaboration; policy and practice influence; work–life stability; strong growth field

Cons: High accountability; complex regulatory environment; audit/transition burnout risk; less direct patient interaction

Personality Traits: Analytical; principled; collaborative; detail-obsessed; diplomatic

Clinical Tools: Encoder software (gl); dual monitors; PHI (gl) encryption keys (gl); ergonomic keyboard (gl); annotated Code of Federal Regulations (gl) binder

Clinical Confession: "Behind every chart, there's a story waiting to be told right."

Character Description

Clara didn't start her career in healthcare.

For twenty years, she worked for the federal government — steady, reliable, predictable. Until one morning, it wasn't. A restructuring. A meeting that lasted eight minutes. A layoff she never saw coming.

She walked out carrying a box, a badge she could no longer use, and a truth she could no longer ignore: she'd always been drawn to healthcare. She'd always been good with numbers. And she was finally free — or forced — to rethink everything.

So she did what people do when they're ready for reinvention: she researched. She asked questions. She got brave.

Clara enrolled in medical coding and health information courses — ICD-10 (gl), CPT (gl), revenue cycle (gl) foundations, even a Q&A prep class she jokingly called "fluency in medical shorthand." She studied at her kitchen table, surrounded by highlighters, old coffee, and a stack of anatomy (gl) flashcards she never let anyone see.

And little by little... she found her alignment.

Today, Clara Chartcheck doesn't wear gloves or carry a stethoscope, yet she safeguards lives just as carefully. Her world is numbers, narratives, and nuance — the digital heartbeat that keeps Hopewell Hospital for Tomorrow's records honest, its reimbursements accurate, and its reputation protected.

In her Coral Spring scrubs, Clara moves between departments like a multilingual interpreter — fluent in clinical, administrative, and financial dialects. She can translate a physician's note into a precise code, a coder's question into a compliance rule, and a hospital policy into a workflow that actually makes sense. She sees the entire map of care — and knows where every path intersects.

Because of her strong leadership background, Clara stepped seamlessly into the role of Associate Director of Health Information Management. And when the Director who hired her — Lena Ledgerly — announced her retirement, Clara was the first name on her succession list. She didn't just get the job... she had earned it.

To Clara, data isn't just information; it's integrity. She teaches her team to treat each chart like a patient's voice on paper.

"Accuracy is advocacy," she reminds them. "We don't just code diagnoses. We code stories."

Her leadership is steady, practical, deeply human. When her HIM team feels overwhelmed by backlogs (gl), she doesn't retreat to her office — she rolls up her sleeves, orders lunch, and abstracts charts (gl) alongside them. Her door is rarely shut; her presence is rarely unnoticed.

Clara's desk is a quiet monument to precision: color-coded folders, tiered Post-its, and a mug labeled Ctrl + Alt + Deliver. People leave her office calmer, clearer, and just a little more confident.

She didn't come to healthcare through a straight line. She came through life. Through setbacks, grit, and the courage to start over.

When Clara talks about alignment, she doesn't mean perfection — she means purpose. She believes a hospital runs on data as clean and trustworthy as an IV line: steady, transparent, life-supporting.

And every day, in her quiet way, she keeps that line open.

Day in the Life

5:12 a.m. — The World Is Quiet, but the Charts Are Not

The sun hasn't even stretched yet, but Clara is already awake.

Her alarm doesn't blare — it pulses, like a gentle heartbeat. She slides out of bed, socks whispering over her hardwood floor as she tiptoes past her sleeping partner and the family's retired greyhound, Maple, who lifts one lazy eyebrow as if to say: Chart audits (gl) already?

Clara kisses Maple's forehead and heads to the kitchen where her cold brew has been patiently waiting overnight. A splash of oat milk. A swirl. A nod of approval.

Before she even sips, she checks her phone:

14 documentation queries (gl) unanswered

3 coding discrepancies (gl) flagged overnight

1 ICU note missing a discharge summary (gl)

Clara smiles. Her kind of puzzle.

She lifts her mug to no one in particular.

"Let's tighten this documentation universe."

6:07 a.m. — The Commute of Quiet Observers

Clara drives to work with a podcast on healthcare fraud (gl) cases playing softly. Most people find this grim. Clara finds it motivating.

Her car smells faintly of lavender and determination.

As she parks, she tucks her hair behind her ear, straightens her Coral Spring scrubs, and breathes in the crisp morning air. She's not a clinician in the traditional sense — no stethoscopes or med carts — but she knows the truth:

No documentation = no care delivered.

No codes = no reimbursement.

No accuracy = no trust.

She marches toward the hospital with purpose.

6:59 a.m. — Dual Monitors, Double Power

Clara flicks on the lights in the Health Information Management suite, and her dual-monitor setup glows like a command center.

Left screen: EHR inbox (gl)

Right screen: Coding interface (gl)

Bottom left: HIPAA (gl) reminders

Bottom right: A tiny succulent named "Audit Annie"

She logs in, and the system practically sighs with relief that Clara is here.

7:43 a.m. — The Case of the Confusing Consult Note

A cardiologist's note catches her eye.

The Assessment section says one thing. The Plan says another. The ICD-10 code (gl) used? Not even in the same galaxy.

Clara raises one eyebrow — the famous Clara Chartcheck Eyebrow of Disapproval™.

She fires off a friendly clinical documentation query (gl) (yes, friendly — Clara refuses to be passive-aggressive).

"Hi Dr. Rao! Quick clarification on Mr. Henson's consult note. Assessment lists NSTEMI (gl), but plan mentions unstable angina (gl). Could you confirm the correct diagnosis (gl)? Thank you!"

No "gotcha." No tone. Just accuracy — served warm.

9:12 a.m. — Coffee #2: The Audit Awakens

Clara joins a brief huddle with Revenue Cycle (gl), Nursing, and even one wandering hospitalist (gl) who swears he's "just here for the donuts."

She presents trends:

• More incomplete discharge summaries (gl) from the trauma unit

• Increase in missing medication reconciliation (gl) notes

• A rise in copy-paste errors (gl) on the overnight shift

Everyone nods. Clara gently, politely, relentlessly makes sure they understand:

"The chart speaks for the patient. We have to let it speak accurately."

They all agree. Even the donut doctor.

11:00 a.m. — A Victory in Coding Land

Clara reopens a previously denied claim (gl) that she knew was coded correctly.

She reviews the policy.

She reviews the documentation.

She attaches the supporting notes.

She writes an appeal letter that could win a Pulitzer for Precision.

When the approval hits her inbox, Clara whispers:

"Justice."

12:20 p.m. — Lunch, but Make It Predictable

Clara eats the same lunch every day: turkey wrap, apple slices, and a small handful of dark chocolate chips.

A few coworkers tease her. Clara simply replies:

"I save my unpredictability for ICD-10 mystery cases."

1:37 p.m. — The Case of the Rogue Abbreviation

A junior resident uses an abbreviation she's never seen before:

"PRB-FN-Q3"

Clara stares at it.

The abbreviation stares back.

She digs through past notes, departmental shorthand lists, archived abbreviations. Nothing.

She messages the resident:

"Hi! Can you clarify what PRB-FN-Q3 refers to? I want to make sure we're coding accurately. Thank you!"

The resident replies:

"Oh — that just means 'patient requested blankets — for nighttime — quantity 3.' I was just making it up."

Clara pauses. Breathes. Then very calmly writes:

"Please do not create abbreviations."

Somewhere in the distance, a compliance binder (gl) whispers "thank you."

3:05 p.m. — A Walk Through the Wards

Clara does something unique for an HIM professional: she rounds.

She believes seeing the flow of care helps her understand the notes better — and helps clinicians see that documentation isn't "paperwork." It's patient care (gl) in a different language.

Nurses wave. A respiratory therapist gives her a thumbs-up. A PA (gl) shouts from down the hall, "HEY CLARA — your query saved us last night!"

Clara blushes.

Her work is often invisible, but moments like this remind her: she protects the integrity of every story in the medical record.

4:22 p.m. — Final Check, Final Click

Back at her desk, she rechecks her dashboard:

- 62 charts reviewed

- 17 coding errors corrected

- 11 documentation queries sent

- 4 denials appealed

- 1 strange abbreviation eliminated from the hospital forever

Audit Annie looks proud. Clara pats the succulent gently.

She logs out, satisfied.

5:01 p.m. — The Drive Home and the "Chart Unwind"

She drives home listening to her favorite playlist: "Songs to Audit By." It has Beyoncé, Mozart, and a surprising amount of early 2000s emo.

Clara pulls into her driveway where Maple greets her like she's been gone for 10 years, not 10 hours.

Her partner hands her dinner — stir fry, hot, flavorful, perfect. They debrief about their days.

Clara says her favorite line, as she does every evening:

"I fixed things today."

Because she did.

9:48 p.m. — One Last Chart (Don't Judge Her)

She's "not working," but she can't help it — she glances at her phone.

A provider responded to her morning query:

"Thanks Clara — corrected the diagnosis."

Clara smiles, satisfied, and finally powers down.

Tomorrow, the charts will rise again.

And Clara Chartcheck will be ready.

The Vital Link — Translating the Story

The Vital Link transforms complexity into confidence. Their alignment lives in accuracy, connection, and trust — proving that data itself can be compassionate. They remind us that every heartbeat, scan, and signature becomes part of a patient's story only when someone like Clara ensures it's told right.

Because in the end, healthcare doesn't just depend on information — it depends on interpretation.

→ Next Up: The Care Crew — the heartbeat of connection.

Chapter 29
SCRUBfit Squad:
The Care Crew

No one heals alone.

Not every hero wears a title that makes headlines — or a badge that commands attention. The Care Crew are the quiet constants, the people who make sure the day actually works. They're the steady hands guiding patients through check-in, the reassuring voice answering "just one more question," and the adaptable teammates who keep a clinic from unraveling when the schedule runs long.

Their gift is versatility. One moment they're taking vitals (gl); the next, they're calming a nervous parent, prepping a procedure (gl), or untangling the day's bottlenecks (gl) so providers can focus on care. They're connectors — bridging front desk and exam room, specialist and patient, systems and stories.

The Care Crew proves that alignment isn't always flashy. It's being the presence patients remember — and the colleague every provider relies on. In a healthcare system that often feels rushed, they remind us that the "little things" — kindness, consistency, attention — are actually the big things.

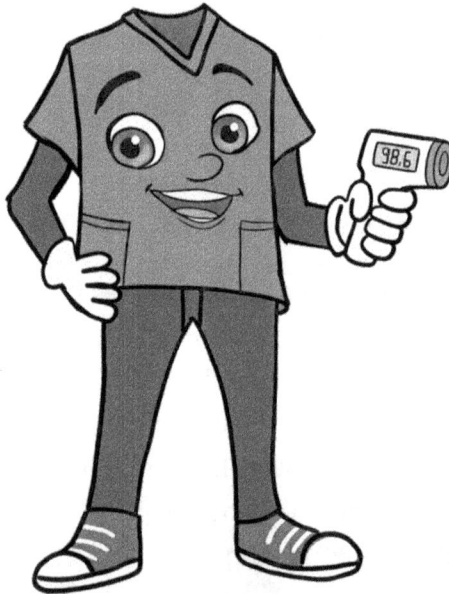

SCRUBfits™

Harper Helpwell, CMA (AAMA)

Harper Helpwell, CMA (AAMA) — "The Care Connector"

Scrub Color: Hunter Green

Primary Role: Medical Assistant

Also Aligns With: Dietitian (RDN) (gl); Certified Diabetes Care and Education Specialist (CDCES) (gl); Certified Health Coach (NBC-HWC) (gl); Clinical Exercise Physiologist (ACSM-CEP) (gl); Public Health Nutritionist (MPH, RDN) (gl); Bariatric Program Coordinator (RDN/RN) (gl); Integrative Nutrition Specialist (RDN, IFNCP/CNS) (gl)

SCRUB*fit*™ Category: The Care Crew

Pros: Patient-facing; versatile skill set; strong job growth; short training timeline (gl)

Cons: Lower pay scale (gl); heavy workload; role varies widely by practice

Personality Traits: Dependable; adaptable; patient-focused; quick learner; empathetic

Clinical Tools: Stethoscope; blood-pressure cuff; EHR (gl); thermometer; exam gloves

Clinical Confession: "Doctors sign the notes, but I'm the one patients tell their stories to first."

Character Description

Harper Helpwell is the backbone of many outpatient practices — moving seamlessly between front-office tasks and hands-on clinical care. Often the first friendly face a patient sees and the last before they head out the door, Harper blends precision with people skills: taking vital signs (gl), updating charts, and easing nerves.

While physicians, NPs, and PAs take the spotlight, Harper thrives in the rhythm of a busy clinic, keeping the flow steady and reducing bottlenecks (gl). Patients feel comfortable, reassured, and informed — the "little questions" get answered, the small fears named.

Harper embodies accessibility (gl) — translating medical tasks into a patient-friendly experience and pivoting from pediatrics (gl) to geriatrics (gl), family practice to specialty clinics. Calm in chaos, steady in uncertainty, Harper brings order to scattered workflows and offers a reliable presence patients can depend on.

Through Harper, the work of many others comes into focus: the precision of dietitians and diabetes (gl) educators, the coaching of health coaches, the insights of public-health nutritionists, and the guidance of bariatric (gl) and integrative (gl) specialists. Harper carries those voices forward — the bridge that ties the entire care spectrum (gl) together.

Day in the Life

4:41 a.m. — When the World Is Heavy but the Heart Still Wakes Light

Harper Helpwell wakes before dawn — not because he's rested, but because healthcare runs on the schedules of everyone except the people who work in it. He rubs his eyes, pulls on navy scrubs, and brews what he generously calls coffee.

His rescue dog, Toast, trots over and drops a toy at his feet like: Sir, we have two minutes for joy before chaos claims you.

Harper sits on the floor for exactly those two minutes, playing tug-of-war with Toast, feeling the small spark of warmth that makes the day possible.

He whispers: "Be kind. Be quick. Be steady. Be human."

Then he stands, grabs his badge, and inhales one long breath. Today, he will help people at their most vulnerable. And he will carry their stories home.

5:28 a.m. — Entering the Clinic, Becoming the Pulse

The outpatient clinic lights hum with a low buzz. Monitors glow in the dim. The printer warms like a creature awakening from hibernation (gl).

Harper walks in, drops his lunch bag into the staff fridge, and begins the ritual: he wipes down exam tables, primes the autoclave (gl), stocks gloves and swabs, checks oxygen tanks, logs vaccine fridge temps (gl), and lays out syringes, BP cuffs (gl), and stethoscopes (gl).

He moves with practiced efficiency — a choreographer preparing a stage. Medical assistants and CNAs are often invisible. But Harper knows: nothing works without him.

6:02 a.m. — The First Patient: A Diabetic Foot Check (gl)

Mr. Rowland arrives early, limping slightly.

Harper smiles warmly. "Morning, Mr. R. I've got you."

He checks vitals (gl), preps supplies, inspects the foot carefully — skin integrity (gl), sensation (gl), temperature, color. He sees the small fissure (gl) near the heel. Not infected yet. But it will be.

"You caught that," Mr. R murmurs.

Harper shrugs gently. "Caring is in the details."

He places the patient in the exam room for the provider and notes everything in the chart. The tiny catch that prevents a major hospitalization (gl). That's Harper's world.

6:56 a.m. — Second Patient: A Teen Getting Vaccines (gl)

A 14-year-old girl sits stiff as a wooden plank.

"I don't do needles," she whispers.

Harper kneels beside her. "Hey, totally normal. Look at me, not the needle. We'll breathe together."

She nods, teary-eyed.

Harper administers the shot with near-invisible precision.

"Done," he says.

Her eyes widen. "No way!"

He smiles. "I only use my ninja speed before 8 a.m."

She laughs — a real one. Courage restored.

7:48 a.m. — Blood Draw Marathon

Three fasting labs (gl) check in at once.

Harper rolls up his sleeves — literally and spiritually — and draws blood smoothly: a butterfly needle (gl) for the elderly patient, a straight needle for the bodybuilder who brags he "never looks away" but absolutely does, and a pediatric gauge (gl) for the nervous seven-year-old clutching a stuffed dinosaur.

Harper's voice is calm, rhythmic. "In... out... perfect. You did great."

He labels tubes, preps courier pickup (gl), and updates documentation (gl) with the speed of a man chased by time itself.

9:03 a.m. — The CNA Part of His Soul Takes Over: Elderly Transfer (gl)

He's called over to help with a patient who uses a wheelchair.

"I've got her," Harper says gently.

He performs a perfect pivot transfer (gl) — safe, stable, dignified. He fixes the patient's sweater, smoothing it over her shoulders the way he once did for his grandmother.

"Thank you," she whispers.

"Always," he replies softly.

10:12 a.m. — The Controlled Chaos Hour: Phones, Providers, and Puzzling Symptoms

The waiting room fills. Phones ring like an alarm system gone feral.

Providers call out: "Harper, can you grab a rapid strep?" "Harper, room 3 needs a neb treatment (gl)!" "Harper, do we have more 22-gauge needles (gl)?" "Harper, what do I need for a Pap kit (gl)?"

He answers all of it. Because he is the circulatory system (gl) of the clinic.

He runs a rapid strep test (gl), sets up a nebulizer (gl), finds the needles, and preps the exam tray. No one notices the speed. Only the smoothness. That's the point.

11:53 a.m. — Lunch: A Burrito and Three Interruptions

He sits. He unwraps his burrito. He takes one bite.

The provider pokes in: "Hey, can you check an elevated BP (gl)?"

He nods. He returns. Takes another bite.

The front desk calls: "We need you for triage (gl)!"

He nods. He returns. Another bite.

A patient knocks softly: "Um... the bathroom is out of paper towels."

He smiles. "On it."

He never resents it. He chose this life because showing up matters. But the burrito does go cold.

12:42 p.m. — Afternoon Wave: Wound Care (gl)

Harper prepares a wound irrigation (gl) setup for a construction worker who stepped on a nail. He explains every step: "This part will sting. This part will help. You're safe."

The patient winces. "You're good at this, man."

Harper shrugs with a grin. "I've been told I have a soothing dad-energy."

"Dude, I'm older than you."

"Exactly."

The patient laughs, and the fear melts.

2:06 p.m. — A Crying Mother and a Feverish Baby

Harper steps into the exam room to find a mother trembling.

"My baby is burning up."

Harper scoops the infant into his arms gently. "Let's check everything together."

Vitals (gl). Pulse ox (gl). Temp. Breathing sounds.

He wraps the baby back into mom's arms. "You got here fast. That's the hardest part. We're going to take great care of her."

Mom's tears slow. Her shoulders drop. Harper's presence is medicine.

3:14 p.m. — The Hard Part: Transporting a Patient to the ED (gl)

A middle-aged man comes in looking unwell. Too unwell.

Harper checks vitals (gl) — BP low, oxygen saturation (gl) concerning, skin color worrying. He signals the provider with a subtle nod. They agree: call EMS (gl).

Harper stays with the patient until the ambulance arrives — hand on the man's shoulder, grounding him through fear.

"You're not alone. I'm right here."

When EMS rolls him out, the man locks eyes with Harper. "Thank you."

Harper nods. He doesn't need more than that.

4:51 p.m. — Final Patient: The Lonely Regular

Mr. Caldwell comes every week for "blood pressure checks."

Harper knows what he really needs: connection.

They chat about baseball, grandkids, the weather, old movies. Harper listens — really listens.

When Mr. Caldwell leaves, he smiles softer, lighter. Human touch without touching. That's Harper's specialty.

5:38 p.m. — Closing the Clinic, Opening the Exhaustion

Harper wipes down rooms, restocks drawers, logs temperatures, signs off charts, and turns off exam lights one by one.

The clinic finally falls silent.

He sits for a moment, overwhelmed but fulfilled. Today he caught a diabetic foot ulcer (gl) early, calmed vaccine fear, did perfect blood draws, transferred patients safely, ran diagnostics (gl), educated families, comforted the anxious, helped save one life, and connected with the lonely.

Harper Helpwell isn't a sidekick. He is the heartbeat of frontline care.

6:11 p.m. — Going Home, Finding Himself Again

Toast greets him at the door like he fought off dragons.

Harper laughs for the first time all day. He kicks off his shoes, sits on the floor, and lets Toast climb into his lap.

He whispers into the soft fur: "Another day of helping people, buddy."

Toast sighs contentedly.

Harper finally breathes.

The Care Crew — The Everyday Glue

The Care Crew is the everyday glue of healthcare. Their alignment lives in adaptability, teamwork, and a willingness to step in wherever needed. Impact doesn't depend on the spotlight — it depends on showing up, shift after shift, with purpose and heart. When their day ends and the lights dim, the story of healthcare continues — carried forward by every color, every role, and every act of alignment across the **SCRUB*fit*™** Squad.

The SCRUBfit™ Squad — More Than Just a Uniform

From the crackling urgency of the ER to the quiet precision of the lab — from the heart-thumping drama of the Adrenaline Team to the behind-the-scenes brilliance of the Diagnostic Division — the **SCRUB*fit*™** Squad is where skill meets style, and every color tells a story. These aren't just healthcare professionals; they're the heartbeat, the muscle, the mind, and the soul of the system. Each wears their scrub color like a badge of honor, carrying a lifetime of training, grit, and purpose. Together, they form a living spectrum of expertise — a team that doesn't just fit their scrubs, but owns them. Every shift. Every challenge. Every win. The **SCRUB*fit*™** Squad shows up, stands tall, and leaves the world better than they found it — because in this crew, the only thing more powerful than the skills in their hands is the heart behind them.

SCRUB*fit*™ — Wear Your Role. Live Your Mission.

Chapter 30

Recalibration Is Inevitable. Alignment Is a Choice.

The Thursday Nights That Changed Everything

Healthcare systems will always recalibrate. The difference between burnout (gl) and alignment (gl) is whether the workforce is redesigned along with them.

I once worked at a great hospital that was on its Journey to Magnet®, and we had a clear workforce reality to address: we had 39 LPNs, and the organization needed a structured way to support academic progression and leadership development rather than leaving it to chance, attrition, or individual heroics.

We could have handled that recalibration the way healthcare sometimes defaults to handling change: raise expectations and let the consequences land on individuals. Get your BSN or hit the road. That approach is simple, fast, and blunt, and it shifts the entire cost of system evolution onto working people.

We didn't do that.

Instead, the organization built a bridge — and the person who deserves real credit for making it happen is **Dr. Joy Solomita, PhD, MSN, RN, MPH, CNAA-BC,** who was our Chief Nursing Officer at the time and is also a Masters Series contributor. She understood that standards without support are just pressure. What she created wasn't a perk and it wasn't performative. It was strategy with resources attached.

The hospital partnered with **George Mason University**, a respected public research university known for strong health, nursing, and graduate education programs and for preparing working professionals to lead in complex, real-world systems. The partnership itself sent a message: this wasn't a shortcut credential or an "easy" pathway. It was a serious academic ladder built with a serious institution.

Together, we built a structured education pathway that matched the reality of adult lives. Nurses could enter at different points — LPN, RN, or BSN — and move forward step by step, with a clear line of sight all the way to an MSN. This wasn't framed as a favor. It was a workforce plan aligned to where the organization was headed and what it needed to become.

And yes, it was impressive.

Classes were held on site, often in our board room. No commute across town, no traffic, no scrambling to make an off-site start time after a shift. Dinner was provided. Tuition was covered. The board room itself was gorgeous — the kind of space that quietly signals, without saying a word, that what happens here matters. Holding graduate nursing education in that room did more than solve logistics; it anchored leadership development inside the organization's center of gravity. It made the message unmistakable: this was not a side project. This was part of how the hospital was building its future.

Not everyone chose to cross that bridge.

Some LPNs did not enroll. Some were indifferent. A few were openly resistant — not quietly opting out, but actively negative about the idea that the system was changing and that they were being asked to change with it. I'll be honest: that always bewildered me. They had an opportunity in front of them that most nurses never get — a reputable university partner, a clear internal ladder, major costs covered, and a practical design that removed many of the barriers working clinicians face.

Over time, I came to recognize what leaders eventually learn to recognize: refusal is not always about ability. Sometimes it's fear. Sometimes it's fatigue. Sometimes it's identity. Sometimes it's a stubborn need to keep the world the way it used to be, because change feels like judgment. You can acknowledge those realities without letting them run the organization.

A recalibrating system has limits. A hospital cannot meet a new set of expectations while keeping a permanently stationary workforce, especially after it has built a viable pathway forward and made the direction of travel clear. The individuals who refused the pathway ultimately did have to leave. I don't describe that as punishment. I describe it as misalignment with the organization's trajectory. The moment the system changes, alignment becomes a two-way agreement: the organization has to build the bridge, and individuals have to decide whether they are willing to cross it.

That is the real lesson of those Thursday nights. The dinner wasn't the story. The beautiful board room wasn't the story. The story was an organization refusing to outsource the cost of change onto individual nurses and then calling that "professionalism." Under **Dr. Joy Solomita, PhD, MSN, RN, MPH, CNAA-BC**, the hospital did the harder thing: it matched the expectation shift with structural support, and it treated education and leadership development as workforce design, not a motivational slogan.

Healthcare will continue to evolve. Standards will change. Expectations will rise. That is not the problem.

The problem is when systems recalibrate and expect people to absorb the impact alone.

Alignment happens when the system changes — and redesigns what produces its outcomes at the same time.

Chapter 31

Mason's Alignment Theory (MAT)

Fix alignment, and you don't just prevent burnout — you reignite purpose.

People often talk about burnout like it's a personal defect or a hydration issue.

("Have you tried more water?")

But the deeper truth is this:

Healthcare doesn't have a talent shortage.

It has an alignment crisis.

Every nurse, tech, therapist, pharmacist, EMT, physician, PA, NP, leader, and support professional started with purpose. No one stumbles into healthcare by accident. They came willing to carry other people's worst days on their shoulders.

But when the person and the place stop matching — when the work you do contradicts who you are — even the most purpose-driven people begin to fray.

Mason's Alignment Theory™ (MAT) reframes burnout, turnover, and disengagement not as failures of resilience, but as symptoms of misalignment between three elements:

- The Person

- The Place

- The Practice

Once you see alignment clearly, you cannot unsee it.

1. The Core Premise

Mason's Alignment Theory™ (MAT) begins with a simple, stubborn truth:

When who you are matches where you are, care improves for everyone.

Alignment lives at the crossroads of three elements:

- **Purpose** — Why you do this work in the first place

- **Place** — The culture, pace, and people around you

- **Practice** — How you're allowed to think, care, communicate, and lead

When these elements move together, you feel it. Work is still hard, but it feels true.

When one drifts, you feel that too:

- Your body gets heavier

- Your patience gets shorter

- Your joy gets quieter

That's not weakness.

That's data.

Your nervous system is sending you a memo:

"This environment no longer matches who you are."

Mason's Alignment Theory™ (MAT) asks you to treat that feeling as information, not failure.

2. The Misalignment Epidemic

We have trained generations of caregivers to adapt, absorb, and endure.

"Be flexible."

"Be a team player."

"Do what the unit needs."

Translation:

"Please bend as far as humanly possible and pretend nothing hurts."

But the numbers don't lie. Turnover, moral injury, mental-health crises, and stress-related illness often trace back to chronic misalignment, including situations such as:

• A nurse built for deep connection ending up in a role built for speed and throughput

• A tech wired for precision landing in a system that rewards volume over accuracy

• A leader driven by growth inheriting a culture welded to "we've always done it this way"

At first, they try harder.

They stay later.

They take more.

Then the inner monologue begins:

- "Maybe I'm not cut out for this."

- "Maybe I made a mistake."

- "Maybe I'm the problem."

Nothing is wrong with them.

Something is wrong around them.

Misalignment is not a personal flaw.

It is a system signal.

3. The SCRUBfit™ Model in Motion

Your SCRUBfit™ profile is the mirror inside Mason's Alignment Theory™ (MAT). It doesn't box you in — it reveals where you're wired to thrive.

Each SCRUBfit™ category describes:

- Your natural pace

- The emotional climate where you flourish

- The types of problems that energize you

- The situations that drain or fuel you

SCRUBfit™ doesn't say, "You can only ever do one job."

It says, "Here is the kind of ecosystem that brings out your best."

When you know your category mix, career choices stop feeling like guesses and start feeling like strategy.

A shift from ED to Trauma ICU.

A move from bedside to Informatics.

A pivot from lab bench to leadership.

These stop being panic pivots.

They become aligned transitions.

SCRUBfit™ in motion means this:

"I'm not just leaving something. I'm moving toward a better fit."

4. The PACES™ Connection

You met PACES™ — the five internal dimensions that shape career alignment — earlier in this book. Mason's Alignment Theory™ (MAT) uses PACES™ as its practical checkpoint.

PACES™ helps you evaluate not only whether you can do a role, but whether you can sustain it.

Each decision is filtered through:

- **Personality** — how you're wired

- **Aptitude** — what you naturally do well

- **Constraints** — what your real life allows right now

- **Experience** — what you bring with you

• **Situation** — where you are in this season of life and career

When you run a job, shift, credential, or pivot through PACES™, decisions stop being driven by pay, pressure, or prestige alone.

Within Mason's Alignment Theory™ (MAT):

• SCRUBfit™ reveals your wiring

• PACES™ evaluates the fit of the path ahead

• Mason's Alignment Theory™ (MAT) explains why certain paths feel right or wrong once you're living inside them

PACES™ turns one question into another:

• "Will this look good on my résumé?"

• "Will this still feel true once the novelty wears off?"

5. The CARESET™ Lens

You were introduced to CARESET™ (gl) earlier as a framework for evaluating the external conditions that shape whether healthcare professionals can thrive. These conditions include:

• Culture

• Autonomy

• Resources

• Expectations

• Structure

• Environment

• Team

Mason's Alignment Theory™ (MAT) zooms that lens out to the system level.

When organizations live CARESET™ — not just laminate it for the break room — alignment becomes possible:

• Workflows respect human limits

• Staffing reflects reality, not fantasy

• Culture reinforces values instead of eroding them

In the architecture of alignment:

• SCRUBfit™ helps you know yourself

• PACES™ helps you choose your path

• CARESET™ helps you evaluate whether the system around you can actually support the care it claims to deliver

Individual alignment and system alignment should point in the same direction.

CARESET™ is how you check whether they do.

6. The Alignment Equation

ALIGNMENT = IDENTITY × ENVIRONMENT × CHOICE

Alignment emerges when three forces move in the same direction together: Identity, Environment, and Choice. These elements form the core of Mason's Alignment Theory™ (MAT), captured in the equation above.

The multiplication symbol matters. It reminds us that alignment is not additive — you cannot compensate for a missing element by maximizing the others. If any one of the three is absent or minimized to zero, the entire equation collapses.

A strong sense of identity cannot overcome a harmful environment.

A supportive environment cannot offset a lack of real choices.

And abundant choices cannot create clarity when identity is still unexamined.

But when all three rise together — when people know who they are, work in conditions that support them, and have genuine choices in how they shape their path — alignment becomes not only possible, but sustainable.

7. The Leadership Imperative

Alignment is not a perk.

Alignment is a leadership responsibility.

Leaders must shift from staffing bodies to designing ecosystems.

The best leaders don't ask, "How's your workload?"

They ask:

• "Does this role still feel like you?"

• "Where do you feel most alive at work?"

• "What kind of environment brings out your best?"

When misalignment becomes actionable data:

• Honest conversations replace quiet resentment

• Thoughtful pivots replace sudden resignations

• Teams begin to see alignment as something you build, not something you hope for

A misaligned clinician doesn't need a pizza party.

They need a different seat at the table — or a different table.

8. The Future of Care

In the decade ahead, healthcare systems won't compete on pay alone.

They will compete on alignment in three key ways:

• The best organizations will behave like adaptive ecosystems

• The best teams will be built intentionally

• The best careers will be crafted, not improvised

Alignment drives retention.

Retention drives quality.

Quality drives trust.

And trust is the quiet currency behind every good outcome.

When healthcare realigns, everyone wins:

• Patients feel safer

• Families feel heard

• Clinicians finally breathe again

Closing Reflection

Alignment isn't about perfect days.

It's about knowing your true north — and refusing to live too far from it for too long.

Mason's Alignment Theory™ (MAT) gives you a language and a map:

- To name what you're feeling

- To understand what's happening beneath the surface

- To choose your next step with clarity instead of fear

Because when who you are matches what you do — and where you work actually fits you — you don't just stay in healthcare.

You become one of the reasons it's worth staying.

Chapter 32

Alignment: The Missing Link in Healthcare

The Real Crisis Isn't Shortage — It's Misalignment

"Get alignment right, and everything else improves. We protect our people and our patients. But it starts with awareness: leaders have to look honestly at whether the systems, expectations, and cultures they're creating are aligned with the values they promote. When alignment is missing at the top, it can't exist at the bedside."

— **Ellen Menard, RN, BSN, MBA** — Senior Vice President of Human Resources & Organization Development; Author of *The Not So Patient Advocate*

Everywhere you look, headlines scream about a "healthcare workforce shortage."

Hospitals say they can't find enough nurses.

Clinics struggle to recruit physicians, techs, and therapists.

Health systems lament "staffing crises."

But here's the truth:

We don't just have a shortage problem — we have an alignment problem.

Alignment means placing the right person, with the right strengths and values, in the right role and environment.

Misalignment is when that same passionate professional ends up in:

• the wrong specialty

• the wrong workflow

• the wrong leadership structure

• the wrong culture

It's not a lack of talent.

It's a mismatch.

And the consequences ripple everywhere.

Why Misalignment Matters

The cost of misalignment is staggering.

Billions are lost every year in turnover, recruitment, retraining, and onboarding. Replacing a single bedside RN costs $40,000–$60,000+ — and that's before counting the toll on morale, team stability, and patient safety.

Multiply that across the tens of thousands of clinicians who leave prematurely, and you're looking at numbers that could fund:

• entire hospitals

- research institutes

- training academies

- or community health ecosystems

But this isn't just about money.

Misalignment costs patients continuity, safety, and compassion.

It costs families the stability of a trusted caregiver.

It costs healthcare workers their calling, their energy, and too often, their health.

A People Problem, Not a Pipeline Problem

Healthcare is not running out of caring people.

As Ellen Menard observes, people burn out not from caring — but from caring in the wrong environment.

I've seen it hundreds of times:

- A nurse who went into pediatrics because she "loves kids," only to discover she comes alive in trauma

- A brilliant diagnostic tech placed in a customer- service-heavy outpatient role where their gifts go unused

- A visionary leader trapped inside a system allergic to change

These are not failures of effort.

Not failures of character.

Not failures of resilience.

They are failures of alignment.

Three Levels of Alignment

Alignment in healthcare lives on three interconnected levels.

1. Individual Alignment

Does the role match the person's strengths, values, pace, and personality?

2. Organizational Alignment

Does the culture — leadership, workload, teamwork, expectations — amplify or suffocate those strengths?

3. Systemic Alignment

Does the broader healthcare environment support sustainable staffing, fair pay, innovative models, and psychological safety?

When alignment exists at all three levels, something remarkable happens:

- Burnout falls

- Retention rises

- Patients feel the difference

How Leaders Can Spot Misalignment

Alignment isn't just an individual issue. It is an organizational one.

If you're leading a team, unit, or system, here are your misalignment red flags:

- **Turnover spikes in the first 1–2 years.**

When 20-30% of new hires leave by year two, it's rarely the individual. It's the fit.

• Morale drops while workload rises.

Burnout is not about "working hard." It's about working hard in the wrong direction.

• Exit interviews repeat themselves.

"I didn't feel supported."

"I couldn't grow."

"No one listened."

That's misalignment speaking.

• Patient experience slips.

Misalignment shows up everywhere — in rushed interactions, delayed responses, inconsistent care.

• Innovation stalls.

When people are exhausted, they stop imagining. They start surviving.

Misalignment drains systems from the inside out.

What Leaders Can Do About It

The good news is this:

Alignment is not luck — it's leadership.

You can build cultures where alignment becomes the norm, not the exception.

1. Listen first.

Hold listening sessions, rounds, and surveys not as formalities but as a way to hear the friction.

2. Create career pathways before burnout forces exits.

Show people where they can grow before they start looking elsewhere.

3. Align values with everyday practice.

If your mission is compassion, innovation, safety, or equity — people must be able to live those values in their day-to-day work.

4. Invest in development.

Tuition reimbursement, certifications, onsite programs — these aren't perks. They're alignment tools.

5. Lead by alignment yourself.

When leaders love their work and embody the mission, staff take their cues from that energy.

"Misalignment is contagious — but so is alignment.

When people feel they are in the right role, in the right place, under the right leadership, they not only stay — they thrive.

And thriving staff create thriving systems."

Chapter 33

Education and Training Pathways

Education as a Foundation

"Feeling connected with the profession begins in the first semester of nursing school. When students have positive experiences with the coursework and faculty mentors, they will enter practice with clarity, motivation, confidence, and collaboration, resulting in a smoother transition into practice and increased retention."

— **Billy Mullins, DNP, RN, NE-BC** — Assistant Professor, The George Washington University School of Nursing

Education is the foundation of every healthcare career — but it isn't just about degrees and credentials. It's about creating pathways that allow people to grow into the roles that fit them best.

For some, that means beginning as a medical assistant or CNA and discovering a passion that leads to advanced nursing practice. For others, it may mean pursuing allied-health fields like laboratory science, radiology, pharmacy, therapy, or public health — where specialized training opens doors to deeply rewarding careers.

One of the strengths of healthcare is that there is no single entry point and no one-size-fits-all path. A high-school student can step into a hospital as a volunteer or nursing aide, while a mid-career professional can retrain through a bridge program or certificate. The pathways are as varied as the people who walk them.

Nursing Pathways

Nursing has some of the most formalized progression routes:

• **CNA — Certified Nursing Assistant.** Often the first step, providing basic care and assisting with activities of daily living.

• **LPN/LVN — Licensed Practical/Vocational Nurse.** Expanded clinical duties, medication administration, and close coordination with RNs and providers.

• **RN — Registered Nurse.** The backbone of patient care, via diploma, associate (ADN), or bachelor's (BSN) routes.

• **BSN — Bachelor of Science in Nursing.** Increasingly the standard in many hospitals, especially Magnet® organizations.

• **MSN — Master of Science in Nursing.** Pathway to advanced practice, education, or leadership.

• **DNP — Doctor of Nursing Practice.** Highest clinical practice degree; focuses on systems leadership, advanced practice, and translating evidence into care.

Each step opens new doors. Not everyone needs to climb to the doctorate level to thrive — the key is choosing the step that aligns with your purpose, pace, and patient population.

Allied-Health Pathways

• **Imaging & Diagnostics.** An X-ray technologist can advance into CT, MRI, or nuclear medicine — and some pursue the radiologist-assistant role.

• **Rehabilitation Therapy.** PTAs/OTAs can bridge to DPT/OTD, then add specialty certifications in neurology, orthopedics, or pediatrics.

• **Pharmacy.** A pharmacy technician can complete pre-pharmacy coursework, earn a PharmD, and move into clinical or leadership roles.

• **Laboratory Science.** Phlebotomists may progress to MLT, then MLS with advanced certification, and eventually into lab management or pathology liaison roles.

• **Respiratory Therapy.** An associate degree can progress to bachelor's and master's levels, with opportunities in education and leadership.

• **Public & Population Health.** Community health workers can continue into bachelor's programs, MPH degrees, and doctoral-level leadership in policy or administration.

• **Health Information & Informatics.** A medical records clerk can advance to RHIT, then RHIA, and further into health-informatics leadership at the graduate level.

Bridge Programs and Flexibility

Healthcare careers often allow learners to advance while working.

Nursing offers LPN-to-RN, RN-to-BSN, and RN-to-MSN options. Imaging professionals can cross-train into new modalities. Respiratory therapists can progress from associate to bachelor's degrees. Lab technicians can pursue advanced certification. Community health workers and health educators can bridge into graduate public-health programs.

These bridge models allow people to earn while they learn — one of the most alignment-friendly features in healthcare education.

Licensure and Compacts

The Nurse Licensure Compact (NLC) allows nurses to practice across participating states with one multi-state license. In allied health, reciprocity is limited but expanding in imaging, therapy, and laboratory science.

Mobility matters: the ability to carry a credential across state lines expands career options without repeating exams or coursework. It gives clinicians more freedom to align with the right role and the right location.

Closing Note

Nursing may have the clearest ladders, but every corner of healthcare offers stackable, buildable pathways. Whether it's a CNA becoming a DNP, a dental hygienist becoming a public-health advocate, or a radiology technologist advancing into new modalities, education is never just a degree.

It's a bridge to alignment.

"Degrees open doors, but alignment decides if you'll want to walk through them."

Chapter 34
Alphabet Soup: Decoding the Letters After the Name

Alphabet Soup: Decoding the Letters After the Name

Healthcare loves letters. On badges, résumés, email signatures, lab coats, and LinkedIn profiles — the alphabet often shows up before the story does. To the untrained eye, these credentials can look like an intimidating bowl of alphabet soup (gl). But once you understand them, those little clusters of letters reveal something powerful: a person's training, expertise, specialty, and path.

And here's the good news — you don't have to memorize every credential to make sense of a healthcare career. You just need to understand why the letters matter and what they say about the person wearing them.

What Credentials Really Mean

Credentials fall into a few major categories:

- **Licensure (gl)** — legally required to practice a profession

- **Certification (gl)** — specialty training beyond the basics

- **Degrees (gl)** — academic education earned through schools or universities

- **Fellowships & Advanced Tracks (gl)** — extended practice beyond initial training

- **Leadership or Quality Credentials (gl)** — for those who guide teams or improve systems

A nurse (RN) (gl) might also hold a master's degree (MSN) (gl), a specialty certification (like CCRN) (gl), and a leadership credential (NE-BC) (gl). A radiologic technologist (gl) may wear the letters RT(R)(ARRT) (gl). A pharmacist (gl) may carry PharmD (gl), and a coding specialist may proudly show RHIA or CCS (gl).

Each set of letters represents hours of study, years of training, standardized exams, and commitment — but they also represent alignment. People tend to pursue credentials that match their natural strengths and the healthcare world where they feel most at home.

Why Students Shouldn't Feel Intimidated

If you're a high school student or someone exploring healthcare for the first time, credentials can look like a foreign language. But remember this:

Everyone in healthcare started exactly where you are — knowing none of the letters.

You don't need credentials to explore healthcare. You only need them when it's time to practice healthcare.

Credentials come later. Curiosity comes first.

And careers grow step by step — CNA → LPN → RN → BSN → MSN → NP is one common nursing path, but there are dozens of variations that fit different personalities, styles, and alignments.

The key is not memorizing letters. The key is understanding yourself.

The Most Common Letters You'll See (and What They Mean)

Here's a quick, student-friendly guide to the credentials you'll see most often.

Licensure List (Healthcare Careers That Are Typically State-Licensed in the U.S.)

Medicine

- Physician (MD / DO)

- Physician Assistant (PA-C)

- Nurse Practitioner (NP / APRN)

- Certified Nurse Midwife (CNM / APRN)

- Clinical Nurse Specialist (CNS / APRN)

- Certified Registered Nurse Anesthetist (CRNA / APRN)

- Registered Nurse (RN)

- Licensed Practical/Vocational Nurse (LPN/LVN)

Behavioral Health

- Psychologist (PhD/PsyD) (licensed)

- Clinical Social Worker (LCSW) (licensed)

- Professional Counselor (LPC/LMHC/etc.) (licensed)

- Marriage & Family Therapist (LMFT) (licensed)

Pharmacy

- Pharmacist (PharmD / RPh)

Therapy & Rehab

- Physical Therapist (PT / DPT)

- Physical Therapist Assistant (PTA) (licensed in most states)

- Occupational Therapist (OTR)

- Occupational Therapy Assistant (OTA) (licensed in many states)

- Speech-Language Pathologist (SLP)

- Audiologist (AuD)

- Athletic Trainer (ATC) (licensed in many states)

Dental

- Dentist (DDS/DMD)

- Dental Hygienist (RDH)

Vision

- Optometrist (OD)

- Ophthalmologist (MD/DO) (under physician above)

Emergency & Prehospital

- Emergency Medical Technician (EMT) (state-licensed/certified depending on state language, but functions as licensure for practice)

- Paramedic (same note as EMT)

Respiratory & Imaging

- Respiratory Therapist (RT/RRT) (licensed in most states)

- Radiologic Technologist (Rad Tech) (licensed in many states; some states regulate via state license + ARRT)

- Radiation Therapist (often licensed where the profession is regulated)

Nutrition

- Dietitian / Nutritionist (RD/RDN is national credential; licensure varies by state — many states license dietitians specifically)

Other Licensed Clinicians (Commonly Included)

- Chiropractor (DC)

- Podiatrist (DPM)

- Veterinary (DVM) (only if you're treating vet medicine as "healthcare" in WCAYS)

- Advanced dental specialties (orthodontist, oral surgeon) (under dentist/physician)

Degrees

- **ASN/ADN — Associate Degree in Nursing (gl)**; entry-level nursing degree that qualifies you to test for RN licensure (gl)

- **BSN — Bachelor of Science in Nursing (gl)**; four-year nursing degree that expands leadership (gl), public health (gl), and hospital-preferred RN preparation

- **MSN — Master of Science in Nursing (gl)**; graduate nursing degree for advanced practice (gl), education (gl), leadership (gl), or specialty roles

- **DNP — Doctor of Nursing Practice (gl)**; practice-focused doctoral degree for advanced clinical leadership (gl) and systems-level improvement (gl)

- **PharmD — Doctor of Pharmacy (gl)**; professional doctorate preparing pharmacists (gl) for medication therapy (gl) and clinical practice

- **MPH / MHA / MBA — Master of Public Health (gl) / Master of Health Administration (gl) / Master of Business Administration (gl)**; graduate degrees focused on population health (gl), healthcare leadership (gl), or business strategy (gl)

Specialty Certifications

- **CCRN — Critical Care Registered Nurse (gl)**; certification for RNs caring for critically ill patients (gl)

- **CEN — Certified Emergency Nurse (gl)**; certification validating emergency nursing knowledge and skills (gl)

- **SANE-A — Sexual Assault Nurse Examiner-Adult/Adolescent (gl)**; certification for forensic (gl) sexual assault care and evidence collection (gl)

- **CNOR — Certified Nurse Operating Room (gl)**; perioperative (gl) nursing certification for the operating room (gl)

- **CCS / RHIA — Certified Coding Specialist (gl) / Registered Health Information Administrator (gl)**; certifications in medical coding (gl), health records (gl), and information management (gl)

Don't worry — you won't be quizzed. These letters will slowly become familiar as you explore your path.

Why Credentials Matter — But Not the Way You Think

You might assume:

"More letters = better."

But the truth is simpler:

Credentials show direction, not superiority.

Someone with a long string of letters isn't "better" — they are simply:

- Trained differently

- Aligned differently

- Certified in different environments

- Following a path that fits their strengths and natural wiring

Credentials tell a story about where someone has been, what they love learning, and what kind of healthcare world feels like home.

The Hidden Meaning in the Letters

Credentials often reveal:

- How much patient contact someone likes

- Whether they prefer calm or chaos (gl)

- If they are analytical, technical, emotional, or relational

- Whether they enjoy leadership (gl)

- How they handle stress and complexity

- What kind of environment they thrive in

For example:

- Someone who loves solving puzzles may become a CCS coder (gl)

- Someone drawn to trauma and rapid decisions might pursue CEN or CCRN

- Someone detail-obsessed may become an RHIA

- Someone who loves one-on-one relationships may go for LCSW (gl)

- Someone with steady hands and technical confidence may choose CNOR

- Someone who thrives in deep calm may choose Hospice or Palliative certifications

Credentials are simply alignment written in letters.

A Note for Students and Second-Career Adults

If you're reading this and thinking, "Do I need credentials to work in healthcare?"

Here is your answer:

No. You need curiosity first. The letters come later.

You earn them one at a time.

Your path will unfold one chapter at a time.

Credentials don't define you — they follow you. They are proof of commitment, not identity.

Healthcare is full of people who started with zero letters and built meaningful, aligned careers step by step.

You can too.

Closing Thought

Learning the alphabet of healthcare is not about memorizing letters. It is about discovering where you belong in the vast, vibrant world of care.

And no matter where your journey leads, remember:

Every letter begins with a single step — and every step begins with knowing yourself.

Chapter 35

Professional Associations & Local Chapters

Why Getting Involved Will Transform Your Career

I cannot emphasize this enough: join your specialty association — and get involved early.

Not someday.

Not "once things calm down."

Not "after I feel more established."

Now.

Healthcare is too complex, too dynamic, and too interconnected to navigate alone. When you plug into your national, state, and local specialty associations, you gain something every clinician needs but far too few actively build: a community that grows with you.

The Power of a Professional Community

When I look back on my own career, the biggest leaps forward didn't happen alone in my office or during annual reviews.

They happened in rooms full of people who cared about the same things I cared about:

• Better patient experiences

• Smarter workforce solutions

• Innovation that actually works

• A healthier, more aligned healthcare culture

Associations create those rooms — and when you show up, your world expands.

1. Your Network Starts Working Even When You're Not

People don't realize how powerful these connections become:

• Job opportunities surface before they're public

• Mentors find you and guide you

• Peers share what's working and what isn't

• You gain colleagues you can call when you hit an unfamiliar situation

• Your name begins circulating in rooms you aren't even in yet

In healthcare, your network is one of your greatest assets. You don't build it by accident — you build it by showing up.

2. Associations Are Where the Most Current Knowledge Lives

Your specialty evolves constantly. Associations are where:

• New trends appear

• New research is discussed

- New tools are beta-tested

- New policies are unpacked

- New best practices are shared generously, with zero ego

When you're part of this flow of information, you make smarter decisions — not just for your career, but for every patient or student you touch.

3. Local Chapters Multiply Your Opportunities

Most associations have local or regional chapters, and they are gold.

These groups:

- Help you build deeper relationships

- Connect you with leaders in your area

- Give you access to volunteer roles that lead to leadership roles

- Help you become known in your local healthcare ecosystem

National membership widens your world. Local membership roots you in community.

My Own Path: Why I Believe So Strongly in This

I'm not telling you this because it sounds good. I'm telling you because I've lived it.

Throughout my career, I've had the privilege of serving on:

- The National Association of Health Care Recruiters (NAHCR) Board of Directors

- Gannett Healthcare Advisory Board

- The Chubb Institute Advisory Board

- The AARP Young Leaders Circle

- Judge for the AARP Best Employers for Workers Over 50 Awards

- Judge for National Nurse of the Year competitions

- Judge for customer/patient experience and innovation for the Stevie Awards

- Judge for the DECA Collegiate Business Award Competition

- And yes — I even served on the Employee of the Month Committee

Let me tell you: if your healthcare organization takes Employee of the Month seriously, buckle up. I've witnessed debates more intense than national elections. ("Does Linda from radiology really demonstrate exceptional teamwork, or are we just swayed by the cookies she brings in?")

I do not share any of that with you to brag. While there are social aspects to these, it's definitely extra effort.

But here's the truth: every one of these experiences expanded my understanding of healthcare and connected me with people who shaped my career in ways I couldn't have predicted.

These weren't "extra activities."

They were inflection points.

Get Involved Early — The Momentum Compounds

If I could give you one piece of early-career advice, it would be this:

Don't wait until you feel ready.

You get ready by participating.

When you engage early, you:

• Accelerate your learning

• Build mentors naturally

• Become visible in your field

• Develop leadership skills before you even realize you're leading

• Strengthen your résumé with real contributions

• Become part of conversations that shape your specialty

Small roles — checking people in at conferences, helping with student events, joining a committee — often lead to major opportunities later.

People remember who shows up.

You Don't Just Receive — You Contribute

The real magic of association involvement is reciprocity.

You benefit, yes... but you also give.

You share what's working. You help your peers rise. You strengthen your profession. You build the culture you want to work in.

When clinicians at every level actively contribute to their

specialty's community, the entire field becomes healthier, smarter, more aligned, and more sustainable.

My Strongest Recommendation

So here it is, simply and clearly:

Join your specialty association.

Join your state society.

Join your local chapter.

And get involved.

These organizations change careers. They changed mine. They will change yours.

And who knows — one day you may find yourself on the Employee of the Month Committee, passionately defending the nominee who organizes the potlucks. (Choose wisely. These decisions ripple through hallways.)

Chapter 36

Masters Series Introduction:

Expert Voices on Healthcare Alignment

You've heard my voice throughout this book — from introducing the **SCRUBf*it*™ Squad** to exploring pathways and leadership. But alignment is not just my perspective. It's a challenge and opportunity that leaders across healthcare are confronting every day.

The Masters Series is where I hand the microphone to them.

These essays and reflections come from executives, educators, innovators, and frontline leaders who have lived the realities of healthcare and helped shape the environments where alignment either thrives or struggles.

Each contribution stands on its own, but together they create a panoramic view of what alignment looks like in education, leadership, culture, safety, and practice. You'll see different angles — from Magnet® journeys to workforce retention, from quality and safety frameworks to innovation in care delivery.

Think of this as a conversation with some of the most experienced minds in healthcare. Their words are here not just as advice, but as a legacy — a record of how leaders today are tackling the misalignment epidemic and pointing us toward a better future.

A Note of Thanks

I am deeply grateful to each contributor who shared their time, wisdom, and experience for this series. Their voices give this book dimension far beyond my own perspective. By opening up about their successes, struggles, and visions for the future, they've helped create a collective conversation about alignment that will outlast any single essay.

To each of you: thank you.

Chapter 37

Masters Series: Learning as the Operating System of Alignment

By: **Diane Adams, MS, LCSW, CPXP**; Chief Learning Officer; Mount Sinai Health System

"Learning is the operating system of alignment."

— Diane Adams, MS, LCSW, CPXP

Learning as the Operating System of Alignment

Alignment in healthcare isn't just a buzzword. It's the daily discipline of keeping people, purpose, and practice moving in sync. For leaders committed to building a true learning organization, that alignment begins with a simple premise: learning is the operating system of a high-reliability organization. When learning becomes part of workplace rhythms — shaping how we collaborate, approach challenges, and care for one another — teams and the individuals within them can grow at the speed of care, and patients will feel the difference.

Health systems ask extraordinary things of their people: rapid adaptation, evidence-based decisions, and collaboration across disciplines, with ever-greater demands ahead as every aspect of care delivery transforms. A true learning culture translates those demands into action by strengthening teamwork, relentlessly driving improvement, and fostering innovation. It also provides the pathways people need to adapt, reskill, and grow in their careers. In a learning organization, career development isn't a perk; it's how people stay, grow, and thrive even as the demands of healthcare intensify.

Alignment of learning shows up in everyday practices. A new nurse moves from orientation to confidence because coaching, simulation, and honest feedback take place where questions are encouraged and feedback is rewarded. An educator equips a team to adopt a practice change and stays to debrief on what worked and what didn't. An experienced clinician mentors and teaches while modeling humility and the courage to ask for help — demonstrating that learning never ends.

None of this is accidental. It comes from intentional architecture: competency frameworks, just-in-time learning, simulation, shared governances that truly share power, and inclusive leadership pathways.

A learning culture is not only about safety and innovation but also about career growth and individual potential. Opportunity must be visible, accessible, flexible, and creative — supported by programs, partnerships, and credentials that help people advance without stepping away from their roles. Equally critical are leaders who play their part and are rewarded for sharing talent so the whole system grows stronger, even when it means a short-term loss for their own team.

The work ahead demands adaptive expertise and learning agility. We have to elevate the loop from "train and measure" to listen → learn → iterate → improve, and repeat. We listen to frontline signals, learn from outcomes, iterate programs quickly, and improve impact — then we listen again.

If we want sustainable excellence, we must shape learning cultures that fit the people who hold the work. That means giving every team member clarity, community, and growth so they can adapt and thrive as delivery models transform. When learning is lived this way, alignment is no longer aspirational. It is the daily reality of healthcare — one patient, one team, one person, one day at a time.

Final Thought

A true learning organization doesn't wait for change; it practices change. The moment learning becomes part of how we breathe, we stop reacting and start evolving. Every improvement, every innovation, every act of compassion flows from the same source: people willing to keep learning together. That is how alignment endures — through curiosity, humility, and shared growth.

Diane Adams serves as Chief Learning Officer for the Mount Sinai Health System, a large academic health system with tens of thousands of employees, multiple hospitals, a school of medicine, and an extensive ambulatory network. In this role, she leads enterprise-wide talent strategy and designs educational solutions that support leadership development, workforce growth, and an outstanding patient and employee experience.

Beginning her career as a licensed clinical social worker, Diane moved into teaching, organizational development, and enterprise learning, drawn to the ways that learning can strengthen both people and systems. She brings to the Masters Series a deep expertise in creating people-centered learning ecosystems, aligning talent development with mission-driven care, and driving measurable cultural and behavioral change across complex organizations.

Here's Mason's Take

When Diane Adams writes that "learning is the operating system of alignment," she gives language to something I've witnessed for years but never quite put into words. It's not a slogan — it's a truth. Learning isn't what happens after something occurs in healthcare; it's the rhythm that holds everything together while it's happening. Diane captures that so elegantly, and it's what makes her leadership at Mount Sinai both practical and visionary.

I've always believed that healthcare is the ultimate classroom — one that never closes, never stops teaching, and never stops demanding curiosity. Diane shows that alignment doesn't begin with structure or strategy; it begins with the willingness to learn, unlearn, and relearn together. When she talks about new nurses finding confidence through coaching, simulation, and honest feedback, you can feel the heartbeat of culture work — real-time growth that creates real-time trust.

What I love most about Diane's approach is that it dignifies learning as leadership. She reminds us that creating a learning culture isn't about building classrooms or modules — it's about building psychological safety. It's about creating spaces where people are encouraged to ask, "What can we learn from this?" instead of "Who's to blame for this?" That single shift in tone can transform an organization from reactive to resilient.

Her idea of intentional architecture resonates deeply with me. Competency frameworks, just-in-time learning, shared governance, inclusive leadership — these aren't checkboxes. They're alignment structures disguised as learning programs. They ensure that excellence isn't personality-driven; it's process-driven. And that's how high reliability takes root.

I also love her candor about talent-sharing — how true leadership means growing people, even when it means letting them move forward. That's generosity as alignment. That's the mark of a mature system — one confident enough to prioritize long-term mission over short-term convenience.

Reading this piece reminds me that learning is the purest form of alignment because it invites humility. It's a quiet acknowledgment that none of us ever arrive — we just evolve, together. Diane's words remind every healthcare leader that the moment we stop learning, we stop aligning.

She's right: when learning is lived this way, alignment is no longer aspirational. It becomes the daily reality of healthcare — one patient, one team, one day at a time.

Chapter 38

Masters Series: Educating Humans in a Digital Healthcare World: Humanics as the Foundation of the Workforce of Tomorrow

By: **Michael J. Avaltroni, Ph.D.**

President, Fairleigh Dickinson University

Educating Humans in a Digital Healthcare World: Humanics as the Foundation of the Workforce of Tomorrow

The healthcare workforce of tomorrow will not be defined solely by new technologies, advanced credentials, or expanded pipelines. It will be defined by people — by how they lead, connect, adapt, and care in a world increasingly shaped by digital systems, artificial intelligence, and rapid innovation. As healthcare becomes more technologically sophisticated, the need for deeply human leadership has never been greater.

At Fairleigh Dickinson University, we believe the defining challenge for higher education is not simply preparing students for healthcare jobs, but educating humans to lead healthcare in a digital world. This distinction is essential. Technical skill alone will not sustain the workforce. What will sustain it is human capability — the ability to integrate technology with judgment, empathy, ethics, and purpose.

This belief has led us to center our institutional strategy around **humanics** as the core value proposition of the university of the future. Humanics is not an add-on, a slogan, or a single program. It is a comprehensive educational framework that places human literacy at the center of healthcare education and workforce preparation. In doing so, it reframes what it means to build the healthcare workforce of tomorrow.

The Healthcare Workforce Crisis Is a Human Crisis

Across the nation, healthcare systems face persistent workforce shortages, escalating burnout, and increasing complexity. At the same time, technology is transforming nearly every aspect of care delivery — from diagnostics and treatment planning to population health management and virtual care. Artificial intelligence promises efficiency, scale, and precision, yet it also introduces ethical dilemmas, new cognitive demands, and the risk of distancing care from the lived human experience.

These pressures have exposed a critical gap in workforce preparation. Many healthcare professionals are technically proficient yet underprepared for the human demands of modern systems: navigating uncertainty, communicating across difference, sustaining empathy under pressure, and making ethically grounded decisions in technology-mediated environments. Too often, individuals leave healthcare not because they lack skill or commitment, but because they experience profound misalignment — between who they are and what the work requires, between the environments they inhabit and the values that drew them to healthcare in the first place.

This misalignment often begins in education. Higher education has historically treated technical training and human development as separate domains, assuming that empathy, adaptability, and judgment would emerge organically through experience. In today's environment, that assumption no longer holds. The healthcare workforce challenge is therefore not only about numbers; it is about **human readiness**. Universities must take responsibility for developing that readiness intentionally.

Humanics: Educating Humans to Lead Alongside Technology

Humanics offers a response equal to this moment. At its core, humanics integrates three essential literacies: technological fluency, human literacy, and systems thinking. Together, they form the foundation for leadership in a digitally enabled healthcare environment.

At Fairleigh Dickinson University, we define humanics through five essential human capabilities: empathy, agility, cultural competence, creativity, and critical thinking. These are not "soft skills." They are **durable human advantages** — the capacities that become more valuable, not less, as technology advances.

Empathy anchors trust and connection in moments of vulnerability. Agility enables professionals to adapt as tools, roles, and systems evolve. Cultural competence ensures care that is inclusive, equitable, and responsive to diverse communities. Creativity fuels innovation and problem-solving across disciplines. Critical thinking grounds ethical judgment in environments saturated with data and algorithms.

By intentionally embedding these capabilities across curricula, experiential learning, and campus life, we are educating students not simply to use technology, but to **lead with humanity within digitally complex systems**. Humanics ensures that technological progress enhances human performance rather than eroding it.

Identity Before Occupation: Preparing Healthcare Leaders, Not Just Workers

One of the most consequential shifts we have made is reframing healthcare education around identity rather than occupation alone. Students are often asked early in their academic journeys to choose a role — nurse, technologist, analyst, administrator — before they have had meaningful opportunities to understand themselves as leaders, collaborators, and decision-makers.

Humanics challenges this sequencing. Before asking students what job they want, we help them explore who they are becoming: how they relate to others, what environments they thrive in, how they respond to ambiguity, and what gives their work meaning. Career pathways then emerge as expressions of identity rather than constraints upon it.

This approach is especially critical in healthcare, where misalignment between personal identity and professional environment is a primary driver of burnout and attrition. When students understand themselves and are supported in aligning their capabilities with the right roles and settings, persistence becomes far more likely. Educating humans first does not weaken workforce preparation — it strengthens it.

Alignment as Strategy: Connecting Education, Work, and Environment

Humanics also reframes how universities design pathways into healthcare careers. Alignment — between identity, education, environment, and work — is not incidental; it is strategic.

At Fairleigh Dickinson University, models such as **Learn While You Earn** are not simply workforce accelerators. They are alignment mechanisms. By integrating education with meaningful employment, students continuously test and refine their sense of fit, purpose, and contribution. Learning becomes iterative and reflective rather than linear and transactional.

Stackable credentials, flexible entry and re-entry points, and lifelong learning pathways further support alignment across the span of a healthcare career. In a world where professionals will navigate multiple roles and transitions, education must be designed to move with them — reinforcing identity, capability, and resilience at every stage.

Teaching Through Technology, Not Around It

Humanics does not resist technology; it situates it properly. Digital tools, data analytics, and artificial intelligence are essential to the future of healthcare. The question is not whether students should learn them, but how.

We teach technology as an amplifier of human judgment, not a substitute for it. Students learn to ask not only what a system can do, but what it should do — and what it cannot replace. Ethical reasoning, bias awareness, narrative understanding, and relational intelligence are taught alongside technical proficiency.

In this model, graduates become translators between human need and technological possibility. This role — bridging data and dignity, efficiency and empathy — will define healthcare leadership for decades to come.

Fairleigh Dickinson University as a Curator of a Healthcare Ecosystem

Our commitment to humanics extends well beyond our campuses. We view the university not as a standalone institution, but as a curator of partnerships and an anchor within a broader healthcare and workforce ecosystem. No single institution can build the healthcare workforce of tomorrow in isolation. The future demands collaboration across education, healthcare delivery, public policy, and community systems.

A powerful example of this ecosystem-building approach is Fairleigh Dickinson University's partnership with Rowan University and the Rowan-Virtua School of Osteopathic Medicine. This collaboration was intentionally designed to strengthen New Jersey's healthcare workforce through aligned pathways rather than fragmented pipelines. The partnership includes accelerated and articulated pathways, dual-degree opportunities such as a Doctor of Osteopathic Medicine/Master of Public Health program, and expanded collaboration across nursing, allied health, informatics, public health, and emerging health professions.

Equally important, the partnership convened nearly one hundred leaders from both institutions — faculty, administrators, and practitioners — to examine how healthcare education must evolve in an era defined by artificial intelligence, demographic change, and workforce strain. These conversations focused not only on capacity, but on human literacy, ethical leadership, and alignment across the continuum of education and practice.

This partnership exemplifies how Fairleigh Dickinson University is working to build a statewide healthcare education ecosystem — one that connects institutions, reduces barriers, expands access, and aligns preparation with real workforce and community needs. It is not about competition; it is about coordination around a shared human-centered purpose.

Campus as a Living Laboratory for Humanics

At Fairleigh Dickinson University, our campuses are not static backdrops for instruction. They are **living laboratories** where education, health, technology, and community intersect. Through initiatives such as FDU HealthPath Forward, we are formalizing the university's role as a hub for interdisciplinary education, workforce development, and healthcare innovation.

Students engage in applied learning environments that mirror the complexity of modern healthcare systems. They work across disciplines, interact with real data and real communities, and practice integrating humanics into decision-making. They learn that healthcare is not merely a set of clinical transactions, but a human system shaped by relationships, environment, and access.

Intergenerational learning, wellbeing-centered design, and community-embedded education further reinforce this understanding. Education itself becomes a determinant of health — supporting resilience, purpose, and long-term wellbeing for students and the communities they serve.

A Distinct Value Proposition for Higher Education

What distinguishes Fairleigh Dickinson University is our explicit, institution-wide commitment to **humanics as the organizing principle** for healthcare education in a digital age. While many institutions are innovating in programs or technologies, fewer are addressing the foundational human question: how do we prepare people to lead with humanity as systems become more automated and complex?

Humanics gives us a clear and compelling value proposition. We educate humans for an era of human-machine partnership. We prepare healthcare leaders who can integrate empathy with analytics, ethics with innovation, and adaptability with purpose. And we do so while curating partnerships that expand opportunity, strengthen workforce pipelines, and build resilient healthcare ecosystems.

Building a Workforce That Can Endure

The healthcare workforce of tomorrow will not be sustained by technical competence alone. It will be sustained by people who understand themselves, feel aligned with their work, and are supported by systems designed for human flourishing.

Universities have a profound responsibility in this moment. We must move beyond narrow definitions of workforce preparation and embrace a broader vision — one that integrates education, identity, and alignment as the foundations of student success and professional endurance.

At Fairleigh Dickinson University, we believe that the future of healthcare depends on our ability to educate students who are not only capable, but resilient; not only knowledgeable, but grounded; not only employable, but enduring. By centering humanics, curating partnerships, and building a statewide ecosystem for healthcare education and innovation, we are working to shape not just the workforce of tomorrow, but the **human leaders** who will sustain it.

In a world increasingly defined by intelligent systems, the most powerful innovation may not be technological. It may be educational — recommitting higher education to its most essential task: developing human beings capable of caring for one another, wisely and well.

Michael J. Avaltroni, Ph.D., is a nationally respected higher-education leader and President of Fairleigh Dickinson University, one of the largest private universities in New Jersey and a major hub for healthcare, business, and professional education. A passionate advocate for access, equity, and student success, Dr. Avaltroni has built his career around the belief that education is the most powerful engine for social mobility and workforce transformation.

Under his leadership, Fairleigh Dickinson University has expanded its footprint in healthcare, nursing, pharmacy, public health, and allied health programs—creating pathways that connect students directly to the hospitals, clinics, and communities they will serve. His work has been especially influential in strengthening partnerships between universities and healthcare systems, ensuring that graduates are not only academically prepared but clinically and professionally ready to meet the demands of modern healthcare.

Dr. Avaltroni is known for blending rigorous academic standards with a deeply human-centered leadership style. He champions first-generation students, adult learners, and working professionals, and he has been a consistent voice for making higher education more affordable, more flexible, and more aligned with real-world careers.

Before becoming President, Dr. Avaltroni served in senior leadership roles across higher education, where he earned a reputation as a forward-thinking strategist and trusted mentor to students, faculty, and emerging leaders. His scholarship and public commentary frequently focus on the future of education, workforce readiness, and the role universities must play in shaping an equitable and sustainable society.

In What Color Are Your Scrubs?, Dr. Avaltroni brings the perspective of a university president who sees, every day, how alignment between education, identity, and career pathways can change the trajectory of a person's life.

Here's Mason's Take on Dr. Michael J. Avaltroni's Contribution

What struck me most about Dr. Avaltroni's contribution is that he names something many people in healthcare *feel* but rarely see articulated so clearly: the workforce crisis is not primarily a technology problem or a pipeline problem — it is a human alignment problem.

In a moment when healthcare conversations are dominated by artificial intelligence, automation, and efficiency, Dr. Avaltroni makes a compelling and necessary pivot. He reminds us that the future of healthcare will not be sustained by tools alone, but by people who know who they are, how they lead, and where they belong within increasingly complex systems. His concept of **humanics** — educating humans to lead alongside technology — is not theoretical. It is deeply practical, especially for a workforce under strain.

What I deeply appreciate is his insistence that *technical skill is not enough*. That truth sits at the heart of *What Color Are Your Scrubs?* Every day, people leave healthcare not because they lack competence, intelligence, or commitment, but because the work environment conflicts with their identity, values, and wiring. Dr. Avaltroni calls this out directly, naming misalignment as an early and often invisible failure of education itself — not a personal shortcoming.

His emphasis on identity before occupation is particularly powerful. Too often, students are pushed to choose a role before they've had the chance to understand themselves. Dr. Avaltroni flips that sequence, arguing that sustainable careers emerge when individuals first explore who they are becoming — how they relate, adapt, think, and care — and then align into roles that fit. This is not just good pedagogy; it is burnout prevention.

Equally important is his view of the university as an ecosystem builder rather than a credential factory. By describing Fairleigh Dickinson University as a curator of partnerships — aligning education, health systems, and communities — he reinforces a central idea of this book: alignment is not an individual responsibility alone. Systems must be designed to support it.

Dr. Avaltroni's contribution grounds *What Color Are Your Scrubs?* in a hopeful truth: that education, when done intentionally, can be one of the most powerful determinants of long-term wellbeing in healthcare. His work reminds us that in a world of intelligent machines, the most critical investment we can make is still in human beings — prepared not just to work in healthcare, but to *endure* within it.

Chapter 39

Masters Series: Private Equity in Healthcare —The Good, The Bad and the Ugly

By: **Scott Becker, JD, CPA**; Partner, McGuireWoods LLP; Founder & Publisher, Becker's Healthcare; Founder, Becker Business Media

Private Equity in Healthcare — The Good, the Bad, and the Ugly

There has been a great deal of attention paid to private equity investing in healthcare over the last several years.

A significant portion of that attention has grown around investments that went poorly. Perhaps the most widely cited example is the investment by a private equity fund in Steward Health Care, which grew into a 34-hospital system and then ultimately entered bankruptcy, with some hospitals closing.

The Steward situation is useful for understanding where private equity investing in healthcare can go wrong. It is not necessarily representative of private equity investing as a whole. (See "The Steward Debacle: Legal and Ethical Risks of the New Breed of Health Care For-Profits," *Health Affairs*, and "Steward implosion provides cautionary tale on private equity in health care," Lown Institute.)

In many discussions about private equity, one overlooked factor is the people side of the equation. Health systems and physician groups are, at their core, human-capital enterprises, and their long-term performance depends on clinicians and staff who feel supported, aligned, and able to do their best work. When debt loads rise or financial pressure intensifies, the first cracks often appear not only in financial metrics but in workforce stability, retention, and morale. The success of an investment often turns on whether leadership can sustain alignment between the mission of the organization and the day-to-day experience of the workforce.

Across organizations that have navigated private equity partnerships most successfully, a common pattern emerges: strong alignment between clinicians, leadership, and mission. These organizations invest intentionally in people — giving clinicians the resources, staffing models, and support structures needed to deliver high-quality care. When that alignment is present, private equity can add significant value through capital, operational expertise, and strategic capabilities. When alignment is absent, even well-funded deals can struggle because the workforce becomes disconnected from the mission and the pressures of the investment thesis.

Private equity in healthcare spans a wide range of sectors, including hospitals and health systems, physician practices, outpatient facilities and services, healthcare technology, dental services, revenue cycle companies, artificial intelligence firms, digital health companies, medical device companies, pharmaceutical services, and biotech organizations.

It is also important to distinguish between healthcare venture capital and private equity. Venture capital typically invests in earlier-stage companies that are not yet profitable or cash-flow positive and may not yet have revenue. Private equity, by contrast, generally invests in companies that already have profits and cash flow. These companies are past the startup phase and may serve as growth platforms for further expansion.

Private equity investments in healthcare can succeed or fail based on many factors, including the company being acquired, market dynamics, management quality, competitive headwinds and tailwinds, and the amount of debt used in the transaction.

By design, private equity transactions use a mix of equity and debt. The company being acquired will almost always carry more debt after the transaction than before. The use of debt is not inherently good or bad. However, when excessive debt is placed on a company, it becomes more fragile — more vulnerable to softening growth, unexpected challenges, or market shifts. One of the most important considerations in healthcare private equity deals is therefore the total debt burden placed on the organization.

When private equity investments go poorly, it is often because declining margins or revenue combine with heavy debt obligations. Income drops while fixed financial commitments remain.

In healthcare, acquiring lower-margin businesses can be especially risky. This is not unique to private equity, but debt magnifies the risk. As private equity firms increasingly invest in areas such as primary care or OB-GYN — where margins have been tightening — the pressure of debt becomes harder to manage, though there are also notable examples of large, successful PE-backed practices in these areas.

Currently, approximately 8% of U.S. hospitals and nearly 7% of physicians are part of organizations with private equity investment. Many of these organizations perform very well. At the same time, flat valuations and multiples in recent years have made it more difficult to buy and then sell these assets within the typical three-to-seven-year private equity investment horizon.

Regulatory scrutiny has also increased, with more states placing limits and review requirements on healthcare transactions involving private equity.

Organizations typically partner with or sell to private equity firms for three main reasons: to access capital, to gain management expertise, or because financial or operational challenges require a transaction. There are nearly 19,000 private equity funds, and their quality and alignment vary widely. Some are excellent partners. Others are not.

Private equity funds also form joint ventures with health systems to operate service lines. In these structures, governance and economics are shared, and each deal must be evaluated on its own terms.

Private equity in healthcare should not be viewed as

categorically good or bad. It depends on the specific circumstances and goals of the organization.

Ultimately, the sustainability of any healthcare investment — private equity or otherwise — depends on maintaining both financial discipline and a culture in which clinicians can thrive and stay aligned with the mission.

Scott Becker, JD, CPA, is a nationally recognized healthcare attorney, media founder, and trusted voice in the business of healthcare. A longtime Partner in the Healthcare Department at McGuireWoods LLP, he has spent decades advising hospitals, health systems, ambulatory surgery centers, private equity firms, and physician groups on strategy, transactions, and regulatory matters. He previously served on the firm's Board of Partners and chaired its national Healthcare Department.

Becker is also the Founder and Publisher of Becker's Healthcare and the Founder of Becker Business Media, which together produce some of the most widely read publications, podcasts, and national conferences in the field. What began as a small newsletter has grown into one of the country's most influential platforms for healthcare leaders.

His work bridges law, media, strategy, and leadership in a way few individuals in healthcare can.

Mason's Take

Scott Becker does something important here: he pulls private equity in healthcare away from headlines and ideology and back to fundamentals. Capital isn't the villain — or the savior. What matters is how it's used, where it's used, and who carries the weight when pressure inevitably shows up.

The strongest thread in this piece is the people side of the equation. Healthcare organizations aren't factories or software platforms. They're human systems built on trust, expertise, and professional identity. When financial structures become too heavy — when debt rises or margins tighten — the first cracks often appear not on a balance sheet, but in morale, retention, and silence. Clinicians disengage. Staff stop speaking up. Alignment frays.

That's the reality I see across healthcare regardless of ownership model: sustainability lives at the intersection of financial discipline and human alignment. You can have capital, strategy, and scale, but if the day-to-day experience of clinicians disconnects from the mission, the model eventually strains.

Scott also highlights something the public conversation often misses: private equity isn't monolithic. Some firms bring operational rigor, resources, and discipline that organizations genuinely need. Others apply pressure without understanding the clinical realities beneath the numbers. The difference is often alignment — between investors, leadership, clinicians, and the work itself.

Debt, as Scott explains, is an amplifier. It doesn't automatically create fragility, but it magnifies what is already there. In lower-margin environments or thinly staffed systems, that amplification can quickly become destabilizing.

In the end, the question isn't whether private equity is good or bad for healthcare. The real question is whether the structure supports a system where clinicians can do good work, feel supported, and stay aligned with why they entered healthcare in the first place. When that alignment holds, capital can be a powerful tool. When it doesn't, no amount of capital is enough.

Chapter 40
Masters Series: Preventing the Little Slights

By: **Peter Cappelli, PhD**; George W. Taylor Professor of Management, The Wharton School; Director, Wharton's Center for Human Resources; Workforce Strategy and Talent Management Authority

With **Michael Cappelli**, St. James Medical School

"Even small lapses in respect have measurable effects on performance."

Preventing the Little Slights

In many workplaces, the way managers and leaders interact with those around them has a powerful effect on performance, morale, and trust. This is especially true in healthcare settings, where authority may be less formal on paper but power differences are deeply felt in daily interactions.

Most people understand that overtly abusive behavior — harassment, shouting, or public humiliation — can damage individuals and organizations. What is less obvious is that much smaller, seemingly insignificant moments can have consequences as well. These are not dramatic incidents, but subtle actions that signal a lack of respect.

These small slights are best understood as failures to show due regard for another person. They are directed at individuals rather than groups, and they do not cause material harm. They are different from simple rudeness or carelessness. Leaving a shared space messy may be inconsiderate, but unless it is intentional and personal, it does not rise to the level of a slight. A slight, by contrast, communicates — often unintentionally — that someone does not matter.

What counts as respect depends on context and on reasonable expectations of how people should be treated. Consider a workplace where supervisors are expected to personally acknowledge an employee's birthday by handing them a card. The expectation is not merely that the card arrives, but that the supervisor takes a moment to deliver it directly. When that moment is missed — when the card is left behind or arrives late — the employee may experience it as a signal that they were not worth even a brief pause in the day.

These moments are often unintentional. Leaders may be busy, distracted, or overwhelmed. But intent matters far less than impact. From the employee's perspective, the question is simple: how hard would it have been to take one minute and acknowledge me?

It is important to be clear about what slights are not. They are not defined by how sensitive a person happens to be. Nor does avoiding slights mean avoiding accountability. Leaders must still address poor performance and unmet expectations. Respect does not mean the absence of consequences. It means that correction and critique do not require embarrassment or dismissal.

This distinction is often confused with the idea of psychological safety. Psychological safety does not imply that every idea is a good one or that performance should go unchallenged. It means that when people are asked to take risks — such as offering ideas or raising concerns — they are not punished or demeaned for doing so.

In healthcare, incivility between clinicians and staff is widely recognized, particularly in interactions involving nurses and other frontline professionals. The most obvious examples — shouting, name-calling, or aggressive behavior — are known to affect patient safety, staff wellbeing, and burnout. Less visible, but just as consequential, are the everyday slights that occur within and across professional roles. These behaviors are not limited to one group or hierarchy; they appear wherever power differences exist.

Although slights are less severe than overt incivility, they still matter. Over time, repeated small signals of disregard can erode trust and silence communication. In environments where professional hierarchies are steep, even routine interactions can discourage people from speaking up. When respect is missing, silence often takes its place.

Healthcare work also varies by context. No one expects formal introductions or social niceties during a medical emergency. But emergencies account for only a small portion of the typical workday. Outside those moments, basic acknowledgment and courtesy are neither burdensome nor optional.

Why should leaders pay attention to these small moments? Beyond concern for stress and wellbeing, there are practical reasons. Healthcare relies on communication that is incomplete, informal, and ongoing. If someone has a minor question about an order, will they ask the person who dismissed them earlier in the day? If they notice an administrative issue that could cause trouble later, will they speak up — or decide it is not worth the interaction?

The good news is that preventing these slights requires almost no effort. They often look like this:

• Not making eye contact or responding when greeted (even when busy, this takes seconds)

• Skipping introductions, which can make rotating staff, travelers, and new graduates feel invisible

• Eye-rolling, sighing, or dismissive body language

• Responding to a question with "You should know this" instead of answering first and then explaining

• Offering only collective thanks when individual contributions were clear

• Dismissing a concern raised by a nurse or mid-level professional without explanation

• Enforcing rules without context or inquiry, particularly with students or trainees

• Allowing patients to devalue physician assistants or other clinicians by failing to set expectations

- Blurring the line between staff social interactions and patient-facing spaces in ways that feel exclusionary

The simplest way to avoid these moments is to recognize power differences. Attending physicians, preceptors, and senior leaders hold real authority over staff, students, and trainees. Everyone involved knows who has that authority. They do not need reminders. They pay close attention to words, tone, and behavior.

While friendliness is often well-intended, treating subordinates as peers can be uncomfortable. Humor that feels casual to a leader may feel compulsory to those below them. A remark that would be harmless among friends carries different weight when it comes from someone with power.

A useful analogy comes from outside healthcare. When a team goes out socially, the leader should attend, participate briefly, and then leave. Staying too long may feel enjoyable to the person in charge, but it often has the opposite effect on others, who remain aware that they are being observed and evaluated.

Perhaps the simplest guideline for avoiding slights is to imagine explaining your words or actions to someone whose judgment you trust. The next best step — though harder — is to imagine being on the receiving end.

And if you find yourself thinking, "I endured this when I was starting out, so others should too," pause — and explain that reasoning out loud. The answer usually becomes clear.

About Peter Cappelli

Peter Cappelli, PhD, is the George W. Taylor Professor of Management at The Wharton School of the University of Pennsylvania and Director of Wharton's Center for Human Resources, one of the world's leading hubs for workforce and talent research. Widely regarded as one of the foremost authorities on workforce strategy, talent management, and organizational performance, Professor Cappelli has spent decades shaping how organizations understand hiring, retention, leadership, and the changing nature of work.

Through his research, advisory work, and bestselling books, Professor Cappelli has helped organizations move beyond simplistic staffing models toward evidence-based approaches that align human potential with organizational design. His work is frequently cited in national media and academic literature for bringing clarity to complex workforce challenges, including skills shortages, employee engagement, and long-term workforce sustainability.

His contribution to the Masters Series brings a rigorously grounded, human-centered lens to healthcare's workforce crisis, offering readers a powerful framework for understanding how small moments of respect, leadership behavior, and structural alignment directly influence performance, trust, and retention across clinical environments.

About Michael Cappelli

Michael Cappelli is in his fourth year of medical school at St. James Medical School.

Mason's Take

Professor Cappelli puts words to something healthcare professionals feel every day but rarely name: respect is not abstract — it is operational. The smallest interactions between people quietly shape whether a workplace becomes a place of safety or a place of silence.

What strikes me most is how little it takes to change the trajectory of a person's day, or even their career. A greeting returned. A question answered without condescension. A moment of acknowledgment. These are not soft gestures. They are the scaffolding that allows trust to exist inside high-pressure environments.

In healthcare, where hierarchies are real and stakes are high, small slights carry extra weight. A nurse who is dismissed may not speak up the next time something feels wrong. A student who feels invisible may decide they don't belong. Over time, those quiet moments accumulate, and what disappears is not just morale — it is safety, innovation, and retention.

That is why alignment is not only about matching people to roles. It is also about matching leaders to the responsibility of the power they hold. When leaders understand how their tone, timing, and attention shape the psychological environment around them, they don't just prevent harm — they create the conditions for people to do their best work.

Respect is not an add-on. It is infrastructure. And as Professor Cappelli shows so clearly, even the smallest cracks in that foundation eventually show up in performance, trust, and patient care.

Chapter 41

Masters Series: Your 5-Year Alignment Map: From Milestones to Momentum

By: **Susan Carroll, FACHE, MBA, MHA**

President, Inova Loudoun Hospital; Senior Vice President, Inova Health System

Your 5-Year Alignment Map: From Milestones to Momentum

I didn't plan every step of my career. But I always had a compass. That compass — my sense of purpose, my values, and my responsibility to those I serve — has guided me through every change and challenge.

Alignment, to me, isn't a destination. It's the discipline of returning to your purpose every time the landscape shifts. It's what carried me from my start in Business Affairs to hospital president. And it's what carried our entire team to this moment: Inova Loudoun Hospital has officially been designated a Level II Trauma Center — and has now achieved its fifth consecutive Magnet® designation.

Both milestones symbolize the same truth: when purpose, people, and process are aligned, excellence becomes repeatable.

Defining Alignment in Action

Alignment isn't about control — it's about coherence. In healthcare, so many moving parts can pull us off-center: regulation, technology, recruitment, reimbursement, burnout. The work never slows down. But alignment allows us to move fast without coming apart.

At Inova Loudoun, we align around one core promise: to provide world-class care close to home. Every expansion, certification, and recognition is a reflection of that compass. Alignment means leading from values rather than reacting to pressure. It means asking why before how. It means having the courage to re-center when success tempts us off-balance.

Level II: What It Means and Why It Matters

When we became a Level II Trauma Center, it wasn't about prestige — it was about proximity. A Level II Trauma Center provides 24/7 access to trauma surgeons, anesthesiologists, critical care, neurosurgery, orthopedics, and emergency surgery — all within minutes.

It delivers nearly the same level of capability as a Level I academic trauma center but focuses fully on clinical outcomes rather than teaching volume. In real life, that means fewer transfers. It means faster intervention. It means families in Loudoun County no longer have to travel elsewhere for the highest level of trauma care. Seconds that used to cost lives now save them.

But alignment made it possible. Every service line had to coordinate; every nurse, physician, and technologist had to calibrate to the same rhythm. Alignment is the hidden architecture of readiness.

At the reception celebrating our designation, I watched our trauma nurses and ED staff — people who've trained, drilled, and sacrificed for years — take in the moment. That night wasn't about a plaque. It was about purpose realized through alignment.

Magnet® Five Times: The Power of Sustained Alignment

Before Level II, there was Magnet® — and it remains the heartbeat of who we are. To have achieved five consecutive Magnet® designations, and now Magnet® with Distinction accompanied by fifteen exemplars, is not just a milestone; it is elite. Fewer than one percent of U.S. hospitals have reached this level of sustained nursing excellence — an honor shared by only a few dozen institutions nationwide.

Each Magnet® era has marked a chapter in our story of alignment: the first proved our potential; the second confirmed our consistency; the third strengthened our systems; the fourth elevated our outcomes — and the fifth, now recognized as Magnet® with Distinction, redefines what's possible and codifies fifteen exemplars as a new standard of excellence.

This journey is a living validation that our culture doesn't just support shared governance, evidence-based practice, and professional autonomy — it breathes them. Magnet® is not a medal we hang on the wall; it's the mirror we hold to ourselves. It asks the hard questions: Are we still living our values? Are we elevating the voices closest to the bedside? Are we aligning every decision to our promise of world-class care, close to home?

Our nurses have taught us that alignment isn't top-down — it's side-by-side. It's the quiet courage to speak up, the collective discipline to improve, and the shared pride in every patient's story. Alignment isn't declared; it's demonstrated — shift by shift, story by story, life by life.

Magnet® at Inova Loudoun isn't a title we keep. It's a standard we keep raising.

Leading Through Growth Without Losing Your Center

Loudoun County remains one of the nation's fastest-growing communities. As the population evolved, so did the hospital — from a small regional facility to a high-performing, full-service institution.

Years ago, we purchased fifty acres of land before we had a need for it. That decision — questioned by some at the time — was alignment in action. We saw where the community was headed and positioned ourselves ahead of it. That foresight now enables expansion without disruption.

But infrastructure isn't the hard part. Maintaining alignment while growing — that's the real leadership test. Growth can fragment people's sense of belonging. My responsibility is to make sure every expansion plan is matched by cultural cohesion.

We don't grow away from our people; we grow with them. That's why I walk the floors, listen more than I speak, and remind our teams: your alignment is our greatest infrastructure.

System Alignment: Local Depth, Regional Reach

My dual role — as President of Loudoun and Senior Vice President for Inova Health System — means I straddle both micro and macro views. I lead locally but must think systemically.

During the height of COVID-19, I also oversaw supply chain and emergency management for the system — two functions that became lifelines when the world's supply routes broke down. Those months redefined leadership under pressure. We built new vendor pipelines overnight, protected caregiver safety amid PPE shortages, and kept hospitals supplied when global inventories ran dry.

That experience changed how I view alignment forever. Because when supply chains collapse, relationships become the true logistics network.

Today, my portfolio focuses on security, emergency management, and patient support services — each function still rooted in that same lesson. Alignment doesn't remove crisis; it gives you a shared language to navigate one.

The Alignment Map: A Framework for Intentional Leadership

Every few years, I revisit what I call my Alignment Map — a five-year cycle of reflection, recalibration, and readiness. It's not a strategic plan; it's a compass check.

• **Purpose Alignment** — Reconfirm your why. Does your work still reflect your values?

- **People Alignment** — Are the right voices shaping decisions, especially from the front line?

- **Performance Alignment** — Are your metrics measuring what truly matters?

- **Process Alignment** — Do your systems support — or suffocate — innovation?

- **Personal Alignment** — Are you leading from clarity, or from exhaustion?

I share this with emerging leaders often. The most dangerous misalignment is the silent one — the slow drift between what you do and why you do it.

Recognition and Renewal

Being named one of Washington, D.C.'s Most Powerful Women this year was deeply humbling. I don't see it as personal power; I see it as collective alignment made visible.

Every recognition reflects the unseen work of hundreds of people pulling in the same direction. At the Level II celebration, I looked out at my team — nurses, surgeons, techs, transporters, environmental services, leaders — and I thought: this is what alignment looks like in real time.

A thousand small commitments converging into one big moment of purpose. That night, I didn't think about the years behind us. I thought about the five years ahead.

Looking Forward: Sustaining Alignment Through Change

Alignment is not permanent; it's a practice. The next era of healthcare will bring new models, technologies, and challenges. We'll need to align faster, listen deeper, and care broader.

If the last five years were about building readiness, the next five are about building resilience.

And as we move forward — with Level II secured and our fifth Magnet® milestone achieved — our compass hasn't changed: lead with integrity, plan with intention, and align every decision to the people who trust us with their lives.

About Susan Carroll

Susan Carroll, FACHE, MBA, MHA, serves as Senior Vice President of Inova Health System and President of Inova Loudoun Hospital, where she leads a 200+-bed community hospital while also overseeing key system-wide functions. In more than two decades at Inova, she has served as president of each of the system's five hospitals — an exceptional span of leadership responsibility across the enterprise.

Carroll holds a Bachelor of Arts in Social Science and Finance from Radford University and dual master's degrees — an MBA and an MHA — from Ohio University. In 2025, *Washingtonian* magazine named her one of the "Most Powerful Women in Washington," recognizing her impact on regional healthcare and community leadership. Her contribution to the Masters Series reflects the vantage point of a system executive who has led at every rung of the ladder while staying deeply rooted in community-based care.

Mason's Take

Inova Loudoun Hospital is doing something that too many organizations talk about and too few actually deliver: proving, year after year, that alignment isn't a slogan — it's a system. Their newest accomplishment, a Magnet® with Distinction recognition that includes fifteen exemplars, signals a new level of nursing excellence that only the most disciplined, values-driven hospitals ever touch. It's rare air — and Inova Loudoun isn't visiting; they're living there.

What strikes me most is how seamlessly this achievement fits into the story Susan Carroll tells. Alignment at Inova Loudoun isn't episodic. It's engineered. It's protected. It's renewed. Becoming a Level II Trauma Center and earning a fifth consecutive Magnet® designation aren't isolated milestones — they're outcomes of a workforce and leadership team moving in the same direction, guided by the same compass, and unwilling to compromise on the quality of care their community receives.

Hospitals don't accidentally achieve Magnet® five times. They don't stumble into Level II Trauma readiness. And they certainly don't produce fifteen exemplars — exemplary performances recognized during the Magnet® appraisal — without a culture that breathes shared governance, data-driven improvement, and authentic listening to the voices closest to the bedside.

Susan's Alignment Map captures what every healthcare leader should be doing: stepping back every few years to recalibrate their purpose, people, performance, processes, and personal clarity. Alignment isn't about perfection; it's about continuous course correction — the willingness to stay tethered to your why even as your environment evolves.

And here's the part that resonates most: growth didn't dilute Inova Loudoun's identity. It sharpened it. They expanded infrastructure without drifting from their center — something that separates organizations that scale with integrity from those that grow into misalignment and eventually collapse under their own weight.

When Susan writes about the Level II celebration — trauma nurses, ED teams, environmental services, transporters, surgeons, leaders — you feel the truth of it: alignment is visible in the room long before it shows up on the résumé.

That's the real lesson here. Excellence isn't a plaque. It's a practice.

Inova Loudoun now stands as one of the few hospitals in the nation to achieve Magnet® at this level, and even fewer to do it with the expanded distinction and fifteen exemplars. That is not just success — that is stewardship. That is leadership. That is alignment in its purest form.

Hospitals everywhere talk about culture. Inova Loudoun proves what it looks like.

Chapter 42

Masters Series: Physician Alignment: The Power of Purpose Over Position

By: **David S. Goldberg, BA, MS**

President and CEO, Mon Health and Davis Health Systems; Executive Vice President, Vandalia Health

Physician Alignment: The Power of Purpose Over Position

When people ask what keeps me up at night, my answer is simple: alignment.

Not revenue, not volume, not the next merger announcement. Alignment — between physicians and their organizations, between mission and strategy, between what we say and how we act. Because when alignment breaks down, everything else starts to fray.

In my years leading Mon Health and now Vandalia Health, I've learned that physician alignment is not a buzzword. It's the bloodstream of any successful healthcare system. If you want to deliver consistent, compassionate, high-quality care, you need clinicians and leaders moving in the same direction — not just in theory, but in heart.

And at its core, that means this: physician alignment is human alignment.

It's about trust, communication, and shared purpose — the same ingredients that make a family, a team, or a community thrive. Without those, strategy collapses into slogans.

The Heart of Alignment

The first thing I tell new physicians joining Mon Health is that we're not just a network of facilities. We're a collection of relationships.

Patients don't experience healthcare as departments or service lines; they experience it as a series of human connections. So if those connections are fractured internally — if our physicians feel unheard, unempowered, or misaligned — patients feel it immediately.

Alignment starts with conversation. I meet with physician leaders regularly — not because it's a checkbox, but because leadership can't be effective from a distance. Every month, I hold an early morning meeting with our medical directors, medical staff leaders, and physician group heads. No agenda too polished, no topic off-limits. We talk about what's working, what's frustrating, and what would make care better for the people of West Virginia.

It's 6:30 a.m., coffee in hand, and what happens in those rooms is the truest form of strategy I know: physicians, nurses, and executives telling the truth to each other. That's where alignment begins.

The Post-Merger Test

When Mon Health merged with Charleston Area Medical Center to create Vandalia Health, we faced a question that defines modern healthcare: how do you scale up without losing your soul?

Every integration tests alignment. It asks people who once operated independently to now think and act collectively. And that's hard — especially for physicians who chose community-based medicine because they value autonomy, personal connection, and local decision-making.

From day one, I made a promise to our teams: We will grow, but we will not homogenize.

The purpose of integration was to share resources, expand reach, and increase access — not to erase the unique character of our hospitals. We standardized what should be standardized (supply chains, technology platforms, financial infrastructure), but we protected what should never be standardized — our relationships, our culture, our physician voice.

We call it **systemness with soul**. It means every physician, whether in Morgantown or rural Nicholas County, feels heard and respected. It means that local medical councils still make decisions about patient flow, quality priorities, and schedules. It means that being part of something larger doesn't mean losing what made you join in the first place.

That's alignment in action — not forcing everyone into the same mold, but helping everyone see themselves in the mission.

Lessons From the Field

If you've ever led physicians, you know they don't align because you tell them to. They align because they believe you're listening, you're transparent, and you share their purpose.

I learned this lesson years ago walking hospital halls during a late-night shift. One of our emergency physicians stopped me and said, "David, every time we talk about alignment, it sounds like corporate speak. But what I really want is to know that my work still matters, that you understand what I see every night."

That conversation changed how I lead. Alignment isn't about compliance. It's about meaning. It's about making sure every physician can answer three questions with confidence:

1 Do I know the mission?

2 Do I believe in it?

3 Do I see myself in it?

When any one of those answers slips, misalignment creeps in — quietly at first, then pervasively.

Alignment as a Two-Way Street

Physician alignment is not about control; it's about partnership. It's not leadership talking at clinicians — it's leadership walking with them.

At Mon Health, that means physicians aren't just implementers of strategy; they help create it. They sit on committees that decide how we reinvest capital, where to expand services, how to improve quality, and what technology to adopt.

We've also been intentional about giving physicians access to real performance data — not as punishment, but as empowerment. When clinicians see metrics connected to outcomes they care about, they engage. When they're left in the dark, frustration grows.

Transparency builds trust. And trust builds alignment.

The Cultural Compact

Alignment has to live in the culture, not just the contract.

You can write the best employment agreements in the world, but if your culture is toxic, misalignment will eat those contracts alive.

That's why we've worked hard to build what I call a **cultural compact** — a mutual understanding between leadership and clinicians:

• We promise to listen and resource.

• You promise to engage and lead.

• We promise to tell the truth, even when it's hard.

• You promise to do the same.

It's not about hierarchy; it's about shared ownership.

We want our physicians to feel like owners, not employees. Owners speak up when something's wrong. Owners mentor others. Owners stay. That sense of ownership doesn't just improve retention — it transforms morale.

When physicians feel aligned, the tone of an entire organization changes. You can feel it in the way teams greet each other, the speed at which problems get solved, and the way patients are treated. It's contagious — in the best possible way.

The Cost of Misalignment

Misalignment is expensive.

It shows up in turnover, in disengagement, in poor patient experience scores, and in slow adoption of best practices. It's not always loud — sometimes it hides in the pauses between words. You hear it when physicians say, "I used to love this place." You see it when meetings turn into debates instead of dialogues.

Replacing a single physician can cost hundreds of thousands of dollars. Rebuilding lost trust can take years. But fixing alignment starts with one consistent act: showing up.

When leaders stop showing up, misalignment grows roots.

The best way to rebuild it is by being visible — rounding, listening, asking questions, and following through. Physicians don't need executives to be perfect. They need them to be present.

What Alignment Feels Like

When physician alignment is strong, everything changes. Communication flows more easily. Silos shrink. Teams start finishing each other's sentences.

At Mon Health, we've seen how alignment fuels innovation. A cardiologist in one hospital develops a new workflow for reducing readmissions, and within weeks it spreads across the region. A surgeon collaborates with our nursing and tech teams to reimagine perioperative safety. A family medicine group designs a pilot for chronic care management that improves diabetic control rates across the network.

That's alignment in action — when good ideas don't need permission to move, only support to scale.

Aligned organizations feel different to patients too. The handoffs are smoother. The tone is calmer. The "we" outweighs the "me."

You can't fake that.

Kindness as Alignment's Compass

I've learned that kindness is the truest indicator of alignment. When people are aligned with their purpose, they have capacity for kindness. When they're not, kindness evaporates first.

In my last essay, I wrote that if you can't give your best on someone's worst day, you might be in the wrong lane of healthcare. The same holds true for leadership. If we can't be kind under pressure, we've lost the plot.

Kindness isn't weakness; it's alignment expressed through behavior. It's what happens when you know you're in the right place, doing work that matters, surrounded by people who share your values.

That's why alignment isn't just a business strategy. It's a moral one.

When physicians are aligned — with the mission, with their teams, with their sense of calling — kindness thrives naturally. And when kindness thrives, quality follows.

Alignment Is Personal

Alignment isn't one size fits all. Some physicians find meaning in the high tempo of acute care. Others find it in the long relationships of primary care, the precision of surgery, or the quiet vigilance of radiology. The point isn't to force everyone into the same rhythm; it's to help each person find where their rhythm fits best within the symphony.

When I speak to medical students or residents, I always remind them: find the environment that aligns with your heart, not just your résumé.

If you're a problem-solver who loves systems thinking, maybe you belong in leadership or informatics. If you're an empath who thrives on connection, maybe community practice is your calling. If you love research, teach. If you love motion, join emergency care.

The only wrong choice is ignoring misalignment and staying stuck in the wrong fit. Because misalignment doesn't just hurt you; it hurts the patients who depend on your full attention.

Leadership in Alignment

True alignment doesn't start in the boardroom. It starts at the bedside, in the clinic, in the places where care is delivered.

As leaders, our job isn't to dictate alignment — it's to earn it. Every day. Through our decisions, our transparency, and our follow-through.

Alignment is not a project. It's a posture. It's how we show up for one another — physician to nurse, administrator to tech, leader to patient.

I've seen what happens when alignment takes hold. Innovation accelerates. Communication simplifies. Culture heals.

And that's what we're trying to build at Vandalia Health: a system where people don't just work for a paycheck or a logo, but for a shared purpose.

Because at the end of the day, no matter how advanced the technology or how complex the merger, healthcare still comes down to trust between people — and alignment is how that trust takes root.

A Final Word

If you strip away the titles and the org charts, physician alignment is about belonging. It's about knowing you are part of something bigger than yourself, and that your contribution matters.

When physicians, nurses, and leaders are aligned, they create care environments where patients feel safe — not just clinically, but emotionally. That's the kind of healthcare people remember.

So let's stop talking about alignment like it's a corporate initiative. Let's start treating it like what it truly is — the soul of our profession.

Because when alignment is strong, kindness follows. And when kindness leads, healing happens.

· · ·

About David S. Goldberg

David S. Goldberg, BA, MS, is President and CEO of Mon Health System and Executive Vice President of Vandalia Health, bringing nearly two decades of senior healthcare leadership experience to his role. He has led hospitals, service lines, and regional networks across competitive markets, including prior senior leadership roles at Allegheny Health Network (Highmark Health) and in home and community services.

Goldberg's leadership is marked by a strong focus on physician partnership, community-based care, and system integration. He is deeply engaged in regional economic development as well as clinical strategy, reflecting a belief that hospitals are not just care sites but economic and social anchors for their communities. His contribution to the Masters Series brings a pragmatic, operations-plus-mission lens to system leadership and growth.

Mason's Take

David Goldberg understands something most people in healthcare only talk about: alignment isn't a management theory — it's a heartbeat. When he writes that "physician alignment is human alignment," you can feel the truth of it. That's the kind of statement that belongs on the wall of every hospital boardroom.

I've watched David lead with quiet authority and visible empathy — the rare kind of executive who still walks the halls, listens before he speaks, and remembers that culture isn't created by memos; it's created by moments. His idea of systemness with soul might be one of the most powerful phrases in modern healthcare. It says you can grow without losing who you are — and that purpose must always outrank position.

What I love most about this piece is how human it is. It's not written from the top down; it's written from the inside out. David doesn't describe alignment as a checkbox or a KPI — he describes it as kindness, belonging, and meaning. That's exactly what we're trying to restore through **SCRUB***fit***™** and through this book: to remind everyone that alignment isn't a slogan. It's how healing happens — between clinicians, between leaders, and between purpose and person.

Chapter 43
Masters Series: The Path I Didn't Plan

By: **Jon Macaskill**

Former U.S. Navy SEAL; Leadership Coach; Host, *Men Talking Mindfulness*

At 18, I had one plan: get into the United States Naval Academy and become a Navy SEAL officer.

I didn't get in.

I had done well academically and athletically, but I put all my eggs in one basket — the United States Naval Academy — and when that door closed, it felt like my entire future had closed with it. I couldn't afford college, and I hadn't lined up scholarships or financial aid. So I enlisted in the Navy at 19 and started again from the bottom, swallowing my pride and telling myself I'd find another way in.

That "detour" became a theme in my life.

From the enlisted ranks, I earned a Naval Reserve Officers Training Corps scholarship to Tulane. I almost took it. Then,

465

one year after being turned down by the Naval Academy, something unexpected happened — I received a Secretary of the Navy nomination and an appointment to the United States Naval Academy. I took it.

And then I hit the wall.

At the Academy, I struggled. First semester, I almost failed out. I wasn't just tired — I was exposed. Surrounded by people who looked like they belonged, I felt like the guy who snuck in through the side door and was about to get caught. I wanted to quit. Instead, I did the less heroic thing, the thing that actually works: I asked for help. I got tutors for calculus and chemistry, rebuilt my foundation, and kept going. The next semester I earned a 3.2, and I stayed above that the rest of my time there.

I still wanted to become a Navy SEAL — but at the time, only sixteen men per class were selected. Going into senior year, I wasn't one of the top sixteen.

That stung.

So I used it.

I worked on everything — fitness, leadership, balance, discipline, the boring details that don't show up in highlight reels. By the end, I was one of the sixteen.

Then came Navy SEAL training — Basic Underwater Demolition/SEAL training — the program that turns candidates into SEALs.

People ask me what it's like, and the honest answer is: it's designed to make you question who you are. It's long days that blur together, constant cold, constant discomfort, constant fatigue. Your body is wrecked, your mind is loud, and the environment keeps asking the same question in a hundred different ways: will you quit, or will you keep moving?

Once again, I struggled.

I wasn't good on the obstacle course and everyone knew it. In a place where weakness is obvious and excuses are useless, that kind of visibility feels brutal. The instructors watched me like I was a problem they were waiting to solve. I could feel the microscope on my back every time I stepped up.

So I went back to what had saved me before: humility and reps.

I found a "tutor." A fellow student showed me the tricks of the obstacle course — the small adjustments that mattered, the hand placements, the pacing, the things you don't learn from just wanting it badly enough. I got better. Not fast... but faster. I graduated. I went to the SEAL Teams.

Professionally, I did well. Personally, I didn't. My first marriage was strained and eventually fell apart. Later, I remarried. Now I have three young kids. I struggle regularly as a dad... but I reset every day. That's real life — you don't "arrive." You recommit.

Along the way, I also developed a deep connection to medicine and caregiving. In the military, I trained in Tactical Combat Casualty Care — emergency trauma care under pressure, when seconds matter and you don't get perfect conditions. I've also been part of a medical and spiritual mission trip to Nepal, where I served as one of the team's "dentists." I got a crash course in injections and pulling teeth, and then did that work for several weeks. There's nothing theoretical about helping someone in pain when you're working outside your comfort zone. You learn how to steady your hands. You learn how to stay calm. You learn how to be useful.

I've also done work with medical schools and have done some teaching for the Hospital for Special Surgery in New York City. I've got additional work lined up with the Anschutz Medical Campus here in Colorado. Healthcare has been part of my life in more ways than people might assume — and it's part of my home life too. My wife is an orthopedic physician assistant, so we live close to the realities of medicine, recovery, and what it takes to carry responsibility for other people.

In 2020, I retired from the military with what I thought was a solid plan.

But my first job failed.

Then I started a business with no idea what I was doing. Honestly... I still don't a lot of the time.

Now, I've found my stride. But I also know I'll lose it again. I'll stumble, maybe even trip.

The point is: life is not linear.

You're going to have setbacks, need help, take second chances, and learn humility. You're going to get knocked down — and realize that falling behind doesn't mean you're done. Sometimes it just means you're being redirected.

Looking back, I don't think the lesson is "never fail." I think the lesson is learning how to find alignment again — between who you are, what you're doing, and the life you're trying to build — even after you've been knocked off course.

And if there's one thing I've learned — in the SEAL Teams, in family life, and in the moments I've worked alongside healthcare teams — it's that the goal isn't to force yourself into the life you first imagined. The goal is to keep moving toward work and environments where you can actually thrive, contribute, and stay whole. That's alignment. And it's something you earn one reset at a time.

Jon Macaskill is a former U.S. Navy SEAL, leadership coach, and host of *Men Talking Mindfulness*, a podcast focused on the mental, physical, and emotional wellbeing of leaders. His work intersects with healthcare through training in Tactical Combat Casualty Care, service on a medical mission trip to Nepal supporting hands-on clinical care, and teaching engagements including the Hospital for Special Surgery in New York City. He has also worked with medical schools and has upcoming engagements through the Anschutz Medical Campus in Colorado.

Jon lives close to the realities of healthcare not only professionally but personally — his wife is an orthopedic physician assistant, and together they are raising three young children. That combination of frontline medicine, leadership under pressure, and life at home informs his perspective on resilience, purpose, and the importance of alignment between who we are, the work we do, and the lives we are trying to build.

Mason's Take

What Jon Macaskill lays out in *The Path I Didn't Plan* is not just a military story — it is a *human one about alignment, resilience, and reinvention.*

To put it in perspective: becoming a Navy SEAL is not a casual goal or a weekend challenge. It begins with rigorous screening and physical standards just to even enter the pipeline, and then progresses into Basic Underwater Demolition/SEAL training — a six-month crucible designed to push candidates to the physical and psychological limits. Navy SEAL training has historically seen attrition rates of 70–80 percent or more, meaning the majority of those who start never finish.

Jon didn't just take on that monumental challenge — he embraced it more than once. He struggled at every turn, from the Naval Academy to SEAL selection and through the grueling days of SEAL training, including the infamous "Hell Week" that crushes even the strongest bodies and minds. What makes his story remarkable isn't that he survived these ordeals — it's that he *kept adapting*, finding help where he needed it, learning from peers, and refusing to quit.

This is where Jon's experience intersects with where so many of us live our lives. Most of us will never wear a Trident or endure a cadre-led evolution on a California beach. But we *do* know disappointment: we've missed opportunities, watched plans fall apart, and struggled with identity when life didn't go the way we thought it would. What separates the stories that become wisdom from the stories that become regret is not never failing — it's how you *respond* when you do. Jon's journey shows us exactly that.

He never gave up on his intentions, even when the path shifted under his feet — and that is why this piece belongs in a book about alignment. Jon didn't just chase a dream. He learned how to lean into the work of becoming himself, again and again. That's the kind of strength that resonates not because it's rare — but because it's universal.

Chapter 44

Masters Series: Magnet® and the Alignment Advantage: How ANCC's Gold Standard Shapes Healthcare Careers

By: **Dr. M. Maureen Lal, DNP, MSN, RN**

Senior Director, Magnet Recognition Program®, ANCC

What Magnet® Really Means

Walk into a Magnet-recognized hospital and you can sense the difference before anyone explains it. The atmosphere feels steady, focused, intentional. Conversations between nurses and leaders sound like collaboration rather than command. Even the pace of care seems synchronized. That feeling is not coincidence — it's what alignment looks like when it comes to life inside an organization.

At its core, the Magnet® Recognition Program, created by the American Nurses Credentialing Center (ANCC), is not an award to display in a lobby. It's a living framework that aligns people, purpose, and practice. It measures not only what outcomes a hospital achieves, but how it achieves them — through empowered nursing practice, shared decision-making, and leadership that listens.

From Name to Nature

"Magnet" began as a way to describe hospitals that naturally attract and retain nurses. Today, Magnet® goes far beyond recruitment. It represents a discipline: the ongoing practice of aligning mission, model, and meaning so every caregiver feels connected to something larger than the shift or the task.

Magnet® hospitals don't just talk about nursing as a pillar of quality; they show that nursing drives quality. Every standard in the framework asks for proof that nurses influence outcomes, participate in decision-making, and advance professionally within a culture that values learning and voice. That is what makes Magnet® rare. It is not built on slogans or glossy branding. It's built on systems that invite nurses into the organization's story — not as spectators, but as authors.

Alignment as a Living System

In healthcare, alignment means more than agreement; it means integration. The Magnet® framework connects the Donabedian Model of structure, process, and outcome into a continuous circle of improvement. It links the bedside to the boardroom so leadership priorities and frontline realities inform each other.

In a Magnet® hospital, decisions aren't just handed down; they're built upward. Nurses serve on councils, bring forward problems worth solving, follow the evidence, and partner to improve patient outcomes. That alignment creates coherence: the organization's mission matches the daily experience of those delivering care. When nurses know their expertise is valued and their perspective is heard, engagement grows naturally. Alignment turns the workplace from a place of endurance into a place of evolution.

Recognition That Renews Purpose

Recognition in a Magnet® culture isn't a ceremony; it's a conversation. It lives in everyday exchanges where leaders and clinicians notice, name, and celebrate excellence in real time.

When leaders intentionally recognize nurses — not with generic praise, but with clear acknowledgment of judgment, compassion, and critical thinking — alignment begins to breathe again. Recognition restores connection. It re-centers people on purpose.

This is why the Magnet® model treats recognition as essential, not optional. Alignment can fade under fatigue; purpose must be renewed through moments of meaning. When people feel seen, they remember why they chose healthcare — and why they choose to stay.

Professional Practice as a Map

Every Magnet® organization defines a Professional Practice Model — its own map of nursing identity, theory, and values. That model guides how care is delivered, how decisions are made, and how outcomes are measured.

In many hospitals, a practice model can feel abstract. In a Magnet® hospital, it becomes a living document. Staff can describe it, illustrate it, and point to how it shapes their work. It's the architecture of alignment, showing how nursing knowledge supports both individual growth and organizational goals.

Shared decision-making is the bloodstream that keeps that model alive. Through councils and committees, ideas circulate; barriers surface and are addressed, allowing innovation to take root. Decision-making here isn't about hierarchy; it's shared responsibility. When bedside insight meets executive strategy, the system learns and adapts faster. Alignment becomes visible — in safer care, smoother communication, and stronger professional relationships.

Transparency, Trust, and a Just Culture

A hallmark of Magnet® leadership is transparency. Leaders share outcomes openly — the triumphs, the setbacks, and the lessons in between. Openness reinforces a Just Culture, where the goal of data is understanding, not punishment.

In that environment, trust becomes a renewable resource. Nurses speak up without fear, ask questions without judgment, and become part of solutions instead of statistics. Transparency transforms accountability into collaboration. When information flows freely, alignment strengthens. Teams start to see data not as a scorecard, but as a mirror reflecting the organization's shared commitment to excellence. The question shifts from "Who caused this?" to "What can we learn from this?" — and that shift is where culture changes.

How Magnet® Shapes Healthcare Careers

For the individual nurse, Magnet® alignment translates into opportunity.

Early-career nurses enter practice in environments that invest in mentorship and continuing education. They learn quickly that their insights matter, even before years of experience accumulate.

Mid-career nurses find pathways that allow them to grow without leaving their purpose behind — specialty practice, education, informatics, care coordination, clinical leadership. They experience an organization that encourages evolution rather than forcing exit.

Advanced-practice nurses and nurse leaders work within a culture already primed for inquiry. They can champion innovation, redesign care processes, and trust their teams to participate in change. Magnet® doesn't just develop nurses; it develops systems where nurses thrive.

This alignment across career stages creates continuity: a rhythm of mentorship, mastery, and meaning that anchors talent and keeps purpose alive.

The Leadership Link

Magnet® leadership is not about title; it's about tone. Leaders model curiosity, humility, and accessibility. They listen to understand, not just to respond. They translate strategy into human terms and ensure improvement feels participatory, not imposed.

The best Magnet® leaders use recognition as feedback and data as dialogue. They build credibility through alignment — showing that the organization's goals and a nurse's goals are the same: safety, compassion, learning, and excellence. In turn, that leadership style attracts professionals who want to grow — those who view healthcare not only as a career, but as a calling worthy of constant renewal.

Why Magnet® Still Matters

Healthcare is always changing — technology advances, roles evolve, expectations rise. What remains constant is the need for alignment: people who know their purpose and organizations that know how to support it.

Magnet® provides a roadmap for both. It codifies what alignment looks like when it's working: leaders who listen, nurses who influence, and outcomes that reflect collaboration instead of coincidence. In that sense, Magnet® isn't merely a recognition program — it's a philosophy of belonging. It teaches that the greatest form of excellence is consistency: when the promise on the wall matches the practice at the bedside.

The Alignment Advantage

When alignment becomes cultural, careers become sustainable. Nurses stay not because of incentives, but because they feel seen, safe, and significant. Teams collaborate more freely because trust replaces hierarchy. Leaders rediscover the joy of shaping environments where others can succeed.

That's the quiet power of Magnet®. It proves that excellence in healthcare isn't an act; it's an ecosystem — one sustained by trust, purpose, and alignment. And when that ecosystem thrives, so do the people within it, one aligned decision, one meaningful recognition, one shared purpose at a time.

Dr. M. Maureen Lal serves as Senior Director of the Magnet Recognition Program® at the American Nurses Credentialing Center, where she helps shape and steward standards for nursing excellence worldwide. A nurse for more than 30 years, she joined the Magnet program in 2010 and has held multiple leadership roles within the organization.

Her work focuses on supporting organizations in creating healthy work environments, meaningful nurse recognition, and cultures of professional practice that elevate both outcomes and engagement. She frequently represents Magnet® in global forums, emphasizing ethics, recognition, and the power of professional nursing standards to transform care. Her contribution to the Masters Series brings a systems-level view of what "excellence" really means in nursing — beyond awards and into everyday practice.

Mason's Take

Every time I walk into a Magnet® hospital, I am reminded that alignment is not an abstract ideal — it is a lived experience. You can feel it in the way nurses speak to one another, in the steadiness of the unit, in the confidence that rises not from hierarchy but from shared purpose. Dr. Lal names something here that many people overlook: Magnet® is not about prestige; it is about coherence. It is the rare moment in healthcare when the mission, the model, and the meaning all face the same direction.

What strikes me most is how deeply human this framework is. At its heart, Magnet® is a promise that nurses will not be treated as interchangeable labor but as partners who shape outcomes, elevate standards, and carry the organization's story forward. In my own work, I argue that people don't burn out because they care too much — they burn out because the places they work stop aligning with who they are. Magnet® is one of the few large-scale systems that interrupts that pattern. It translates alignment into structures nurses can touch: shared governance that actually shares, recognition that actually restores, leadership that actually listens.

And when that alignment holds — when identity, environment, and choice all point in the same direction — you can feel the shift. Nurses stay. Teams stabilize. Purpose returns. Dr. Lal captures that beautifully. Magnet® isn't a destination. It is a discipline. A way of building workplaces where the promise on the wall finally matches the practice at the bedside. And for anyone charting a healthcare career, that difference is everything.

Chapter 45

Masters Series: Aligning the Future of Nursing — From Bedside to Virtual

By: **Patricia J. Mook, DNP, RN, NEA-BC, CAHIMS, CAVRN, FAONL**

Senior nurse executive with enterprise-wide leadership in nursing operations, professional development, and clinical education; Adjunct Faculty, UAB School of Nursing

Aligning the Future of Nursing — From Bedside to Virtual

When I began my career, "virtual nursing" wasn't in our vocabulary. Nursing was something you did in person — by the bedside, through touch, tone, and time spent. Every detail mattered: the way a patient gripped your hand, the rhythm of a breath, the look in someone's eyes when reassurance finally landed.

Today, nursing looks and feels different — but its essence hasn't changed. Our tools have evolved, our environments have expanded, and our reach has grown beyond walls and zip codes. Technology, once viewed with skepticism, has become one of our most powerful allies in restoring balance to the profession. This shift isn't about moving away from what nursing has always been. It's about expanding it — aligning the heart of nursing with the realities and possibilities of modern care.

When Nursing Really Began to Change

During the height of the COVID-19 pandemic, our teams faced exhaustion unlike anything we'd ever experienced. Hallway lights glowed through the night, monitors chimed nonstop, and we carried the weight of both science and sorrow. Amid the chaos, one truth became undeniable: we had to find a way to keep nurses connected — to their teams, their patients, and their purpose — even when distance became a matter of safety.

That was the seed of transformation. We began experimenting with new care models — pairing experienced nurses working remotely with bedside teams through secure video, shared documentation platforms, and real-time data monitoring. At first, it felt unconventional. Could a nurse not physically in the room still make a meaningful impact? The answer, we quickly learned, was a resounding yes.

Virtual nurses began supporting admissions, managing discharges, completing chart reviews, and monitoring for subtle early warning signs. They became the ever-present second set of eyes, anticipating needs before alarms sounded. Bedside nurses, freed from layers of administrative strain, could stay closer to the work that mattered most.

It wasn't just efficiency we discovered — it was renewal. I watched seasoned nurses who had once contemplated retirement rediscover their spark. I saw early-career nurses gain confidence knowing an expert was just a video call away. And perhaps most strikingly, I saw teams who had been running on fumes begin to breathe again. It became clear that we weren't only rethinking workflow; we were redefining alignment.

Defining a New Kind of Practice

As this new model matured, it became evident that we needed more than enthusiasm — we needed standards. We needed to describe, define, and credential what virtual nursing was becoming. Together with national nursing leaders, we worked to outline the core competencies that make virtual practice distinct: clinical surveillance, data literacy, ethics, communication, teamwork, and the ever-elusive skill of maintaining presence through a screen.

That collaboration led to the creation of the Certified Acute-Care Virtual Registered Nurse (CAVRN) credential through the Medical-Surgical Nursing Certification Board — the first of its kind in the nation. It wasn't about adding a title to a name badge; it was about affirming that this new practice met the same rigor, safety, and accountability as bedside care.

Developing that framework required hundreds of hours of discussion and debate. What does "virtual critical thinking" look like? How do we measure empathy across a camera? What ethical standards must guide remote decision-making? Each question forced us to articulate what we intuitively knew — that nursing is less about where we stand and more about how we serve.

The process reminded me of nursing's long tradition of adaptation and validation of knowledge. From the shift to electronic records to the emergence of new specialties, our profession has always evolved to meet need with integrity. The CAVRN certification became one of those symbols of that commitment: not a replacement for bedside nursing, but a recognition that connection takes many forms.

Alignment Over Replacement

Virtual nursing is not about replacement — it's about redistribution. For decades, the profession has faced an imbalance: too few nurses at the bedside, too much administrative burden, and too little flexibility for nurses navigating life changes, caregiving responsibilities, or late-career transitions.

Virtual nursing can help correct that imbalance. It allows experienced nurses to remain active in the workforce, guiding and mentoring from new vantage points. It opens opportunities for continuity, wisdom-sharing, and patient safety that transcend geography.

We've seen what happens when alignment replaces exhaustion. Bedside nurses spend more time in meaningful patient interaction and experience less cognitive burden. Virtual nurses, working in tandem, provide constant vigilance and support. Families sense the teamwork — two nurses caring from two places, united by one purpose.

That's what alignment looks like in practice: matching every nurse's strength with the setting that allows them to thrive.

Technology With a Human Pulse

I've always believed technology should amplify our humanity, not compete with it. Nursing is, and always will be, a relationship profession. Whether a nurse is at the bedside or behind a monitor, the intention is the same — to notice what others might miss.

Our virtual nurses don't just watch screens; they watch people and stories unfold. They notice the patient who hesitates before answering, the voice that sounds more winded today than yesterday, the subtle facial change that suggests discomfort before vital signs ever shift.

Technology extends our reach, but it's intuition, critical thinking, and compassion that make our presence meaningful. The virtual nursing frameworks emerging today ensure that even as we modernize, we never mechanize the human spirit of care.

Leadership for a Connected Future

To lead nursing today is to lead through uncertainty. Innovation happens faster than policy, and transformation can feel uncomfortable. But leadership is about seeing possibilities where others see disruption — and guiding teams to alignment rather than resistance.

When I look at nurses who have embraced virtual practice, I see pioneers. They're proving that care can be personal without being physical. A nurse in one geography can coach a novice in another through a complex admission. A centrally located team can monitor post-op patients in rural hospitals where resources are scarce. A retired nurse can stay engaged, providing oversight and education from home.

This is leadership on a new plane — one that extends expertise without erasing proximity's power. The ethical charge remains: to ensure this evolution stays equitable, evidence-based, and centered on the people we serve. Leaders today must understand that alignment is not static — it's dynamic. Our responsibility is to continuously match nurses' skills and seasons of life to the environments where they will make the greatest impact.

The Hybrid Horizon

The future of nursing will be hybrid: part physical, part virtual, fully human. I imagine care teams where bedside and virtual nurses move seamlessly between roles — partners in vigilance and empathy. AI may soon anticipate needs, but it will be nurses who interpret meaning. Dashboards may project data, but it will be nurses who sense the nuance. Whether sitting at a patient's bedside or at a command center, the essence of nursing remains the same: presence, advocacy, and alignment with purpose.

Hybrid care models are also unlocking something profoundly human — sustainability. When nurses work in roles that honor their energy and expertise, burnout gives way to belonging. Flexibility doesn't fragment the workforce; it fortifies it. When nurses feel aligned — with their work, their teams, and their values — they stay longer, perform better, and pass on what they know. That's not just a staffing solution; it's a cultural solution.

The Heart of Alignment

Alignment is more than an organizational strategy — it's the soul of resilience. It's what happens when a nurse's work reflects their why. For some, alignment means returning to the bedside after time away. For others, it means mentoring virtually, teaching, leading, or innovating. Alignment is deeply personal, yet collectively powerful. When leaders make alignment a priority, the ripple effects reach patients, families, and communities alike.

We stand at an inflection point in our profession. Nursing has always adapted — from paper charting to EHRs, from open wards to intensive units, and now from proximity to presence across digital spaces. What's different now is intentionality. We're not just adapting to change — we're architecting it. We're building a model where technology carries empathy forward, and every nurse, no matter where they practice, can find purpose without losing connection.

Patricia J. Mook, DNP, RN, NEA-BC, CAHIMS, CAVRN, FAONL is a nationally respected nurse executive, educator, and pioneer in virtual nursing practice. With enterprise-wide leadership experience across nursing operations, professional development, and clinical education, she has spent her career designing systems that allow nurses to thrive while delivering safe, high-quality care at scale. In addition to her executive leadership work, she serves as Adjunct Faculty at the University of Alabama at Birmingham School of Nursing, where she helps prepare the next generation of nursing leaders for a rapidly evolving healthcare landscape. Dr. Mook played a central role in defining professional standards for virtual nursing and in the creation of the nation's first Certified Acute-Care Virtual Registered Nurse (CAVRN) credential through the Medical-Surgical Nursing Certification Board. Her work bridges technology, workforce sustainability, and professional identity, ensuring that innovation strengthens — rather than replaces — the human heart of nursing. In the Masters Series of *What Color Are Your Scrubs?*, Dr. Mook offers a powerful vision of how alignment, flexibility, and purpose will shape the future of the nursing profession.

Mason's Take

Dr. Patricia Mook reminds us that nursing's evolution has never been about replacing people with technology — it's about re-centering people through technology. What she describes isn't just a shift in workflow; it's a living example of alignment at scale. Virtual nursing doesn't replace the bedside; it supports it, protects it, and makes it more sustainable. It gives nurses choices that honor seasons of life, energy, and expertise, and it creates a team-based model where vigilance and care can be delivered from two vantage points without diluting the human core of the work.

What stands out most in Dr. Mook's vision is the insistence that technology must carry a human pulse. Screens don't replace presence; they extend it when the framework is built with rigor, ethics, and real accountability. The CAVRN credential represents that seriousness — not a trend, not a workaround, but a professional standard designed to keep safety, trust, and nursing judgment at the center of modern care.

As leaders and educators, the challenge now is to treat innovation as an invitation — to design systems that keep nursing human while nursing becomes more hybrid. Alignment is not nostalgia for what nursing was; it is the compass that keeps the profession grounded as it grows. Dr. Mook shows that when we match nurses to environments where they can thrive, we don't just improve staffing. We restore belonging, stabilize teams, and protect the future of nursing itself.

Chapter 46

Masters Series: Breaking the Silence — Why Safety Must Be Part of Your Scrubs

By: **Stephanie O'Bryon, DNP, RN, NEA-BC**

Nurse Executive; Advocate for Safe, Just, and Compassionate Workplaces; Adjunct Professor, Northeastern University

"No one should bleed for caring."

— Stephanie O'Bryon, DNP, RN, NEA-BC

Breaking the Silence — Why Safety Must Be Part of Your Scrubs

If you're drawn to healthcare, chances are it's because you want to help people — to comfort, to heal, to make a difference. But there's a truth you deserve to know before you ever put on your scrubs: sometimes, the people who give the most care face the most harm.

Across hospitals, clinics, and long-term care facilities, violence toward healthcare workers — especially nurses — has become shockingly common. A slammed door. A shove. A scream in your face. Sometimes it's a patient in crisis.

Sometimes it's a family member. Occasionally — heartbreakingly — it's even a co-worker.

And for too long, too many of us have whispered the same toxic phrase: "It's just part of the job."

It isn't. It never should be. And you, as the next generation of caregivers, can help stop it.

The Reality We Can't Ignore

Healthcare workers are five times more likely to experience workplace violence than people in any other industry. The American Nurses Association reports that up to eight out of ten nurses will be verbally or physically assaulted at some point in their careers — and most never report it.

Why? Because we're trained to prioritize others. To downplay our pain. To move on. But violence — verbal or physical — leaves marks that don't always fade: fear, anxiety, sleepless nights, and doubt.

And yet, there's hope. Awareness is rising, and a new wave of professionals is demanding better.

How We Got Here

1 The Caregiver Paradox. Healthcare attracts the helpers — the ones who keep showing up. But that same compassion can make us hesitate to protect ourselves.

2 Overcrowded, Understaffed, Overwhelmed. Emergency departments, behavioral units, long waits, and stressed families create tension — and caregivers often absorb it first.

3 Silence Feels Safer. Reporting violence can feel like

making trouble, especially for new employees, students, or trainees.

4 The Old Mindset. For years, "the patient is always right" became a shield for unacceptable behavior. But patient care and personal safety aren't opposites — they're partners.

Here's the Good News: There Are Answers

You're entering healthcare at a moment of awakening. Hospitals, schools, and professional associations are finally saying out loud: safety is part of quality care. And while the problem is real, so are the solutions. You have more power than you think — both now and in the career you're building.

1. Know Your Worth — and Your Rights

You have the right to feel safe at work. No one — patient, family member, or colleague — has the right to harm or harass you. As you start clinicals or your first job, learn your organization's violence prevention policies. Know where panic buttons are located. Know how to report. Know who your allies are. And if anyone ever tells you to "let it slide," remember this: silence protects no one. Your voice can protect the next nurse, tech, or student who walks into that same room.

2. Learn the Language of Prevention

Violence rarely appears out of nowhere — it escalates. Learn to recognize early warning signs:

• Staring or glaring that feels threatening

• A raised or mocking tone

• Pacing, clenching fists, or muttering

- Rising anxiety or frustration

These cues are teachable, and they save lives. The sooner you recognize them, the sooner your team can intervene — often before anything physical ever happens.

3. Training Is Power

Don't settle for a single "de-escalation" video during orientation. Ask for real, hands-on, simulation-based training. If it isn't offered — ask why not. Some hospitals now run Code Gray drills, practicing how to calmly and safely manage violent or escalating situations. These simulations build confidence and teamwork. They remind you: you're not alone.

4. Choose Workplaces That Walk Their Talk

As you evaluate potential employers, pay attention not just to pay — but to culture. Ask these questions:

- How does your organization handle workplace violence?

- Are there safety officers on every shift?

- Do you provide peer support after incidents?

- How do leaders respond when staff are harmed?

If they stumble or change the subject, that tells you everything you need to know. You deserve to work where your safety matters as much as your skill.

5. Support Each Other

Violence isolates. It makes good people feel powerless and alone. But connection changes everything. If you see a colleague shaken after an encounter — don't ignore it. Check in. Walk them to the break room. Offer to report the incident together. When one of us is harmed, all of us are impacted. When one of us speaks up, all of us grow stronger.

6. Take Care of Your Own Healing

If something happens to you, it's okay to need help. Talk to someone — your manager, your mentor, your counselor, or your EAP. Trauma doesn't disappear by pretending it's not there. As one nurse told me, "It took me a long time to realize I couldn't pour from an empty cup — but also that the cup was mine to protect."

7. Use Your Voice — Even Early in Your Career

Many hospitals now have Safety Councils or Violence Prevention Committees. Students and new grads are often invited to join. These are the rooms where change begins — where data becomes policy, and policy becomes protection. Your ideas matter. Your stories matter. Your perspective — the fresh eyes of someone who still believes healthcare can be better — is exactly what's needed.

8. Bring Hope, Not Fear

This chapter isn't meant to scare you away. It's meant to prepare you — and to remind you that change is already happening. Hospitals are redesigning units for safety. States are passing laws to protect healthcare workers. And leaders are learning that a truly healing environment must also heal the healer.

You're entering a profession that's rewriting its own rules. And you get to help write the next chapter.

If You Remember Nothing Else, Remember This

- Violence is never part of the job.

- Reporting is not weakness — it's leadership.

- Asking for help is not unprofessional — it's human.

- Your voice can change what happens next.

One day, a new nurse or tech will walk into a safer hospital because you spoke up. That's how real change happens — one person at a time, choosing courage over silence.

The Future You're Helping to Build

Picture this: you finish a 12-hour shift. Instead of exhaustion mixed with fear, you feel tired — but proud. Your hospital celebrates another week without a single violent incident. Your manager thanks you for filing reports that made the difference. Your team protects each other — and patients notice.

That's what safety looks like. That's what alignment feels like. That's the kind of healthcare you deserve to be part of.

Final Thought

Healthcare is a calling — but it should never cost you your safety or your peace. The world needs caregivers with courage — people who will not only heal bodies but help heal a broken system. Because the next time someone says, "It's just part of the job," someone else — maybe you — will have the strength to say, "Not anymore."

Stephanie O'Bryon, DNP, RN, NEA-BC is a seasoned nurse executive and emergency care leader with more than three decades of experience advancing patient care, workforce resilience, and operational excellence in high-acuity environments. She serves as an Assistant Vice President overseeing multiple adult emergency departments within one of the nation's leading integrated health systems in the Carolinas, supporting care delivery across a vast regional footprint that includes 900+ care locations.

Known for steady, people-first leadership in complex settings, Dr. O'Bryon's work centers on building clinical environments where teams can perform at a high level while remaining supported, developed, and sustained over time. Her leadership spans quality and safety, workforce development, and the operational design required to keep emergency services strong when volume, complexity, and urgency collide.

In addition to her executive leadership, Dr. O'Bryon is an Adjunct Professor at Northeastern University, contributing to the preparation of future nurses and healthcare leaders through real-world perspective, high standards, and practical mentorship.

Dr. O'Bryon is nationally recognized for her expertise in nursing leadership, emergency services, workforce development, and organizational transformation. She brings a rare combination of operational insight, systems thinking, and educator perspective to her work, consistently advocating for environments where clinicians are supported, empowered, and able to deliver exceptional care without sacrificing their well-being.

Her leadership philosophy centers on alignment—between people, purpose, and practice—and on building healthcare systems that are resilient not just in crisis, but every day.

Mason's Take

Dr. Stephanie O'Bryon's message is one I wish every nursing student, recruiter, and executive could hear. *"No one should bleed for caring"* stopped me cold — because she's right. For too long, we've normalized harm in a profession built on healing. And it's time to break that silence.

I've met countless nurses who wear invisible scars from moments they never reported — moments that changed how safe they felt in the very place they came to help. Stephanie gives those nurses a voice, and she gives future caregivers a map. She's saying what so many have felt: our duty to care cannot include sacrificing our dignity or safety.

What I love about this piece is how it reframes safety as alignment. It's not a checklist or a compliance task — it's a human right. When healthcare environments protect their people as fiercely as they protect their patients, that's alignment realized. And when new nurses are taught that reporting isn't weakness but leadership, we begin to heal the culture that created the silence.

Stephanie's leadership reminds me that courage is contagious. Her blueprint — learn the warning signs, speak up, protect one another, and demand better — turns hope into action. This is how systemic change starts: one person refusing to accept "just part of the job" as the price of compassion.

Every time I read about or witness a caregiver stand up, report, or debrief after an incident, I think of her words. Because she's right — safety isn't optional. It's part of your scrubs.

Chapter 47

Masters Series: Finding Your Path in a Profession with a Thousand Doorways

By: **Patti Rager, RN, MSN, MBA**

Former President & Publisher, *Nursing Spectrum* / *NurseWeek* (Gannett Healthcare Group)

I didn't set out to become a publisher or a president. I was a nurse who loved the work and was curious about where nursing could take me. The pivotal moment? I answered one of those tiny "confidential box" ads in the back of *The Washington Post* — the kind you circled with a pen and mailed in with a cover letter and hope. I thought I was applying for a Chief Nursing Officer — Vice President of Patient Care Services position. No LinkedIn, no applicant-tracking portals, no algorithm judging my keywords. Just paper, postage, and a decision to bet on myself.

That unlikely door opened to something altogether different: an opportunity to lead *Nursing Spectrum*, and later, the national integration with *NurseWeek*. I didn't know it then, but that small act of courage would change the trajectory of my career — and amplify the voices of nurses across the country.

We published stories that reflected what nurses were really living — the triumphs, the heartbreaks, the lessons from every shift — not what others assumed they needed to hear. We gave nurses a national platform and a common language. Over time, I realized that what we were building wasn't just a publication; it was a movement, one that made nurses feel visible and valued in ways that policy and pay often didn't.

When *Nursing Spectrum* became part of Gannett Healthcare Group and merged with *NurseWeek*, the mission grew — but so did the responsibility. Suddenly we were connecting nurses from coast to coast, curating continuing education, and producing live events that united clinicians and leaders under one banner: pride in the profession. Those were some of the most challenging and rewarding years of my life.

"At our peak, *Nursing Spectrum's* twelve regional biweekly magazines reached more than one million registered nurses — delivered at no cost — giving bedside voices a national platform for education, jobs, and community."

If you're reading this and wondering where your next doorway is, I'll start here: healthcare is not one hallway with a single promotion ladder. It's a city of neighborhoods. Clinical practice will always be our heartbeat, but the map includes publishing and media, education, informatics, consulting, policy, and innovation. Your preparation matters, but so does your curiosity — spotting where your passions intersect with the system's unmet needs.

My own education — an MSN paired with an MBA — gave me two lenses I used every day. The MSN lens kept me grounded in evidence and patient outcomes. The MBA lens taught me to read a P&L, build a business case, and navigate growth and change. Together, they helped me translate nursing values into enterprise decisions. That's what leadership really is: translation — turning the language of care into the language of strategy so nurses are heard at every table.

Opportunities Everywhere

Care Delivery, Reimagined. Inpatient units, EDs, ORs, ambulatory clinics, and home health remain vital — yet each is morphing. Virtual nursing, hospital-at-home, and command-center models are expanding how care is coordinated. Nurses who bridge settings become the glue for continuity.

Quality & Safety. For those who love systems thinking, this space is your frontier. If you can interpret data and inspire safer practice, you'll always be in demand.

Education & Professional Growth. Whether you teach in a simulation lab or mentor new grads, helping others "click" is one of the profession's most meaningful roles. I spent years in publishing because I saw how a single article, course, or event can change practice at scale.

Informatics & Innovation. Nurses who keep technology humane — who understand the workflow and the why — are reshaping the future of care delivery.

Across every path, the through line is the same: nurses are translators, bridge-builders, and implementers. We adapt. We operationalize. We find the tripping hazards and remove them so care flows.

A Few Lessons Along the Way

Follow the friction. The things that frustrate you most may be pointing to your future. Solve one problem well, and you'll never be without opportunities.

Stack your credentials with intent. Education should sharpen your next chapter, not decorate your résumé.

Build a portfolio, not just a job history. The evidence of what you've improved — your before-and-after stories — will carry you farther than any title.

Say yes to the mic. Teaching, speaking, or writing clarifies your thinking and magnifies your influence.

Learn to read the business. Great care must be sustainable care.

Network like a neighbor, not a tourist. Purpose multiplies when we stay connected.

When I think back to that "confidential box," I smile. It wasn't glamorous. It was small, easy to miss — and life-changing. Opportunity rarely announces itself; it whispers. It invites. Sometimes it comes disguised as something else entirely, like a CNO posting that leads you to build the largest nurse-media platform in the nation.

If a tiny ad in a newspaper could redirect my life, a single, intentional action can redirect yours. Healthcare needs your curiosity, your courage, and your refusal to accept "that's just how it is." There's a neighborhood in this profession with your name on the mailbox. Find it — and then hold the door open for the next nurse who's still scanning the classifieds for a sign.

Patti Rager, RN, MSN, MBA is a nationally recognized nursing and healthcare media leader whose career helped shape how the profession tells its story. As President and Publisher of *Nursing Spectrum, NurseWeek,* and nurse.com at Gannett Healthcare Group, she guided one of the largest and most influential nursing-focused publishing platforms in the United States, elevating the voices of nurses long before workforce storytelling became a national priority. Her leadership brought visibility to frontline clinicians, expanded professional development resources, and strengthened the bridge between nursing practice, policy, and public understanding.

In retirement, Patti continues to champion the power of narrative in strengthening the nursing profession. She remains an advocate for workforce development, mentorship, and leadership pathways that honor both the art and science of nursing. Her contribution to the Masters Series reflects her deep understanding of how aligned stories shape aligned careers — and how giving nurses a platform to be seen and heard can transform not only individual trajectories, but the culture of healthcare itself.

Mason's Take

I had the honor of nominating Patti Rager for a Lifetime Achievement Award when I served on the Board of Directors of the National Association for Health Care Recruitment (NAHCR). It was one of those moments that felt less like an award and more like a thank-you the profession needed to say out loud.

Patti is one of the finest professionals — and one of my favorite people — in healthcare. Her leadership elevated an entire generation of nurse communicators and career innovators. She has that rare blend of intelligence, humility, and humor that makes everyone around her better.

Even in retirement, she and her husband, Ed, continue to serve as Court Appointed Special Advocates (CASAs), standing up for children who need a voice. That's alignment in its purest form: when purpose doesn't retire — it just finds new ways to serve.

Chapter 48

Masters Series: The Moment I Almost Walked Away

By: **Dr. Marco Scarci**

Internationally Recognized Thoracic Surgeon; Medical Author

No Surgeon Stands Alone

I nearly quit in theatre that day.

You won't hear many surgeons admit that.

But in the middle of a marathon case—with a patient whose cancer had tangled itself around every vital structure in the chest—I came close.

The plan looked straightforward on paper. A scheduled lung cancer resection. But when I opened the chest, reality crashed in.

The tumour was everywhere. Encasing arteries. Clinging to nerves. Wrapped tight around the bronchus. Every move risked disaster.

For a moment, I stared at the operative field and thought: this can't be done. Not safely. Not today.

I felt the weight of expectation—the patient, their family, everyone hoping for a cure.

My hands paused. My mind raced through options. None seemed safe enough. I heard my own breathing, the beep of the monitors, the tense silence of the team.

Then something remarkable happened.

My theatre nurse cut through the fog. "Let's take it step by step. We're with you."

My anaesthetist grounded me with quiet certainty. "The patient is stable. We have time. Let's think."

My registrar pulled up the most recent CT scan and held it beside the operative field, mapping the unseen onto what lay open in front of us.

The scrub nurse organised trays for every possible instrument. Each member of the team offered a lifeline.

We talked through the options like a chess match. Could we mobilise the artery before touching the tumour? Might it be safer to divide the bronchus first? Was there a way to peel the mass off the nerve with minimal trauma?

Minute by minute, the fog lifted. The impossible started to look... possible.

We adapted the plan on the spot. We worked methodically, with each pair of eyes spotting what I couldn't see from my angle.

After hours that felt like days, the tumour was finally free. Margins clear. Bleeding controlled. No structures lost that didn't absolutely have to go.

I remember stepping away from the table—sweat-soaked and exhausted—but more than that, relieved.

We hadn't just saved the patient's life. We'd proved something fundamental.

The best surgeon is never a solo hero.

No matter how many years of training, how many awards, how many cutting-edge fellowships—it's the team. The theatre nurse who keeps you steady. The anaesthetist who gives you time. The registrar who catches the detail you miss. The radiographer who responds in seconds when new images are needed.

Alone, I would have called it off. Together, we found a way.

I've learned that surgical skill is only half the equation. The rest is humility. And trust. And the courage to admit you don't have all the answers.

If there's one thing I want every doctor, every patient, every family to know, it's this:

Surgery is never a solo act. It's a symphony.

And the best outcomes come from listening to every note.

Marco Scarci, MD, FRCS(Eng), FCCP, FACS, FEBTS is a consultant thoracic surgeon based in London, England, with specialist expertise in complex chest surgery, including lung cancer and minimally invasive (keyhole) thoracic procedures. He is a consultant at Imperial College Healthcare NHS Trust and has held senior posts across leading UK and international centres, including Papworth Hospital (Cambridge) and University College London Hospital, as well as serving as Director of Thoracic Surgery at San Gerardo Hospital in Monza, Italy.

His training spans Malta, the Essex Cardiothoracic Centre, and Guy's & St Thomas' in London, with an additional thoracic surgery fellowship at the University of Toronto.

Across his work, Mr Scarci is known for advancing patient-centred thoracic care and for advocating the reality behind high-stakes surgery: exceptional outcomes are built by teams —through preparation, situational awareness, and trust in every role around the table.

Here's Mason's Take

What Dr. Marco Scarci just showed us is the quiet truth behind nearly every great outcome in healthcare: alignment saves lives.

We love the myth of the brilliant solo surgeon — the steady hand, the flawless decision-maker, the heroic moment. But real medicine doesn't happen in isolation. It happens inside systems. Inside rooms filled with people whose roles are different but whose purpose is shared.

When Dr. Scarci paused in the middle of that marathon case, it wasn't weakness. It was the human nervous system doing exactly what it does when the stakes are impossibly high. What broke the paralysis wasn't more personal brilliance — it was environmental support. A nurse who grounded him. An anesthetist who bought him time. A registrar who surfaced data. A scrub nurse who anticipated what would be needed next.

That is alignment in action.

In my work, I call this the difference between who you are and where you are allowed to be human. Even the most talented clinician will struggle in an environment that isolates them, pressures them to perform, and punishes uncertainty. But put that same person inside a team that shares load, communicates clearly, and respects every voice — and suddenly the impossible becomes manageable.

Dr. Scarci didn't succeed because he was a hero. He succeeded because he was surrounded by one.

And that's the lesson healthcare keeps trying to tell us:

You don't prevent burnout or errors by asking people to be stronger.

You prevent them by building systems that don't require anyone to be alone.

Chapter 49

Masters Series: Aligning Hospitals, Aligning Careers: A Journey Through Mission, Merger & Meaning

By: **Knox Singleton, MHA**

Former CEO, Inova Health System; Healthcare Executive-in-Residence & Board Member

Alignment is not hierarchy — it's harmony

When I first walked into a hospital hallway, I felt both awe and alarm. The energy: purpose, urgency, life. The reality: fragmented silos, duplicate efforts, care gaps. Over time, I learned that alignment — between institutions, clinicians, and communities — is as essential as medicine itself.

My career began at Hershey Medical Center (gl) after earning a master's degree from Duke University (gl) in 1973. Academic hospitals teach precision; community hospitals teach pragmatism. At Hershey, I learned how decisions in boardrooms echo in hallways and patient rooms. A teaching hospital has all the right ingredients — expertise, technology, research — but alignment determines whether those ingredients create health or chaos.

That realization became the compass for the rest of my professional life.

From Movement to System

In 1983 I joined the Fairfax Hospital Association (gl) (FHA) as executive vice president for operations. The next year, I became president. FHA had been founded by citizens in 1956 who refused to accept long drives for care. By 1961, they had opened Fairfax Hospital (gl) and soon built Mount Vernon Hospital (gl) and Fair Oaks Hospital (gl) from scratch to serve rapidly growing neighborhoods. It was a movement rooted in service, not scale.

When I arrived, those hospitals were operating independently, each with its own culture and systems. We needed to think like a network without losing the spirit of local ownership. That tension — unity versus autonomy — would define my next three decades.

Mergers Without Alignment Are Empty Conquests

Healthcare loves growth. But growth without alignment creates distance instead of reach. When we built or merged, our mission was to harmonize, not homogenize.

Each campus brought something irreplaceable. Alexandria Hospital (gl) had earned national recognition for its "Alexandria Plan," which redefined how emergency departments were staffed. We kept that identity alive after its 1997 merger. Mount Vernon kept its neighborhood feel and rehabilitation expertise. Fair Oaks cultivated a suburban innovation ethos. Loudoun Hospital (gl) joined in 2004, extending our reach westward as Northern Virginia boomed.

To outsiders, this looked like expansion. Inside, it was integration — aligning culture, standards, and systems so that a patient could walk into any campus and feel both the local touch and the Inova consistency.

We built cross-campus leadership councils and rotation programs so leaders would understand the organization beyond their own walls. We shared clinical pathways and data dashboards years before it became common language in healthcare. If Fair Oaks cut infection rates, Mount Vernon learned how within a week.

That is alignment in motion.

Alignment and the People Who Live It

A system is just a mirror of its people. Every nurse, physician, and technologist faces the same alignment test that institutions do: Do my values and my environment belong together?

Over the years, I watched hundreds of careers flourish when values and roles matched. A respiratory therapist who thrives on precision finds joy in intensive care. A social worker driven by community connection flourishes in outreach clinics. Alignment at the individual level is as vital as alignment at the institutional level. Without it, we burn out our best people and wonder why our systems fail.

That's why we invested in career pathways and mentorship long before it became a retention strategy. I believed that when people see their own purpose reflected in the organization's purpose, they don't just stay — they lead.

Alignment is relational. It shows up in how we listen during rounds, how we resolve conflict, and how we recognize quiet excellence. Culture isn't taught in orientation; it's transmitted in moments of respect.

Continuity as a Strategy

In 1984, few expected anyone to stay in a CEO role for three decades. By the time I retired in 2018, I had served 33 years — long enough to see our early values tested, challenged, and ultimately proven.

Continuity does not mean complacency. It means staying long enough to learn from your own decisions. Over that time, Inova grew from a handful of community hospitals to a regional system serving more than two million people each year. We built trust by delivering predictable excellence and by keeping our promises through change.

Leadership continuity also allowed us to take measured risks — like our move into personalized medicine and genomics through the University of Virginia (gl) partnership in 2016. That initiative converted a former corporate campus into a personalized health research center — a symbol of what happens when academic and community institutions align.

The Throughline: Mission Before Metrics

Every strategic plan faces the same temptation: measure what's easy and forget what matters. We reversed that order: first mission, then metrics.

We asked three questions whenever faced with a decision:

1 Will this improve access and quality for our community?

2 Can it be scaled system-wide so every Inova patient benefits?

3 Does it strengthen trust within our workforce and our region?

If the answer to all three was yes, we moved. If not, we paused or walked away. Alignment requires that discipline.

We also built systems for feedback long before surveys were standard. Employee forums fed directly into executive rounds; patients helped design new service lines. Alignment cannot be mandated — it must be co-authored.

Lessons for a New Generation

To today's healthcare professionals: your career will mirror the system you join. If you pick a culture that moves faster than its mission, you'll feel the friction immediately. If you find one that matches your values, you'll find flow even in hard days.

Here's what I wish someone had told me early on:

• Mission first, merger second. If your alignment is weak, no contract will bind it.

• Culture outlives strategy. People remember how you made them feel, not the PowerPoint you showed them.

• Continuity creates credibility. When leaders stay long enough to see outcomes, trust deepens.

• Choose environments that fit you. Skills get you in; alignment keeps you whole.

• Harmony beats hierarchy. Leadership is not about control; it's about connection.

The future of healthcare won't be decided by the biggest systems or the brightest technologies. It will be decided by how well we align our intentions with our actions — from the executive suite to the student nurse.

When institutions and individuals find that rhythm together, care becomes continuity and trust becomes culture. That is alignment at its finest.

Knox Singleton served for more than 30 years as Chief Executive Officer of Inova Health System, guiding its evolution into a nationally recognized, innovation-driven nonprofit health network. Under his leadership, Inova expanded its clinical programs, deepened its community partnerships, and advanced a forward-thinking approach to population health and system integration.

A long-time advocate for mission-driven care, Singleton has held influential roles on boards and advisory groups, helping shape national conversations around healthcare access, quality, and workforce development. He is widely regarded as a visionary strategist and mentor to emerging leaders. His contribution to the Masters Series reflects decades of experience at the intersection of leadership, governance, culture, and community impact.

Mason's Take

In an era defined by rapid turnover, Knox Singleton's thirty-three-year tenure at Inova Health System stands as a masterclass in continuity. His leadership transformed Inova from a local hospital group into a national model of aligned, integrated healthcare delivery.

Inside Northern Virginia, Inova earned the lighthearted nickname "The Cabbage Patch." The joke carried truth: it delivered more babies — and more overall care — than almost any system its size. Under Singleton, volume became not a vanity metric but a reflection of trust. At its peak, Inova sustained one of the nation's highest delivery counts, maintained strong financial surpluses, and reinvested those gains into mission-driven care.

Singleton's genius was subtle: he made scale feel personal. He preserved local culture while aligning every facility to a shared mission of access, consistency, and compassion. His legacy proves that alignment is not about assimilation — it's about orchestration.

Today, the systems he built still anchor Northern Virginia's healthcare ecosystem. For anyone studying leadership longevity, operational harmony, or the art of mission-driven scale — Knox Singleton remains a north star. He didn't just build a network. He built a legacy.

Chapter 50

Masters Series: Working with a Lifelong Vision for Quality & Safety

By: Joy B. Solomita, RN, BSPA, BSN, MPH, MSN, PhD, NEA-BC

Nurse Executive | Systems-Level Nursing Leader | Culture, Quality & Patient-Experience Strategist

"Quality is not a department — it's a shared commitment that begins with vision and ends with accountability."

Nurse Executive and Advocate for Excellence in Care

Understanding Healthcare Quality Metrics: Beginning a Career Through the Lens of Alignment

Every healthcare career—no matter the discipline, credential, or specialty—ultimately converges on the same shared purpose: improving the quality and safety of patient care. Whether you are a student stepping into your first clinical rotation or a seasoned professional entering a new environment, the ability to understand quality metrics is not simply a technical skill. It is a form of alignment—between who you are, how you practice, and the outcomes your organization is accountable for.

Quality metrics are the common language spoken by the Centers for Medicare and Medicaid Services (CMS), regulators, insurers, hospitals, and teams. They are the visible reflection of how well an organization's identity matches its environment. They shape reputations, financial stability, patient trust, and workforce morale. Most importantly, they shape daily decisions and behaviors at the bedside.

If you want a fulfilling and aligned healthcare career, you need to understand the metrics that define excellence.

The CMS Star System: A National Mirror of Performance

CMS assigns hospitals a rating from one to five stars. The rating is built from weighted, publicly reported quality metrics with both clinical and cultural significance:

- Mortality (22%)

- Readmissions (22%)

- Safety of care (22%)

- Patient experience (22%)

- Timely and effective care (12%)

Together, these metrics form a blueprint of organizational alignment. They reflect whether systems are designed well, whether teams communicate effectively, and whether leaders and clinicians share a commitment to practices that improve patient lives.

In 2024, national results were distributed across the five-star range:

- 1 star (5.9%)

- 2 stars (12.8%)

- 3 stars (17.8%)

- 4 stars (16.4%)

- 5 stars (8.2%)

- Not Applicable (38.9%)

Most organizations strive for four or five stars because higher ratings correlate with stronger outcomes, better patient trust, and often financial incentives.

What these numbers reveal is not just performance.

They reveal alignment—or the lack of it.

HCAHPS: The Voice of the Patient as a Quality Metric

The Hospital Consumer Assessment of Healthcare Providers and Systems (HCAHPS) survey is the nation's standardized measure of patient experience. The 2025 version includes 32 questions covering:

- Nurse communication

- Physician communication

- Hospital environment

- Your care in the hospital

- Overall rating

- Patient background questions

These results feed into the CMS star rating and determine national percentile rankings. When a hospital reports nursing care at a specific national percentile, that benchmark comes from HCAHPS.

In alignment language, HCAHPS tells us whether the environment supports the behaviors patients value:

- Kindness

- Clarity

- Responsiveness

- Teamwork

- Safety

Excellence here is not an accident. It is the outcome of culture.

Knowing Your Metrics: The Foundation of Professional Alignment

Beyond federal measures, every hospital sets internal quality goals. Common goals include:

- Hospital-acquired infections

- Sepsis bundle adherence

- Patient experience targets

- Readmission rates

- Mortality reduction

Some organizations adopt federal thresholds. Others set more ambitious goals. Either way, you cannot align your work with your environment unless you know what the measures are and how you contribute to them.

One of the wisest moves early in your career is to ask:

"What quality metrics define success for my unit and my role?"

This is alignment in action—understanding how your identity as a professional connects to the expectations around you.

The Formula for Improvement and the Role of Alignment

Years of studying leadership, quality, and change in healthcare reveal a consistent truth: improvement is not driven by force. It is driven by alignment—of vision, people, relationships, standard work, and accountability. When these five elements align, improvement becomes sustainable.

1. A Clear Vision for Quality

Every quality journey begins with vision. The Institute of Medicine's landmark report *To Err Is Human* (1999) exposed the reality of preventable harm and reshaped how healthcare systems think about safety.

But vision cannot live in a department alone. If quality is not shared across the organization—executives, managers, physicians, nurses, technicians, therapists, and support staff—the work collapses into paperwork rather than lived practice.

Vision creates alignment by asking:

"What do we stand for—and are we willing to change to live up to it?"

2. Hiring for Alignment, Not Just Skill

People shape culture more than policies ever will. Hiring for excellence means selecting individuals who bring not only competence but also values aligned with the organization's commitment to safety and quality.

Effective hiring practices include:

• Group interviews

• Peer interviews

• Behavioral scenarios

• Evidence-based selection

The question is not only *Can they do the job?*

It is *Do they fit the work, the culture, and the expectations tied to quality?*

Misalignment here creates ripple effects that no amount of training can fix.

3. Building Relationships That Influence Practice

Even the best-quality initiatives fail without strong relationships. Influence is not about authority—it's about clarity, credibility, and collaboration. You must understand what motivates others and articulate the specific behaviors that drive results.

Alignment is relational. When people understand the "why," the "what," and the "how," they are far more likely to walk toward the goal with you.

4. Creating Standard Work That Is Clear and Actionable

Standard work is the bridge between vision and behavior. Yet organizations often assume that "everyone knows what to do." In reality, practices vary widely across departments and individuals.

An example for improving patient experience may include:

• Bedside shift report

• Hourly rounds

• One sit-down conversation per shift

• Review MyChart results with the patient

• Reinforce discharge teaching with the patient

Clear behaviors create clear results.

5. Accountability: The Hardest and Most Essential Element

Accountability is alignment under pressure. Teams drift when accountability weakens—whether because of leadership turnover, unclear priorities, or loss of focus.

Accountability must live everywhere:

• Leaders to teams

• Teams to leaders

• Individuals to each other

• Everyone to the patient

When accountability dissolves, results erode within months. Sustained excellence requires holding the line together.

Navigating Obstacles: Where Alignment Is Tested

Every healthcare environment faces obstacles that challenge quality improvement—and reveal misalignment. Common obstacles include:

- Leadership turnover

- Staffing instability

- Lack of change-management knowledge

- Competing commitments

- Poor communication

- Underutilized technology

Clear communication is alignment in practice. Documentation tools, reporting systems, and AI-driven alerts can be powerful resources—but only if staff know how to use them.

Bringing It All Together: Alignment as a Professional Calling

No matter your discipline—nursing, therapy, diagnostics, medicine, administration, support services—your work is part of the quality ecosystem.

Alignment emerges when your identity as a professional matches the expectations of your environment and the choices you make each day.

When you understand:

- The metrics

- The vision

- The culture

- The standard work

- The relationships

- The accountability

...you become a leader of quality, regardless of your job title.

Your journey in healthcare will be long, challenging, and deeply meaningful. But when you anchor your practice in alignment—purpose, clarity, accountability, relationships, and vision—you not only contribute to better outcomes; you become part of a safer, stronger, more compassionate healthcare system.

Quality is not a department.

It is a way of thinking, a way of showing up, and a way of aligning who you are with the care every patient deserves.

Final Thought

When we align the right people, with the right preparation, in the right systems, we create excellence that sustains itself. That lifelong vision has guided my career—and I hope it will guide yours.

Joy Solomita, PhD, MSN, RN, MPH, CNAA-BC is a nationally respected healthcare executive, workforce strategist, and executive consultant with decades of experience shaping nursing leadership, professional practice, and organizational culture across major U.S. health systems. A former Chief Nursing Officer and Chief Nurse Executive, Dr. Solomita has led complex clinical enterprises through periods of transformation, growth, and cultural change—always with a steadfast focus on people, purpose, and outcomes.

Dr. Solomita is widely recognized for her ability to bridge strategy and humanity in healthcare leadership. Her work centers on strengthening the nursing workforce, advancing leadership development, and designing systems that allow clinicians to thrive rather than burn out. As an executive consultant, she partners with boards, CEOs, and senior leadership teams to align mission, culture, and workforce strategy in ways that are both sustainable and deeply human.

A prolific speaker, mentor, and thought leader, Dr. Solomita brings a rare combination of academic rigor, operational expertise, and lived leadership experience. Her voice reflects a deep understanding that the future of healthcare depends not only on innovation and efficiency, but on honoring the professionals who deliver care every day.

Mason's Take

Watching Joy lead was watching alignment in motion—precision and grace. She walks units, listens to staff, and translates metrics into human meaning. She never hides behind data; she humanizes it.

Three lessons stayed with me:

• Metrics without meaning create compliance, not excellence—and culture is what makes the numbers move

• Quality is relational before it is operational—trust has to come before systems

• Accountability without kindness becomes surveillance

When I run her leadership through **CARESET™**, the message sharpens: compassion and compliance aren't trade-offs. They're the same commitment, lived daily.

Chapter 51

Masters Series: Caring Science as a Pathway to Career Alignment

By: **Jean Watson, PhD, RN, AHN-BC, FAAN**

"Caring Science is alignment science."

— Jean Watson, PhD, RN, AHN-BC, FAAN

Why Watson, Why Now

In a moment when healthcare systems are grappling with burnout, turnover, and a fraying sense of purpose, Jean Watson's *Caring Science* offers more than a philosophy — it's a practical operating system for alignment. Watson reframes nursing as a healing profession grounded in a *relational ontology* (we are formed in relationship, not isolation) and a *unitary view of personhood* (mind-body-spirit within environment), restoring the *why* of nursing to the daily *what*.

The Core: Transpersonal Caring & the Caritas Processes®

At the heart of *Caring Science* is the **transpersonal caring relationship** — a nurse's presence that goes beyond task and ego to honor the whole person. This is articulated through the

10 Caritas Processes® — Embrace (loving-kindness); Inspire (faith-hope); Trust (transpersonal presence); Nurture (authentic relationship); Forgive (healing environment); Deepen (creative self); Balance (learning); Co-Create (caritas field); Serve (humanity); and Open (spaciousness/unknowns).

These aren't slogans; they are applied commitments that align inner values with outward practice.

Alignment, Defined the Watson Way

Career alignment in nursing means your role, unit culture, and leadership context match your values and strengths. *Caring Science* operationalizes that match: it connects personal purpose (*Caritas* intentions) with professional behaviors (*caritas-informed* practices) and organizational design (*caring-healing* cultures). The Watson Caring Science Institute© explicitly frames its mission around education, practice, research, and leadership that produce deep individual and cultural system change — in other words, alignment that scales from the nurse to the whole system.

Evidence Signals: What Changes When Caring Leads

• **Nurse Well-Being & Burnout:** Caritas-based and related workplace interventions are associated with improved well-being, resilience, and reduced burnout — key preconditions for retention and aligned practice.

• **Professional Identity & Presence:** Scholarship continues to evolve the *transpersonal Caritas relationship* construct, reinforcing the knowledge base that supports authentic nurse-patient presence and purpose.

- **Educational Alignment:** Programs integrating Watson's theory teach whole-person care as core identity, not "extra," helping students form aligned professional selves from day one.

- **Organizational Adoption:** Health systems that declare *Caring Science* as their nursing model (e.g., incorporating Caritas Coaching® and caring-healing environments) formalize alignment in policy, practice, and professional development.

- **Downstream Outcomes:** Broader workforce literature shows that misalignment (manifesting as chronic overload, poor leadership fit, or toxic culture) drives errors, lower satisfaction, and turnover — costly at both human and financial levels — making alignment an operational imperative.

Caritas → Career Alignment: A Practical Map

- **Embrace (Loving-Kindness) → *Fit to Mission & Values:*** Nurses select units and organizations that authentically honor compassion — not just in posters but in staffing, breaks, and debrief norms.

- **Trust (Transpersonal Presence) → *Role-Person Match:*** Roles that allow presence (e.g., oncology, palliative, cardiac rehab, primary care) better fit nurses who derive meaning from deep relationships.

- **Nurture (Authentic Relationship) → *Team Culture Alignment:*** Preceptors, mentors, and charge nurses trained in *Caring Science* cultivate psychological safety and growth — key for early-career retention.

• **Forgive (Healing Environment)** → *Work Design Alignment:* Units intentionally design caring-healing spaces and micro-rituals (shift huddles with gratitude, pause practices) to buffer stress and sustain purpose.

• **Balance (Learning)** → *Professional Growth Alignment:* Caritas-aligned CE, reflective practice, and coaching reinforce identity formation and prevent skills-purpose drift.

• **Co-Create (Caritas Field)** → *Leadership Alignment:* Leaders adopt a caring ethic (transformational/servant styles) linked to lower burnout, stronger engagement, and retention.

From Philosophy to Daily Practice: A 5-Move Blueprint

1 State the Why (Caritas Intentions): Begin shift huddles with a 30-second Caritas intention (e.g., "We will hold loving-kindness for ourselves and our patients today.")

2 Design for Presence: Protect two "presence pockets" per nurse per shift — brief, uninterrupted care moments — so practice matches values.

3 Coach the Coaches: Train preceptors and charge RNs as Caritas Coaches®; embed reflective practice and micro-debriefs to transmute stress into learning.

4 Make Culture Visible: Post unit-level Caritas commitments and track one behavior metric (gratitude pauses, mentor touches) and one outcome metric (fatigue or intent-to-stay).

5 Align the Pipeline: In schools and residencies, assess for values fit and teach *Caring Science* as a core competency — not an elective soft skill.

What Leaders Should Measure (Simple, Sticky Indicators)

- *Meaning-in-Work Index:* Short pulse (3–5 items) mapping Caritas presence, team belonging, and purpose clarity.

- *Caritas Practice Frequency:* Track unit rituals (gratitude/centering/debriefs).

- *Resilience & Burnout Trends:* Use brief, validated tools quarterly; pair with stay interviews.

- *Early-Career Retention:* Monitor 6–24-month retention where Caritas Coaching® is implemented.

Final Thought

Caring Science restores the sacred to the scientific. When nurses realign their practice through the 10 Caritas Processes®, they rediscover both their purpose and their power. It reminds us that alignment begins not with policy, but with presence — one authentic moment of caring at a time.

© 2025 Jean Watson

Global Icon of Nursing Philosophy, Healing & Holistic Care

Dr. Jean Watson is one of the most influential nurse theorists in modern history and the originator of the Theory of Human Caring, a framework that reshaped nursing practice around compassion, presence, and healing relationships. Her work, often referred to as Caring Science, has become foundational in nursing education, research, and leadership across the globe.

A Distinguished Professor and Dean Emerita at the University of Colorado College of Nursing, Dr. Watson has authored landmark texts, mentored generations of nurse leaders, and founded the Watson Caring Science Institute to advance research and systems-level transformation rooted in humanistic care. Her contribution to the Masters Series brings philosophical depth and moral clarity—an insistence that even as healthcare modernizes, the heart of healing must remain profoundly human.

Here's Mason's Take

Jean Watson changed the way I see alignment — not as structure, but as spirit. Her *Caring Science* gave nursing a language for love, presence, and purpose that no organizational chart could ever capture. When she says, *"Caring Science is alignment science,"* she's not just being poetic; she's giving healthcare its compass back.

For me, Watson's Caritas framework connects directly to everything we're building with **SCRUB*fits*™** and *The Healthcare Career Misalignment Epidemic*. She offers the missing piece — the why behind every what. Her belief that we are formed in relationship, not isolation, explains exactly why misalignment hurts so deeply. It's not just burnout; it's spiritual disconnection.

What I love most about Watson's approach is its simplicity wrapped in depth. Ten Caritas Processes®, each one practical and profound, like an internal checklist for the soul. *Embrace. Inspire. Trust. Nurture. Forgive. Deepen. Balance. Co-Create. Serve. Open.* They sound like poetry, but they are instructions for leadership, teaching, and healing — an operational model for the heart.

When I read her work, I see alignment everywhere: in the charge nurse who pauses before a code to breathe and center, in the preceptor who turns a mistake into a teachable moment, in the manager who writes a gratitude note instead of an email correction. Watson teaches that alignment is presence in motion.

Her influence runs through this entire project. *Caring Science* is the philosophical ancestor of the alignment movement we're naming in this book. It's what turns caring into culture, and culture into retention. It's why nurses stay — not just for a paycheck, but for a purpose they can feel in their bones.

Jean Watson reminds me that the science of alignment begins with a single human act: caring enough to connect.

Chapter 52

Masters Series: Your Surgical Tribe: The Alignment No One Talks About

By: **Chip Taunt, DO**

The Jumpstart — 45-Second Lesson in Alignment

Last week in the OR, we hit one of those gray-zone moments —something unexpected, something that didn't match the textbook, something that required judgment, not just skill. My partner, scrubbed in, called out for my opinion. I didn't have a confident answer.

So I texted two global thought leaders in revision (gl) total joint (gl) surgery and periprosthetic (gl) joint infection.

Both replied within minutes.

Their answers gave us clarity, but more importantly, they reminded me of something we rarely acknowledge in medicine:

Alignment isn't just internal.

Alignment is communal.

And your tribe (gl) is part of your clinical alignment.

Your hands did the surgery.

But your tribe guided your judgment.

That 45-second exchange was a mirror:

Your tribe is shaping you, whether you know it or not.

The Hidden Variable in Surgical Alignment

We talk endlessly about burnout, technique, robotics, implants, protocols, AI decision support—but not this.

The people you surround yourself with quietly calibrate (gl) your:

• confidence

• caution

• risk tolerance

• clinical philosophy

• identity as a surgeon

When you face a difficult revision (gl) or an unexpected finding, you're not just drawing from your residency, your training, or your CME.

You're drawing from the alignment created by your tribe.

The best decisions come from surgeons whose internal compass aligns with the collective compass of a high-quality tribe.

The worst decisions often come from surgeons aligned with the wrong tribe—or none at all.

Alignment isn't just who you are.

It's who you're with.

Most Surgeons Don't Choose Their Tribe. But the Aligned Ones Do.

Most tribes form by accident:

- who trained with you

- who works in your OR

- who happens to show up for cases

- who texts back fastest

- who shares gossip instead of insight

But clinical alignment doesn't happen accidentally.

It happens deliberately.

The surgeons who consistently deliver the best outcomes have one trait in common:

They intentionally align with the right minds, the right standards, the right ethics, and the right energy.

"People like us do things like this" isn't just cultural.

It's clinical alignment in action.

Your tribe defines:

- what "good enough" means

- what "aggressive" means

- what "reckless" means

- what "evidence-based" means

- what "patient-centered" means

- what "aligned practice" looks like

Your tribe is the architecture of your alignment.

If you inherit your tribe, your alignment is random.

If you choose your tribe, your alignment is intentional.

Two Alignment Questions Every Clinician Must Ask

1. Is your tribe aligned with excellence—or aligned with fear?

Do your colleagues center their thinking around:

- surgical mastery

- innovation

- patient outcomes

- truth

- growth

Or do they center around:

- liability

- politics

- income protection

- self-preservation

Fear-based alignment shrinks you.

Excellence-based alignment expands you.

2. Does your tribe stretch your alignment—or soothe it?

Some colleagues make you feel good.

Others make you feel more precise, more curious, more honest, more aligned with your best self.

There's a difference.

Comfort validates your current self.

Challenge aligns you with your future one.

Technology Will Surge Ahead — But Your Tribe Will Still Be Your Alignment Anchor

We're entering an era of:

- smarter implants

- predictive analytics (gl)

- real-time AI guidance

- more precise navigation

But here's the truth all seasoned surgeons know:

All the tools in the world won't compensate for misalignment.

And alignment comes from people, not robots.

Your tribe refines your judgment.

Your tribe sharpens your instincts.

Your tribe keeps your identity centered.

Your tribe keeps your alignment true.

Even in a high-tech world, alignment is still deeply human.

My Tribe, My Alignment

My tribe isn't just friends.

It isn't just the social circle.

It isn't the golf foursome (well, maybe one).

My tribe is made of individuals whose judgment I trust enough to influence mine—and who trust me enough to let me influence theirs.

They are my alignment anchors.

They shape my thought process.

They raise my standards.

They keep me calibrated.

And not one of them entered my professional orbit by accident.

Final Word — The Alignment You Choose Determines the Surgeon You Become

Whether you're a surgeon, a nurse, a student, a PA, or a future healthcare leader, the truth is the same:

Alignment is the new burnout prevention.

Alignment is your safety system.

Alignment is your identity.

And your tribe is part of your alignment.

Choose carefully.

Curate intentionally.

Protect fiercely.

Because the clinician you become will always reflect the tribe you trust and the alignment you build.

Charles J. "Chip" Taunt Jr., DO is a nationally recognized, board-certified, fellowship-trained orthopedic surgeon specializing in hip and knee replacement at Michigan Orthopedic Center in Lansing, Michigan. His practice focuses on delivering excellent outcomes with the shortest, safest recovery possible, and he has become the go-to surgeon for complex cases—component loosening (gl), material failure, infection, instability, fractures, and metal hypersensitivity (gl) that other surgeons refer in.

Beyond the operating room, Dr. Taunt is a teacher and leader. An Associate Clinical Professor of Surgery at Michigan State University, he trains orthopedic residents, interns, and medical students, and lectures around the country on advanced hip and knee replacement techniques. Professional organizations and trade publications have highlighted him as an "orthopedic surgeon leader to know," reflecting both his clinical expertise and his role in shaping best practices in joint reconstruction. His path runs through Des Moines University College of Osteopathic Medicine, an orthopedic residency in Michigan, and an adult reconstruction (gl) fellowship at the University of Chicago—training that positioned him to work at the intersection of precision surgery and second chances.

Here's Mason's Take

What Dr. Chip Taunt names here is the part of alignment most people never see — the communal wiring behind clinical judgment. We tend to think alignment is a private journey:

personality, pace, wiring, environment. But Chip is right. In healthcare, your alignment is also shaped by the people who surround you when the stakes are highest.

Your tribe becomes your calibration system.

Surgeons talk about technique, nurses talk about ratios, leaders talk about strategy — but very few talk about the invisible influence of the people you trust. A strong tribe sharpens your thinking. A careless one dulls it. An aligned tribe elevates your decisions. A misaligned tribe erodes them.

Chip's message is universal:

Your tribe is not a social circle — it's part of your clinical identity.

And whether you're a student choosing your first credential, a nurse finding your voice, or a surgeon navigating gray-zone moments, the same truth applies:

Alignment isn't just who you are. It's who you stand with. Choose your tribe with the same intention you choose your career.

Chapter 53
Healthcare Career Hotlist

Spotlight: The Top 25 Healthcare Roles to Watch Through 2034

Healthcare isn't slowing down—it's evolving. Over the next decade, the U.S. Bureau of Labor Statistics (gl) projects the healthcare and social-assistance sector will add 2 million+ new jobs, more than any other industry. That growth is fueled by aging populations (gl), telehealth (gl) expansion, new care models, and one unstoppable truth: people will always need people who care.

These twenty-five roles represent the most promising, resilient, and purpose-driven careers shaping healthcare through 2034. Each one offers opportunity—but alignment is what turns opportunity into longevity. The goal isn't just to land a job that's in demand; it's to find the one that matches your heartbeat.

A Note on the Numbers

Even national data has its quirks. The Bureau of Labor Statistics (gl) can tell you how fast a job is growing, but not how fast your heart beats when you walk into work. They measure projections (gl)—not passion.

(And they've yet to publish a chart on how many nurses survive on caffeine (gl) and purpose alone.)

Mason's Reflection

Lists reveal where opportunity lives, but only alignment shows where you belong. These 25 roles prove that healthcare's future is still human—built on curiosity, compassion, and courage. Data can forecast trends, but purpose decides destiny. When your pace, personality, and principles line up with your profession, you don't just work—you shine.

"Maybe it isn't this exact career that fits you—but something inspired by it."

And remember—alignment doesn't always mean the obvious path. Every one of these careers creates ripple effects—needs that spark new needs. The demand for nurses drives innovation in staffing, education, and patient-care technology. The rise of respiratory therapy opens doors for engineers, designers, and sales professionals creating safer equipment. Pharmacists inspire tech specialists developing smarter dispensing systems; physical therapists influence entrepreneurs building AI-driven (gl) rehab tools. Healthcare is changing at the pulse of progress, and every beat creates a new rhythm of opportunity. The secret is thinking creatively enough to hear your note in that rhythm—and playing it your way.

1. Nurse Practitioner (NP)

Autonomous (gl), trusted, and rapidly growing—NPs lead the charge in primary care (gl), urgent care (gl), and telehealth (gl).

Mason's Take

Nurse practitioners thrive at the intersection of science and soul. They make critical decisions while never losing the human connection that grounds them. Alignment here is about independence without isolation, confidence balanced with compassion. It's the career for those who want responsibility and relationship in equal measure. You don't just treat symptoms—you change systems.

2. Physician Associate (PA)

Versatile clinicians (gl) bridging medicine and collaboration.

Mason's Take

PAs are connectors—between patients and physicians, between expertise and empathy. They flourish where teamwork fuels trust. Alignment means being flexible, curious, and collaborative in every encounter. You're never "the assistant"; you're the amplifier of care. Every shift is a masterclass in shared purpose.

3. Registered Nurse (RN)

The backbone of every healthcare setting, from bedside to boardroom.

Mason's Take

Nurses are the heartbeat of healthcare. They bring structure to chaos, compassion to crisis, and calm to the storm. Alignment here thrives on adaptability—you can serve in a trauma bay, a clinic, or a classroom. No two paths look alike, and that's the beauty of it. Nursing isn't a job; it's a lifelong conversation between skill and spirit.

4. Medical and Health Services Manager

Strategists turning complexity into coordination.

Mason's Take

These leaders prove that spreadsheets can save lives. They align people, policy, and purpose behind every patient outcome. If you find satisfaction in systems (gl), this is your canvas. True alignment means making efficiency feel human. When operations work, healing follows.

5. Physical Therapist (PT)

Experts in movement, mobility (gl), and measurable hope.

Mason's Take

PTs rebuild more than muscles—they rebuild momentum. They understand progress as both science and spirit. Alignment here is persistence paired with patience. You learn to celebrate inches as victories and setbacks as lessons. Every day you remind someone that recovery is still possible.

6. Occupational Therapist (OTR/L)

Champions of independence who transform rehabilitation (gl) into real life.

Mason's Take

OTRs are healthcare's inventors. They design paths back to purpose using creativity as medicine. Alignment means loving details that restore dignity—small motions, big meaning. You see potential where others see limitation. Your therapy sessions don't just heal—they empower.

7. Speech-Language Pathologist (SLP)

Guardians of communication and confidence.

Mason's Take

SLPs give people their voices back. They teach patience, perseverance, and presence all at once. Alignment here lives in empathy—you cheer every syllable like a standing ovation. It's a role for listeners who believe in progress at the pace of courage. You don't just treat speech; you restore identity.

8. Respiratory Therapist (RRT)

Specialists in the science of breath and the art of calm.

Mason's Take

RTs are the quiet heroes of every code blue (gl) and every recovery. They measure oxygen but deliver peace. Alignment is steadiness under stress and compassion under pressure. You hold life in your hands—literally—and never take a single breath for granted. This is purpose you can feel in your own lungs.

9. Radiologic and Diagnostic Imaging Specialist (RT[R])

Seeing what others can't through precision and perspective.

Mason's Take

Imaging pros are storytellers in grayscale. They reveal truth pixel by pixel. Alignment means precision with empathy—each scan represents a person, not just an image. You thrive on accuracy, curiosity, and quiet impact. Sometimes the most powerful healing begins with being seen clearly.

10. Pharmacist

The last checkpoint before treatment becomes therapy.

Mason's Take

Pharmacists are detail warriors and patient advocates rolled into one. They turn chemistry (gl) into clarity and safety into standard. Alignment here is about vigilance, patience, and heart-led precision. You see the whole person behind every prescription label. In a world of speed, you make careful feel courageous.

11. Dentist

Architects of confidence and oral health.

Mason's Take

Dentistry is artistry with anatomy (gl). Alignment here means precision and prevention working hand in hand. You transform anxiety into assurance with skill and empathy. Every smile restored is a story rewritten. It's not just enamel—it's esteem.

12. Dental Hygienist

Frontline defenders of prevention and education.

Mason's Take

Dental hygienists are teachers disguised as technicians. They keep communities healthier one cleaning, one conversation at a time. Alignment is found in patience and prevention—you stop problems before they start. You're proof that small acts create lifelong impact. Your tools sparkle because your mission does.

13. Optometrist

Vision specialists who help people see clearly—in more ways than one.

Mason's Take

Optometrists reveal clarity where blur once lived. Alignment means blending science with lifestyle—each prescription reframes a life. You measure millimeters but deliver miles of difference. Empathy here looks like patience behind every lens. You don't just improve sight—you expand perspective.

14. Dietitian and Nutritionist

Masters of balance—on the plate and in the plan.

Mason's Take

Dietitians decode the link between nourishment (gl) and healing. Alignment thrives on curiosity, counseling, and care that lasts beyond discharge. You educate, empower, and sometimes rehabilitate habits more than diets. Every meal plan is an act of advocacy. You feed hope as much as health.

15. Medical Laboratory Scientist (MLS)

Detectives of diagnosis who see the unseen.

Mason's Take

Lab scientists are the quiet voices behind every accurate diagnosis. They work in the hum of machines yet anchor the heartbeat of medicine. Alignment here favors precision, patience, and pride in detail. You turn data into direction for the whole team. Your microscope might be small—but your impact is huge.

16. Surgical Technologist

The right hand of every operation.

Mason's Take

Surg techs live where trust meets timing. Alignment means grace under the brightest lights and focus that never flinches. You prepare, anticipate, and assist with unshakable calm. Every instrument you hand off represents safety. You might not speak during surgery—but your presence speaks volumes.

17. Anesthesiologist Assistant (AA)

Masters of focus and physiology (gl), ensuring comfort and control.

Mason's Take

AAs balance science, vigilance, and serenity. Alignment thrives in calm precision—you monitor what matters most when moments get critical. You work seamlessly in teams yet carry solo accountability. It's a role for thinkers who find peace in pressure. Your success is measured in stability—and gratitude that often arrives in silence.

18. Certified Registered Nurse Anesthetist (CRNA)

Calm expertise under pressure, personified.

Mason's Take

CRNAs transform anxiety into assurance with every breath they guide. Alignment here is courage fused with control. You balance independence with impeccable teamwork. The operating room may run on anesthesia, but it's powered by trust in you. Few roles embody "steady hands, steady heart" like this one.

19. Medical Assistant

The Swiss Army knife (gl) of outpatient (gl) care.

Mason's Take

Medical assistants keep clinics humming. Alignment means loving variety and thriving in the flow of patient after patient. You bridge front office and back, compassion and coordination. You see every part of the care journey—and you make each one smoother. Efficiency, empathy, and energy are your superpowers.

20. Phlebotomist

Turning needles into reassurance and fear into trust.

Mason's Take

Phlebotomists master the art of gentle precision. You face nerves, literal and emotional, every day. Alignment here means empathy with technique—comfort first, collection second. You prove that care starts long before results are printed. You draw courage as much as blood.

21. Home Health and Personal Care Aide

Care that meets people where they are.

Mason's Take

Aides are the unsung heroes of comfort and continuity. Alignment lives in empathy, reliability, and respect for independence. You witness the private victories of recovery and aging. Each visit matters more than most people realize. You remind patients that dignity belongs at home too.

22. Massage Therapist

Restoring balance through touch, science, and intuition.

Mason's Take

Massage therapists translate anatomy (gl) into empathy. Alignment means listening with your hands and healing with your presence. You work in wellness, rehab, and renewal. Every session is both art and anatomy in motion. You prove that recovery can feel like relief.

23. Genetic Counselor

Navigating heredity (gl), hope, and hard conversations.

Mason's Take

Genetic counselors are guides through uncertainty. Alignment here means blending evidence with empathy—science delivered softly. You explain the unexplainable and hold space for complex emotions. Your insight changes futures, but your kindness changes moments. You stand at the intersection of data and destiny.

24. Mental Health Counselor / Therapist

Healing minds to sustain bodies.

Mason's Take

Therapists turn listening into leadership. Alignment is compassion with boundaries, hope with realism. You witness people at their most honest and help them meet themselves with grace. It's not easy work—but it's sacred work. You hold space where the rest of us find strength.

25. Public Health Professional

Designing systems that keep communities well.

Mason's Take

Public-health (gl) pros think upstream—preventing crises before they reach the bedside. Alignment means believing that data can save lives and that education can change generations. You balance spreadsheets with storytelling and policy with purpose. You measure success in fewer emergencies, not more headlines. It's leadership that scales compassion.

From Hotlist to Heartwork

You've just met a lineup of roles that prove healthcare is bigger—and more human—than job titles and scrubs. Each entry in this Hotlist is more than a career option; it's a doorway. Some open into the fast-paced pulse of emergency care, others into the quiet rhythm of data, education, or healing touch. Together, they form the heartbeat of a system that needs every kind of talent—and yours might be next.

Maybe you found yourself circling one role again and again. Maybe a few surprised you. That's good. Curiosity is the first sign of alignment. The truth is, every fulfilling healthcare career begins with a spark: a question, a moment of empathy, a sense that your skills could ease someone's burden.

So, as you close this section, don't think of it as an ending. Think of it as a launchpad. Use what you've discovered here to chase clarity, not perfection. Explore. Shadow. Volunteer. Ask questions. Keep listening to that inner pull that says, "This matters."

Because when your work aligns with your values, it's no longer just a career—it's care, in motion.

Stay curious. Stay kind. StaySm:)in'.

Chapter 54
Field of 185 Careers

Welcome to the Field of 185 Healthcare Careers

Healthcare is often painted in broad strokes (gl): doctors, nurses, maybe a therapist or pharmacist. But the truth is far more vibrant (gl) and layered (gl). From the operating room to the boardroom, from bedside compassion (gl) to behind-the-scenes analytics (gl), there are hundreds of roles that keep the system alive.

This list isn't just about job titles and salaries. It's about alignment (gl). Each career is broken down with a clear description, education pathways (gl), salary ranges, shortage indicators (gl), and my personal take on who tends to thrive in that role. It's built for dreamers at the starting line, mid-career professionals looking to pivot (gl), and seasoned clinicians who want to realign (gl) their work with their values.

Think of the Field of 185 as your career atlas (gl). Not every path will be for you — and that's the point. Use these pages to spark curiosity (gl), confirm your instincts (gl), or open doors you didn't know existed. Healthcare is one of the few industries where your personality, values, and life circumstances (gl) can be matched with a role that truly fits.

Dive in with an open mind. Somewhere in these 185 is the role where your scrubs, your skills, and your sense of purpose (gl) finally line up.

1. Registered Nurse (RN)

Description: Provides direct patient care, coordinates treatments, educates patients and families, and serves as the backbone of healthcare teams in hospitals, clinics, and community settings.

Education/Training: ADN or BSN (increasingly required). Licensure via NCLEX-RN (gl). Specialty certifications (ACLS (gl), CCRN (gl), CEN (gl)) often add value.

Salary Range: $62,000–$115,000+ depending on region, specialty, and shifts.

Shortage Indicator: Significant and persistent. Demand peaks in critical care (gl), ED (gl), and rural areas.

Pathways & Notes: ADN-to-BSN bridges common; BSN often required for Magnet® (gl) hospitals. Graduate pathways lead to NP (gl), CRNA (gl), or informatics (gl).

Cost-of-Living Lens: Travel nurse (gl) and PRN (gl) shifts can substantially increase income.

Quote: "The right nurse notices what others miss."

Here's My Take: RNs are the Swiss Army knife of healthcare. If you like variety, intensity, and connection, this role keeps you in the heartbeat of care and opens countless doors.

2. Nurse Practitioner (NP)

Description: Advanced practice clinician diagnosing, prescribing, and managing care across populations (family, psych, acute, pediatric, etc.).

Education/Training: MSN or DNP; national certification (AANP (gl) / ANCC (gl)); state APRN (gl) license.

Salary Range: $100,000–$160,000+.

Shortage Indicator: High, especially in primary care, mental health, and rural settings.

Pathways & Notes: Post-master's certifications allow pivots (gl) (e.g., FNP (gl) → PMHNP (gl)).

Cost-of-Living Lens: Independent practice (gl) states boost autonomy (gl) and earnings.

Quote: "Access expands when advanced practice leads."

Here's My Take: NPs thrive when they're given space to make the call. If autonomy (gl) and evidence-based (gl) medicine are your jam, this is it.

3. Physician (Family Medicine)

Description: Generalist physician caring for all ages—prevention, chronic disease, acute issues, and coordination.

Education/Training: MD (gl) / DO (gl); residency (gl); board certification (gl).

Salary Range: $220,000–$300,000+.

Shortage Indicator: One of the highest shortages, especially rural.

Pathways & Notes: Subspecialize (gl) in sports medicine, addiction (gl), or geriatrics (gl).

Cost-of-Living Lens: Loan forgiveness (gl) may be available in rural practice.

Quote: "Continuity (gl) is a medicine of its own."

Here's My Take: For mission-driven clinicians who want long-term relationships and the satisfaction of watching families thrive across generations.

4. Physician Assistant (PA-C)

Description: Diagnoses, treats, and performs procedures in collaboration (gl) with a physician; scope (gl) spans specialties.

Education/Training: Master's in PA studies; certification via PANCE (gl); state license.

Salary Range: $105,000–$155,000+.

Shortage Indicator: High demand in surgery, hospital medicine, and primary care.

Pathways & Notes: Flexible specialty switching.

Cost-of-Living Lens: Surgical call (gl) and hospitalist (gl) shifts can add significant income.

Quote: "Versatility (gl) is the PA superpower (gl)."

Here's My Take: PAs shine when you want variety without the rigid walls of residency (gl).

5. Pharmacist (PharmD)

Description: Ensures safe and effective medication use, manages therapies, monitors kinetics (gl), supports stewardship (gl), and counsels patients.

Education/Training: PharmD required; residencies (gl) (PGY1 (gl) / PGY2 (gl)) common for clinical roles; state licensure.

Salary Range: $120,000–$165,000+.

Shortage Indicator: Moderate overall; strong in inpatient, ambulatory care (gl), ID (gl), and oncology (gl).

Pathways & Notes: Board certifications (gl) (BCPS (gl), BCIDP (gl), BCCCP (gl)) unlock subspecialties (gl). Informatics (gl) pathways exist.

Cost-of-Living Lens: Health-system (gl) roles may include pensions (gl) and schedule balance.

Quote: "Right drug, right dose (gl), right now."

Here's My Take: Perfect for detail-driven professionals who like clinical puzzles and direct impact without always being bedside.

6. Pharmacy Technician

Description: Prepares medications, manages inventory, supports sterile compounding (gl), and keeps automation (gl) flowing.

Education/Training: Certification (gl) (CPhT (gl)) increasingly standard.

Salary Range: $38,000–$62,000+.

Shortage Indicator: Steady across hospitals and specialty compounding (gl).

Pathways & Notes: Pyxis (gl) / Omnicell (gl) super-user (gl); sterile compounding (gl) focus.

Cost-of-Living Lens: Hospitals often balance pay with stronger benefits.

Quote: "Pharmacy runs on tech precision (gl)."

Here's My Take: A great entry point for those who want healthcare exposure with room to grow into more administrative (gl) roles.

7. Respiratory Therapist (RRT)

Description: Manages airways (gl), ventilators (gl), and oxygen therapies (gl); key in codes (gl), ICUs (gl), and NICUs (gl).

Education/Training: Associate or Bachelor's in RT; RRT credential (gl); state license.

Salary Range: $60,000–$98,000+.

Shortage Indicator: Critical shortage, especially ICUs (gl) and neonatal (gl) care.

Pathways & Notes: Specialize (gl) in ECMO (gl) or transport (gl).

Cost-of-Living Lens: Premiums (gl) for nights/weekends boost earnings.

Quote: "When breath is fragile, skill is everything."

Here's My Take: For clinicians who thrive under pressure and love blending tech with human connection.

8. Radiologic Technologist (RT[R])

Description: Conducts diagnostic (gl) X-rays (gl), portable imaging (gl), and OR (gl) C-arm (gl) studies.

Education/Training: Accredited (gl) RT program; ARRT (gl) certified; state license.

Salary Range: $55,000–$90,000+.

Shortage Indicator: Stable but strong need nights/trauma (gl).

Pathways & Notes: Ladder (gl) to CT (gl), MRI (gl), IR (gl), or PACS (gl) admin (gl).

Cost-of-Living Lens: Cross-training (gl) increases pay.

Quote: "Positioning (gl) is half the diagnosis (gl)."

Here's My Take: Great for hands-on learners who want patient contact with technical problem-solving.

9. CT Technologist

Description: Provides cross-sectional (gl) imaging (gl), stroke (gl) protocols (gl), and trauma (gl) imaging (gl).

Education/Training: ARRT(R) (gl) with CT (gl) certification (gl).

Salary Range: $70,000–$110,000+.

Shortage Indicator: High, especially in 24/7 stroke (gl) centers.

Pathways & Notes: Step-up (gl) role from RT(R) (gl). Bridges (gl) to IR (gl) or leadership.

Cost-of-Living Lens: Call pay (gl) is a significant supplement (gl).

Quote: "Seconds matter when vessels (gl) close."

Here's My Take: Best for fast-acting techs who thrive on urgent answers and teamwork.

10. MRI Technologist

Description: Specializes (gl) in advanced magnetic (gl) imaging—neuro (gl), cardiac (gl), musculoskeletal (gl).

Education/Training: ARRT (gl) + MRI credential (gl); MRI safety (gl) training required.

Salary Range: $72,000-$115,000+.

Shortage Indicator: Consistently high due to safety (gl) barriers (gl) and skill intensity.

Pathways & Notes: Cardiac (gl) MRI and academic centers are high-growth niches (gl).

Cost-of-Living Lens: Subspecialty (gl) certification boosts leverage (gl) in negotiations (gl).

Quote: "Clarity without radiation (gl)—precision (gl) with patience."

Here's My Take: For patient communicators who can balance precision (gl) with calmness.

11. Diagnostic Medical Sonographer

Description: Performs ultrasounds (gl) (OB/GYN (gl), vascular (gl), echo (gl), abdominal (gl)) with operator dependence (gl).

Education/Training: Accredited (gl) program; ARDMS (gl) or CCI (gl) credentialing (gl).

Salary Range: $68,000-$110,000+.

Shortage Indicator: Growing need in vascular (gl) and OB (gl).

Pathways & Notes: Adding cardiac (gl) or vascular (gl) specialties (gl) multiplies job options.

Cost-of-Living Lens: PRN (gl) roles can help offset housing costs.

Quote: "The image is only as good as the hands."

Here's My Take: For those with steady hands, empathy, and spatial reasoning (gl).

12. Medical Laboratory Scientist (MLS)

Description: Performs complex (gl) clinical testing (gl) that drives 70%+ of medical decisions.

Education/Training: Bachelor's in MLS; ASCP (gl) certification (gl).

Salary Range: $60,000–$95,000+.

Shortage Indicator: Significant shortages, especially in blood bank (gl).

Pathways & Notes: LIS (gl), microbiology (gl), transfusion (gl), quality leadership.

Cost-of-Living Lens: Stipends (gl) for nights/holidays can matter.

Quote: "Invisible work, visible outcomes."

Here's My Take: If you love science experiments but want real-world stakes (gl), this is your lab.

13. Phlebotomist

Description: Collects blood and other specimens (gl) with accuracy and care.

Education/Training: Certificate (gl) or on-the-job; national cert (gl) (CPT (gl)) helpful.

Salary Range: $34,000–$50,000+.

Shortage Indicator: Steady demand; hospital roles especially strong.

Pathways & Notes: Stepping stone (gl) into MLS, nursing, or other clinical careers.

Cost-of-Living Lens: Health systems often offer better benefits vs. small labs.

Quote: "Gentle hands build trust."

Here's My Take: Ideal for those entering healthcare who want patient contact from day one.

14. Emergency Medical Technician (EMT)

Description: Provides basic life support (gl), rapid transport (gl), and scene stabilization (gl).

Education/Training: EMT certificate (gl); state licensure.

Salary Range: $35,000–$52,000+.

Shortage Indicator: Persistent in urban and rural EMS (gl).

Pathways & Notes: Ladder (gl) to Paramedic (gl), critical care transport (gl), or ED (gl) tech.

Cost-of-Living Lens: Municipal (gl) and fire-department benefits often matter.

Quote: "First on scene, first to steady the chaos."

Here's My Take: Best for adrenaline seekers who want immediate impact in emergencies.

15. Paramedic

Description: Advanced prehospital (gl) clinician—IVs (gl), advanced airways (gl), EKGs (gl), trauma (gl).

Education/Training: Paramedic certificate (gl); NREMT-P (gl); state license.

Salary Range: $48,000–$80,000+.

Shortage Indicator: Strong demand; community paramedicine (gl) models expanding.

Pathways & Notes: Bridges (gl) into flight medic (gl) or education.

Cost-of-Living Lens: Call pay (gl) and overtime (gl) add up.

Quote: "Decisions in minutes that matter for years."

Here's My Take: For decisive clinicians who thrive under sirens and flashing lights.

16. Surgical Technologist

Description: Preps instruments (gl), maintains sterile field (gl), supports surgeons intra-op (gl).

Education/Training: CST (gl) preferred.

Salary Range: $48,000–$78,000+.

Shortage Indicator: OR (gl) demand high.

Pathways & Notes: CSFA (gl) (first assist (gl)) pathways exist.

Cost-of-Living Lens: Call pay (gl) can significantly supplement (gl) income.

Quote: "Anticipation is the art of the OR (gl)."

Here's My Take: Perfect for precision-driven individuals who love choreography (gl) and tech.

17. Operating Room Nurse (CNOR)

Description: RN (gl) circulator (gl) / scrub nurse (gl) ensuring safety, advocacy (gl), documentation (gl), and coordination (gl) during surgery.

Education/Training: Periop (gl) training; CNOR (gl) certification valuable.

Salary Range: $80,000-$125,000+.

Shortage Indicator: Persistent; long orientation (gl) periods increase demand.

Pathways & Notes: Robotics (gl) and cardiac surgery (gl) are common specialties.

Cost-of-Living Lens: OR (gl) call stipends (gl) can be major boosts.

Quote: "In the OR (gl), safety is sacred."

Here's My Take: For those who want to be the patient's voice when they can't speak.

18. ICU Nurse (Critical Care RN)

Description: Manages critically ill (gl) patients requiring high monitoring (gl), drips (gl), vents (gl), and advanced interventions (gl).

Education/Training: ICU (gl) orientation (gl); CCRN (gl) common.

Salary Range: $88,000–$135,000+.

Shortage Indicator: Strong and ongoing.

Pathways & Notes: CRNA (gl), ACNP (gl), ECMO (gl) pathways are common.

Cost-of-Living Lens: Night/weekend pay can matter.

Quote: "Details decide outcomes."

Here's My Take: ICU nurses thrive when precision and vigilance (gl) meet compassion.

19. Emergency Department Nurse (ED RN)

Description: Triage (gl), stabilize (gl), and manage crises (gl) in a fast-paced setting.

Education/Training: CEN (gl), TNCC (gl), ACLS (gl) common.

Salary Range: $80,000–$130,000+.

Shortage Indicator: High; tied to volume and boarding (gl) pressures.

Pathways & Notes: Trauma centers (gl), rapid response (gl), flight nursing (gl).

Cost-of-Living Lens: Shift differentials (gl) and overtime (gl) are common.

Quote: "Prepared for anything, attached to nothing."

Here's My Take: A calling for those who thrive on unpredictability (gl) and speed.

20. Labor & Delivery Nurse (L&D RN)

Description: Provides maternity care (gl) before, during, and after delivery.

Education/Training: Certifications (gl) such as NCC-EFM (gl) and NRP (gl).

Salary Range: $78,000–$125,000+.

Shortage Indicator: Steady, variable by region.

Pathways & Notes: Maternal-fetal medicine (gl) and NICU (gl) pathways are common.

Cost-of-Living Lens: Call shifts can add flexibility.

Quote: "Where science meets beginnings."

Here's My Take: If you love being present for life's first cries, this is the unit where science and humanity intersect.

21. Physical Therapist (PT)

Description: Restores function (gl) and mobility (gl); supports rehab (gl) across settings.

Education/Training: DPT (gl); state license.

Salary Range: $78,000–$115,000+.

Shortage Indicator: Consistent need in rehab (gl) and home health (gl).

Pathways & Notes: Specialization (gl) (OCS (gl), NCS (gl)) options exist.

Cost-of-Living Lens: Productivity models (gl) vary—negotiation (gl) matters.

Quote: "Motion is medicine."

Here's My Take: For clinicians who love measurable (gl) progress and coaching patients back to life.

22. Occupational Therapist (OTR/L)

Description: Helps patients regain daily living skills (gl) across settings.

Education/Training: MOT (gl) or OTD (gl); licensure required.

Salary Range: $76,000–$112,000+.

Shortage Indicator: Strong across inpatient rehab (gl), SNFs (gl), and pediatrics.

Pathways & Notes: Hand therapy (gl) pathways are common.

Cost-of-Living Lens: School-based OTs (gl) often trade pay for schedule stability.

Quote: "Independence is the goal; creativity is the path."

Here's My Take: A great match for inventive clinicians who love function (gl) as much as strength.

23. Speech-Language Pathologist (SLP)

Description: Treats speech, language, and swallowing (gl) disorders (gl) across the lifespan (gl).

Education/Training: Master's in SLP; CCC-SLP (gl); licensure.

Salary Range: $72,000–$110,000+.

Shortage Indicator: High, particularly in rehab and pediatrics.

Pathways & Notes: VFSS (gl) / FEES (gl) swallowing studies (gl).

Cost-of-Living Lens: PRN (gl) and per-diem work can supplement (gl) income.

Quote: "Finding voices—and safe swallows (gl)."

Here's My Take: If you want to give people back their voice and dignity, this role fits beautifully.

24. Medical Assistant (MA)

Description: Ambulatory (gl) role supporting clinic flow (gl) and basic clinical tasks.

Education/Training: Certificate/diploma; certification (gl) such as CMA (gl) or RMA (gl).

Salary Range: $36,000–$52,000+.

Shortage Indicator: Steady across outpatient (gl) settings.

Pathways & Notes: Ladder (gl) into other clinical roles is common.

Cost-of-Living Lens: Tuition perks (gl) can be meaningful in large systems.

Quote: "Clinic flow (gl) is a team sport."

Here's My Take: A great entry role for organized multitaskers (gl).

25. Health Information Manager (RHIA)

Description: Directs integrity (gl) and privacy (gl) of medical records, coding (gl), CDI (gl), and analytics (gl).

Education/Training: Bachelor's in HIM (gl); RHIA (gl) credential (gl).

Salary Range: $78,000–$120,000+.

Shortage Indicator: Strong demand tied to EHR (gl) optimization (gl) and compliance (gl).

Pathways & Notes: Revenue cycle (gl), compliance (gl) officer (gl), analytics (gl).

Cost-of-Living Lens: Remote (gl) / hybrid (gl) roles expand options.

Quote: "Clean data, clean decisions."

Here's My Take: For those who like systems, policy (gl), and structure—this role turns data into the foundation of patient care.

26. Certified Nursing Assistant (CNA)

Description: Provides direct patient support—bathing, feeding, turning (gl), vital signs (gl), emotional comfort. Backbone of bedside (gl) care.

Education/Training: State-approved CNA (gl) course + certification exam (gl).

Salary Range: $32,000–$46,000+.

Shortage Indicator: Very high; long-term care (gl) and hospitals struggle to retain CNAs (gl).

Pathways & Notes: Many bridge (gl) into nursing (gl) (LPN (gl)/RN (gl)) while working. Tuition assistance (gl) common.

Cost-of-Living Lens: Unionized (gl) hospitals or large systems often pay above market.

Quote: "Compassion delivered one basic need at a time."

Here's My Take: CNAs (gl) are the hands and heart of care. Perfect for those who want immediate patient connection while building toward advanced roles.

27. Licensed Practical Nurse (LPN) (gl) / Licensed Vocational Nurse (LVN)

Description: Provides patient care in clinics (gl), LTC (gl), and hospitals under RN (gl)/MD (gl) supervision (gl).

Education/Training: 12–18 month program; NCLEX-PN (gl) exam (gl).

Salary Range: $48,000–$68,000+.

Shortage Indicator: High in LTC (gl) and rehab (gl) facilities.

Pathways & Notes: LPN-to-RN (gl) bridge programs widely available.

Cost-of-Living Lens: Salaries lower than RN (gl) but education costs are significantly less.

Quote: "Nursing skills without delay."

Here's My Take: A practical entry point for bedside (gl) caregivers who want to work quickly while advancing education over time.

28. Certified Registered Nurse Anesthetist (CRNA)

Description: Provides anesthesia (gl) for surgeries and procedures (gl); independent or team-based practice (gl).

Education/Training: RN (gl) + ICU (gl) experience → DNP (gl) or DNAP (gl) in nurse anesthesia (gl); board certification (gl) (NBCRNA (gl)).

Salary Range: $190,000–$260,000+.

Shortage Indicator: High; rural (gl) hospitals heavily reliant (gl) on CRNAs (gl).

Pathways & Notes: One of the highest-paying nursing roles. ICU (gl) RN (gl) background is essential.

Cost-of-Living Lens: Rural (gl) and independent practice (gl) states offer autonomy (gl) and premium pay (gl).

Quote: "Every heartbeat under anesthesia (gl) counts."

Here's My Take: Best for ICU (gl) nurses who want autonomy (gl), responsibility, and a high-reward path.

29. Certified Nurse Midwife (CNM)

Description: Provides prenatal (gl), labor (gl), delivery, and postpartum (gl) care; women's health across the lifespan (gl).

Education/Training: MSN (gl)/DNP (gl) midwifery (gl) program; AMCB (gl) certification (gl).

Salary Range: $100,000–$145,000+.

Shortage Indicator: Growing, especially in underserved (gl) maternity deserts (gl).

Pathways & Notes: Expanding integration (gl) with OB (gl) teams and birth centers (gl).

Cost-of-Living Lens: Rural incentives (gl) and community practice (gl) ownership boost viability.

Quote: "Birth with skill, dignity, and presence."

Here's My Take: For those passionate about maternal (gl) health and patient advocacy (gl)—it's medicine at life's edge and beginning.

30. Certified Nursing Informatics Specialist

Description: Translates clinical practice (gl) into EHR (gl) design, optimization (gl), and training.

Education/Training: BSN (gl); MSN (gl)/DNP (gl) with informatics (gl) focus; ANCC (gl) Informatics Nursing Certification (gl).

Salary Range: $88,000–$135,000+.

Shortage Indicator: Strong with ongoing EHR (gl) rollouts (gl)/upgrades (gl).

Pathways & Notes: Bridges clinical care with IT (gl), analytics (gl), leadership (gl).

Cost-of-Living Lens: Hybrid (gl)/remote options allow COL (gl) arbitrage (gl).

Quote: "Turning clicks into care."

Here's My Take: Perfect for nurses who love tech and process improvement (gl) but still want to touch patient outcomes indirectly.

31. Clinical Nurse Specialist (CNS)

Description: Advanced practice (gl) nurse focusing on quality, outcomes, and specialty (gl) practice improvement (gl).

Education/Training: MSN (gl) or DNP (gl); certification (gl) in specialty (gl) (e.g., oncology (gl), peds (gl)).

Salary Range: $100,000–$140,000+.

Shortage Indicator: Growing in Magnet® (gl) hospitals and large systems.

Pathways & Notes: Strong role in evidence-based (gl) practice, education, and QI (gl).

Cost-of-Living Lens: Salaries influenced by specialty (gl) (oncology (gl), critical care (gl)).

Quote: "Practice changes because CNSs (gl) lead it."

Here's My Take: For RNs (gl) who geek out on protocols (gl), outcomes, and teaching others while staying clinically grounded.

32. Case Manager Nurse (RN, CCM)

Description: Coordinates patient transitions (gl), discharge planning (gl), and resource management (gl).

Education/Training: RN (gl); CCM (gl) certification (gl) preferred.

Salary Range: $78,000–$110,000+.

Shortage Indicator: Strong with growing focus on readmission (gl) reduction.

Pathways & Notes: Many move into utilization review (gl), quality, or leadership.

Cost-of-Living Lens: Remote/hybrid options available in many systems.

Quote: "The right plan shortens the stay and strengthens recovery."

Here's My Take: For nurses who love connecting dots between patient, payer (gl), and provider (gl) while advocating for the patient's best outcome.

33. Public Health Nurse

Description: Focuses on prevention (gl), education, and community health (gl) initiatives (gl).

Education/Training: BSN (gl); MPH (gl) beneficial.

Salary Range: $68,000–$95,000+.

Shortage Indicator: Growing with public health crises (gl) and community health (gl) focus.

Pathways & Notes: Opportunities with health departments (gl), NGOs (gl), schools.

Cost-of-Living Lens: Lower pay vs. acute care (gl), but strong retirement/pension (gl) benefits in public systems.

Quote: "Population health (gl) starts with public health."

Here's My Take: Great for mission-driven nurses who want to improve lives upstream (gl).

34. School Nurse

Description: Provides healthcare, medication (gl) management, and health education in school settings.

Education/Training: RN (gl); BSN (gl) preferred; state school nurse credential (gl) in some regions.

Salary Range: $52,000–$78,000+.

Shortage Indicator: Growing need with student health complexities (gl).

Pathways & Notes: Summers off; pivotal (gl) in chronic (gl) condition (gl) management (gl) (asthma (gl), diabetes (gl)).

Cost-of-Living Lens: Salary often lower, but schedule/lifestyle balance unmatched.

Quote: "The first responder (gl) for the youngest lives."

Here's My Take: Best for nurses who love kids, education, and predictable schedules.

35. Home Health Nurse

Description: Provides care in patients' homes—wound care (gl), IV (gl) therapy (gl), chronic (gl) management (gl).

Education/Training: RN (gl); home health certification (gl) helpful.

Salary Range: $70,000–$100,000+.

Shortage Indicator: Very high with aging population (gl).

Pathways & Notes: Autonomy (gl) heavy; time management essential.

Cost-of-Living Lens: Mileage reimbursement (gl) and flexible scheduling offset base pay.

Quote: "Care doesn't end at discharge—it begins again at home."

Here's My Take: Perfect for self-directed nurses who like independence and one-on-one care.

36. Hospice Nurse

Description: Provides palliative (gl) and end-of-life (gl) care focused on comfort, dignity, and family support.

Education/Training: RN (gl); CHPN (gl) certification (gl) valuable.

Salary Range: $70,000–$102,000+.

Shortage Indicator: Strong; hospice programs growing rapidly.

Pathways & Notes: Emotional resilience (gl) is critical; leadership and case management roles common.

Cost-of-Living Lens: Travel to homes adds variable expenses; mileage stipends (gl) help.

Quote: "Dignity at life's final chapter."

Here's My Take: For those who value presence, empathy, and holistic (gl) care when cure is no longer the goal.

37. Dialysis Nurse

Description: Specializes (gl) in care for patients with kidney failure (gl) requiring hemodialysis (gl) or peritoneal dialysis (gl).

Education/Training: RN (gl); dialysis-specific (gl) training; CDN (gl) or CNN (gl) certifications (gl).

Salary Range: $75,000–$110,000+.

Shortage Indicator: Strong and persistent with CKD (gl) prevalence (gl).

Pathways & Notes: Roles in outpatient (gl) centers, inpatient (gl) dialysis, education.

Cost-of-Living Lens: Predictable clinic schedules offset lower acute care (gl) pay.

Quote: "Life flows through clean blood."

Here's My Take: Great for detail-driven nurses who want predictable hours and deep patient relationships.

38. Flight Nurse

Description: Provides critical care (gl) transport (gl) in helicopters and fixed-wing (gl) aircraft.

Education/Training: RN (gl); CCRN (gl)/CEN (gl)/CFRN (gl); 3–5 years critical care (gl)/ED (gl) required.

Salary Range: $85,000–$130,000+.

Shortage Indicator: Specialized (gl) demand; high turnover (gl) from burnout (gl).

Pathways & Notes: Extremely competitive (gl); roles often require EMT (gl)/paramedic (gl) training.

Cost-of-Living Lens: Hazard pay (gl) and rural (gl) flight programs can significantly raise compensation.

Quote: "Care at 5,000 feet."

Here's My Take: For adrenaline-seekers who thrive in autonomy (gl) and extreme conditions.

39. Forensic Nurse (SANE-A, SANE-P)

Description: Provides trauma-informed (gl) care and forensic (gl) exams (gl) for survivors of violence and abuse.

Education/Training: RN (gl); SANE (gl) training/certification (gl).

Salary Range: $70,000–$108,000+.

Shortage Indicator: High need, especially in rural (gl) and underserved (gl) regions.

Pathways & Notes: Overlaps with advocacy (gl), law enforcement (gl), legal testimony (gl).

Cost-of-Living Lens: Programs often grant stipends (gl)/on-call premiums (gl).

Quote: "Healing and justice can walk together."

Here's My Take: A calling for those with empathy, resilience (gl), and advocacy (gl) spirit.

40. Wound Care Nurse (CWCN)

Description: Specializes (gl) in wound, ostomy (gl), and continence (gl) care; consults across settings.

Education/Training: RN (gl); WOCN (gl) certification (gl).

Salary Range: $82,000–$120,000+.

Shortage Indicator: Strong due to aging and diabetic (gl) populations.

Pathways & Notes: Autonomy-rich consultative (gl) role; overlaps with quality improvement (gl).

Cost-of-Living Lens: Many roles offer hybrid hospital/outpatient (gl) flexibility.

Quote: "Healing starts at the skin."

Here's My Take: For detail-oriented nurses who love solving complex (gl) physical challenges.

41. Infection Preventionist (RN (gl)/MPH (gl)/MT

Description: Monitors, prevents, and manages infection control (gl) programs.

Education/Training: RN (gl), MLS (gl), or MPH (gl) background; CIC (gl) certification (gl).

Salary Range: $85,000–$125,000+.

Shortage Indicator: High; role expanded post-pandemic (gl).

Pathways & Notes: Opportunities for leadership, system-wide oversight (gl), policy (gl).

Cost-of-Living Lens: Hybrid models common; compensation varies by hospital size.

Quote: "One policy can stop a thousand infections."

Here's My Take: Best for evidence-driven professionals who love surveillance (gl), prevention (gl), and safety.

42. Occupational Health Nurse

Description: Promotes and protects worker health—injury prevention (gl), wellness, OSHA (gl) compliance (gl).

Education/Training: RN (gl); COHN-S (gl) certification (gl) optional.

Salary Range: $74,000–$110,000+.

Shortage Indicator: Growing need with employer wellness programs.

Pathways & Notes: Roles in corporations, manufacturing (gl), government.

Cost-of-Living Lens: Often salaried with strong pension/benefit packages.

Quote: "Healthy workers build healthy companies."

Here's My Take: Great for nurses who want predictable hours, prevention (gl) focus, and advocacy (gl).

43. Nurse Educator (Academic)

Description: Teaches nursing students in academic programs; develops curricula (gl) and evaluations (gl).

Education/Training: MSN (gl) or doctoral degree (gl) (PhD (gl)/DNP (gl)); academic experience.

Salary Range: $80,000–$120,000+.

Shortage Indicator: High; faculty shortages (gl) limit student admissions.

Pathways & Notes: Tenure-track (gl), research (gl), administration (gl) opportunities.

Cost-of-Living Lens: Lower salary than practice, but academic lifestyle and pensions (gl) balance.

Quote: "Nurses who teach, multiply their impact."

Here's My Take: For clinicians who love shaping the next generation.

44. Clinical Nurse Educator (Staff Development)

Description: Provides orientation (gl), ongoing training, and competency (gl) assessments (gl) for hospital/unit (gl) nurses.

Education/Training: RN (gl), BSN (gl); MSN (gl) preferred; education certification (gl) beneficial.

Salary Range: $78,000–$112,000+.

Shortage Indicator: Moderate; specialty educators in high demand.

Pathways & Notes: Career ladder (gl) to system education director.

Cost-of-Living Lens: Salaries vary by hospital size/complexity (gl).

Quote: "Every skill taught saves a patient unseen."

Here's My Take: Perfect for nurses who love teaching peers and improving practice (gl).

45. Nurse Researcher

Description: Designs and conducts studies to advance evidence-based (gl) practice.

Education/Training: PhD (gl) or DNP (gl); research (gl) training.

Salary Range: $85,000–$125,000+.

Shortage Indicator: Steady; academic centers drive growth.

Pathways & Notes: Opportunities for grants (gl), publications (gl), policy (gl) influence.

Cost-of-Living Lens: Salaries vary widely between academia (gl) vs. industry.

Quote: "Evidence drives care forward."

Here's My Take: Best for nurses who want to change care at scale, not just bedside (gl).

46. Nurse Administrator (CNO (gl)/Director)

Description: Oversees nursing practice (gl), staffing (gl), budgets (gl), strategy (gl).

Education/Training: BSN (gl); MSN (gl)/MBA (gl)/DNP (gl) often required; leadership certification (gl).

Salary Range: $120,000–$250,000+.

Shortage Indicator: Strong demand for transformational (gl) leaders.

Pathways & Notes: CNO (gl), COO (gl), CEO (gl) trajectories (gl) possible.

Cost-of-Living Lens: Salaries scale with hospital/system size.

Quote: "Leadership amplifies every nurse."

Here's My Take: For vision-driven leaders who want to shape culture, quality, and alignment.

47. Chief Nursing Informatics Officer (CNIO)

Description: Executive role overseeing integration (gl) of clinical workflows (gl) with health IT (gl) systems.

Education/Training: MSN (gl)/DNP (gl) with informatics (gl); leadership experience.

Salary Range: $150,000–$250,000+.

Shortage Indicator: Growing in large systems.

Pathways & Notes: Works closely with CIO (gl)/CMIO (gl) on strategy.

Cost-of-Living Lens: Urban (gl) systems offer highest comp (gl), remote work possible.

Quote: "Clinical voice at the digital table."

Here's My Take: For nurse leaders who want to marry tech with clinical practice at the highest level.

48. Chief Nursing Officer (CNO)

Description: Top nursing leader guiding practice, strategy, and culture across organizations.

Education/Training: BSN (gl), MSN (gl)/DNP (gl); executive experience.

Salary Range: $180,000–$400,000+.

Shortage Indicator: High in systems aiming for Magnet® (gl)/Pathway (gl) status.

Pathways & Notes: Trajectory (gl) often includes COO (gl) or CEO (gl) roles.

Cost-of-Living Lens: Salaries scale with size of system and scope (gl).

Quote: "Culture starts at the CNO (gl) desk."

Here's My Take: A role for leaders who want to turn vision into reality systemwide.

49. Director of Quality Improvement

Description: Oversees hospital/system QI (gl), patient safety (gl), and regulatory (gl) compliance (gl).

Education/Training: RN (gl)/MD (gl)/MPH (gl)/MHA (gl); CPHQ (gl) certification (gl) common.

Salary Range: $110,000–$185,000+.

Shortage Indicator: Strong with regulatory (gl) and reimbursement (gl) shifts.

Pathways & Notes: Bridges (gl) to VP (gl) of Quality, COO (gl), CMO (gl).

Cost-of-Living Lens: Salaries higher in academic/urban (gl) centers.

Quote: "Quality is everyone's job, but leadership owns the standard."

Here's My Take: For detail-oriented leaders who see care through systems lenses.

50. Patient Safety Officer

Description: Focuses on preventing harm through reporting systems, RCA (gl), and safety culture (gl).

Education/Training: RN (gl)/MD (gl)/PharmD (gl)/MPH (gl); CPPS (gl) certification (gl).

Salary Range: $105,000–$165,000+.

Shortage Indicator: Strong; regulators (gl) pushing safety culture (gl).

Pathways & Notes: Often combined with quality or risk management (gl) leadership.

Cost-of-Living Lens: Large health systems support higher comp (gl); hybrid roles possible.

Quote: "Safety is not negotiable."

Here's My Take: Ideal for leaders passionate about Just Culture (gl) and protecting patients through prevention (gl).

50. Patient Safety Officer

Description: Focuses on preventing harm through reporting systems, RCA (gl), and safety culture (gl).

Education/Training: RN/MD/PharmD/MPH; CPPS (gl) certification.

Salary Range: $105,000–$165,000+.

Shortage Indicator: Strong.

Pathways & Notes: Often combined with quality or risk management (gl) leadership.

Cost-of-Living Lens: Hybrid roles possible.

Quote: "Safety is not negotiable."

Here's My Take: Ideal for leaders passionate about Just Culture (gl) and protecting patients through prevention (gl).

51. Risk Manager (Healthcare)

Description: Identifies, evaluates, and mitigates risks to patients, staff, and organizations. Manages liability claims, compliance (gl), and legal reporting.

Education/Training: RN/MPH/JD/MHA; CPHRM (gl) certification valuable.

Salary Range: $95,000–$155,000+.

Shortage Indicator: Strong with increasing malpractice (gl) and regulatory scrutiny.

Pathways & Notes: Bridges into patient safety (gl) or executive leadership.

Cost-of-Living Lens: Larger health systems and insurers pay more.

Quote: "Anticipating tomorrow's risks protects patients today."

Here's My Take: A role for systems-thinkers (gl) who want to prevent problems before they hit the headlines.

52. Clinical Documentation Improvement Specialist (CDI) (gl)

Description: Reviews medical records to ensure accurate coding (gl), billing, and clinical representation of care.

Education/Training: RN, RHIA (gl), or coding (gl) background; CCDS (gl) or CDIP (gl) certification.

Salary Range: $82,000–$115,000+.

Shortage Indicator: Growing with CMS (gl) scrutiny and DRG (gl) payment models.

Pathways & Notes: Pathway to revenue cycle (gl) leadership, compliance (gl), or informatics (gl).

Cost-of-Living Lens: Many roles are hybrid/remote.

Quote: "Clear documentation drives clear care."

Here's My Take: Ideal for detail-oriented clinicians who love chart detective work.

53. Health Information Technician (RHIT) (gl)

Description: Maintains, organizes, and ensures accuracy of health records; coding (gl), release of information (gl), and compliance (gl).

Education/Training: Associate's in HIM (gl); RHIT (gl) credential.

Salary Range: $50,000–$75,000+.

Shortage Indicator: Steady with EHR (gl) expansion.

Pathways & Notes: Ladders into HIM (gl) management or coding (gl) leadership.

Cost-of-Living Lens: Hybrid/remote jobs can help offset modest base pay.

Quote: "Every chart is a patient's story."

Here's My Take: A great behind-the-scenes entry role for organized, accuracy-loving professionals.

54. Medical Coder (CCS (gl) / CPC (gl))

Description: Translates diagnoses and procedures into standardized codes for billing, reimbursement (gl), and compliance (gl).

Education/Training: Certificate or Associate's; AHIMA (gl) or AAPC (gl) credentials (CCS (gl), CPC (gl), CCA (gl)).

Salary Range: $55,000–$80,000+.

Shortage Indicator: High; remote coders in demand.

Pathways & Notes: Risk adjustment (gl) and other specialties can add value.

Cost-of-Living Lens: Remote roles allow flexibility.

Quote: "Accuracy in coding pays for accuracy in care."

Here's My Take: A perfect match for those who love puzzles, patterns, and working independently.

55. Compliance Officer (Healthcare)

Description: Oversees adherence to laws, regulations (gl), and standards (gl), including HIPAA (gl), billing, and accreditation (gl).

Education/Training: RN/JD/MHA/MPH; CHC (gl) certification.

Salary Range: $110,000–$180,000+.

Shortage Indicator: Strong across hospitals and health plans.

Pathways & Notes: Directs compliance (gl), risk (gl), or privacy (gl) programs.

Cost-of-Living Lens: Salaries scale significantly in large academic centers.

Quote: "Compliance is the backbone of trust."

Here's My Take: Best for detail-driven leaders who enjoy policy (gl), law, and ethics (gl) in healthcare.

56. Privacy Officer (HIPAA Specialist)

Description: Protects patient data, oversees HIPAA (gl) compliance (gl), and manages privacy breaches (gl).

Education/Training: HIM (gl), IT (gl), legal, or RN background; CHPC (gl) credential helpful.

Salary Range: $90,000–$140,000+.

Shortage Indicator: Growing with cyber threats (gl) and EHR (gl) reliance.

Pathways & Notes: Bridges into compliance (gl), IT (gl) security (gl), or leadership.

Cost-of-Living Lens: Hybrid/remote models common.

Quote: "Every byte (gl) of privacy matters."

Here's My Take: For guardians of patient trust who thrive on detail and vigilance (gl).

57. Healthcare IT Specialist

Description: Supports EHR (gl) systems, network security (gl), and clinical applications (gl).

Education/Training: Bachelor's in IT (gl) or healthcare informatics (gl); certifications (Epic (gl), Cerner (gl), CompTIA (gl)).

Salary Range: $72,000–$115,000+.

Shortage Indicator: Very strong; digital health (gl) expanding rapidly.

Pathways & Notes: Growth into system analyst (gl), informatics (gl), or IT (gl) leadership.

Cost-of-Living Lens: Remote work widens opportunities.

Quote: "When tech works, care flows."

Here's My Take: A role for tech-savvy pros who want to blend IT (gl) with meaningful patient impact.

58. Clinical Systems Analyst

Description: Customizes and optimizes clinical information systems for providers.

Education/Training: RN/PharmD/IT (gl) degree; Epic (gl) / Cerner (gl) certification.

Salary Range: $85,000–$135,000+.

Shortage Indicator: Growing with EHR (gl) optimization demands.

Pathways & Notes: Bridges to CNIO (gl), CIO (gl), or system leadership.

Cost-of-Living Lens: Premium salaries for Epic-certified (gl) professionals.

Quote: "Systems must serve the clinician, not the other way around."

Here's My Take: For clinicians who can translate bedside needs into IT (gl) solutions.

59. Genetic Counselor

Description: Assesses hereditary (gl) risks, provides counseling (gl), and guides testing (gl) decisions.

Education/Training: Master's in Genetic Counseling (gl); ABGC (gl) certification.

Salary Range: $85,000–$120,000+.

Shortage Indicator: Strong; demand outpaces supply.

Pathways & Notes: Expanding roles in oncology (gl), prenatal (gl), and pharmacogenomics (gl).

Cost-of-Living Lens: Higher pay in academic and specialty centers.

Quote: "Our DNA tells a story—counselors help you read it."

Here's My Take: A great fit for science lovers with strong communication skills.

60. Clinical Psychologist

Description: Provides psychological (gl) testing (gl), therapy (gl), and consultation (gl) across settings.

Education/Training: PhD (gl) or PsyD (gl); licensure (gl) required.

Salary Range: $85,000–$135,000+.

Shortage Indicator: Strong, especially for child/adolescent (gl) and health psychology (gl).

Pathways & Notes: Neuropsych (gl) and primary care (gl) integration (gl) are common specialties.

Cost-of-Living Lens: Private practice (gl) can offset COL (gl) but requires business skills.

Quote: "The mind is medicine too."

Here's My Take: For deep listeners and problem-solvers who want to heal from the inside out.

61. Psychiatrist

Description: Physician (gl) specializing in diagnosing and treating mental illness (gl), often prescribing medications (gl).

Education/Training: MD (gl) / DO (gl) + psychiatry (gl)

residency (gl); subspecialty (gl) fellowships (gl) (child (gl), addiction (gl)).

Salary Range: $230,000–$350,000+.

Shortage Indicator: Severe national shortage.

Pathways & Notes: Telepsychiatry (gl) expanding reach and flexibility.

Cost-of-Living Lens: High demand in underserved (gl) regions with incentive packages (gl).

Quote: "Brains need doctors too."

Here's My Take: For those who want to heal both medically and therapeutically at once.

62. Psychiatric Nurse Practitioner (PMHNP) (gl)

Description: Provides psychiatric (gl) evaluations (gl), therapy (gl), and medication (gl) management.

Education/Training: MSN/DNP with psych focus; national board certification (gl).

Salary Range: $120,000–$170,000+.

Shortage Indicator: Extremely high demand.

Pathways & Notes: Roles in outpatient clinics and telehealth (gl).

Cost-of-Living Lens: Telehealth (gl) allows COL (gl) flexibility and broad reach.

Quote: "Minds matter—and need medicine."

Here's My Take: Great for nurses who want high-demand autonomy (gl) and deep patient relationships.

63. Mental Health Counselor (LPC (gl) / LCSW (gl))

Description: Provides therapy (gl), crisis intervention (gl), and counseling (gl) for individuals, couples, and families.

Education/Training: Master's in counseling (gl), psychology (gl), or social work (gl); state licensure (gl) (LPC (gl), LCSW (gl), LMFT (gl)).

Salary Range: $55,000–$85,000+.

Shortage Indicator: High, especially for crisis services (gl).

Pathways & Notes: Private practice (gl), community health (gl), and teletherapy (gl).

Cost-of-Living Lens: Salaries can be higher in private practice (gl) but benefits may be weaker.

Quote: "Listening saves lives."

Here's My Take: For helpers who want to restore mental health and resilience (gl) one conversation at a time.

64. Substance Abuse Counselor

Description: Provides counseling (gl) and recovery (gl) support for addiction (gl) treatment.

Education/Training: Bachelor's or Master's in counseling (gl) or social work (gl); state certification/licensure (gl).

Salary Range: $50,000–$78,000+.

Shortage Indicator: Strong with opioid crisis (gl) and SUD (gl) prevalence (gl).

Pathways & Notes: Roles in corrections (gl) and community programs.

Cost-of-Living Lens: Public sector often pays less but offers job stability.

Quote: "Hope is the most powerful medicine."

Here's My Take: A meaningful path for those who believe recovery (gl) is always possible.

65. Clinical Social Worker (MSW (gl) / LCSW (gl))

Description: Provides therapy (gl), advocacy (gl), discharge planning (gl), and case management (gl).

Education/Training: Master's in Social Work (gl); LCSW (gl) licensure (gl).

Salary Range: $65,000–$95,000+.

Shortage Indicator: High, especially in healthcare and community services.

Pathways & Notes: Specializations (gl) in medical (gl), psych (gl), peds (gl), or geriatrics (gl).

Cost-of-Living Lens: Hospital vs. nonprofit pay varies widely.

Quote: "Systems change because social workers push them."

Here's My Take: A calling for advocates (gl) who balance therapy (gl) with systemic (gl) impact.

66. Marriage and Family Therapist (MFT) (gl)

Description: Provides therapy (gl) for couples, families, and relational (gl) systems.

Education/Training: Master's in MFT (gl) or counseling (gl); LMFT (gl) license (gl).

Salary Range: $60,000–$90,000+.

Shortage Indicator: Strong.

Pathways & Notes: Roles in private practice (gl), health systems, and schools.

Cost-of-Living Lens: Private practice (gl) can bridge COL (gl) gaps with flexible scheduling.

Quote: "Families are the first healing system."

Here's My Take: Great for those passionate about relationships and systemic (gl) healing.

67. Behavioral Health Technician

Description: Provides frontline support in psych (gl) units, group homes (gl), and rehab (gl) centers.

Education/Training: High school diploma; certification programs available.

Salary Range: $38,000–$52,000+.

Shortage Indicator: Steady openings due to high turnover (gl).

Pathways & Notes: Entry point to nursing (gl), social work (gl), or psych NP (gl).

Cost-of-Living Lens: Higher pay in inpatient psychiatric (gl) hospitals.

Quote: "Presence is the intervention (gl)."

Here's My Take: Perfect for entry-level caregivers who want experience in behavioral health (gl).

68. Recreational Therapist (CTRS) (gl)

Description: Uses recreation (gl), play, art, and exercise to support rehab (gl) and mental health.

Education/Training: Bachelor's in recreational therapy (gl); CTRS (gl) credential.

Salary Range: $50,000–$78,000+.

Shortage Indicator: Stable but specialized (gl).

Pathways & Notes: Roles in rehab (gl), psych (gl), peds (gl), and geriatrics (gl).

Cost-of-Living Lens: Salaries modest, but impact can be high.

Quote: "Healing comes through play, too."

Here's My Take: For those who believe fun and function can heal together.

69. Art Therapist

Description: Uses art to promote emotional healing, coping (gl), and communication.

Education/Training: Master's in art therapy (gl); licensure (gl) varies by state.

Salary Range: $52,000–$80,000+.

Shortage Indicator: Growing in psych (gl) and oncology (gl) programs.

Pathways & Notes: Often combined with counseling (gl) and therapy (gl) roles.

Cost-of-Living Lens: Salaries may be supplemented (gl) by grants (gl) or private practice (gl).

Quote: "When words fail, art speaks."

Here's My Take: Ideal for creative healers who want to give patients new voices.

70. Music Therapist

Description: Uses music interventions (gl) to support physical, emotional, cognitive (gl), and social healing.

Education/Training: Bachelor's or Master's in music therapy (gl); MT-BC (gl) credential.

Salary Range: $50,000–$78,000+.

Shortage Indicator: Growing in peds (gl), oncology (gl), and hospice (gl).

Pathways & Notes: Private practice (gl), school, and hospital roles.

Cost-of-Living Lens: Many therapists blend practice with teaching or performing.

Quote: "Music heals in ways medicine can't."

Here's My Take: For musicians at heart who want to turn talent into therapy (gl).

71. Child Life Specialist

Description: Helps children cope (gl) with hospitalization (gl) through play, education, and support.

Education/Training: Bachelor's in Child Life (gl) or related; CCLS (gl) certification.

Salary Range: $55,000–$82,000+.

Shortage Indicator: Strong in peds (gl) hospitals.

Pathways & Notes: Opportunities in leadership and advocacy (gl).

Cost-of-Living Lens: Nonprofit (gl) salaries can be modest; mission-driven benefits may offset.

Quote: "Childhood shouldn't pause for hospitalization (gl)."

Here's My Take: For playful, empathetic professionals who believe in protecting joy during illness.

72. Genetic Nurse (APRN / BSN)

Description: Provides counseling (gl), testing (gl) coordination (gl), and education for patients with genetic conditions (gl).

Education/Training: BSN or APRN (gl); genetic nurse credential (gl) (CAGC (gl)).

Salary Range: $80,000–$115,000+.

Shortage Indicator: Growing with genomics (gl) integration (gl).

Pathways & Notes: Research (gl) and precision medicine (gl) roles.

Cost-of-Living Lens: Academic centers often lead in pay for genetics nurses.

Quote: "Genes guide care—nurses guide patients."

Here's My Take: Perfect for nurses who love science, precision, and communication.

73. Biomedical Scientist

Description: Conducts lab research (gl) on disease mechanisms (gl), treatments, and technologies.

Education/Training: Bachelor's/Master's/PhD (gl) in biomedical science (gl).

Salary Range: $70,000–$120,000+.

Shortage Indicator: Strong in biotech (gl) sectors.

Pathways & Notes: Career paths in pharma (gl) and biotech (gl).

Cost-of-Living Lens: Higher pay in industry than academia.

Quote: "Science moves medicine forward."

Here's My Take: Best for researchers who love discovery (gl) more than direct patient care.

74. Biostatistician

Description: Designs and analyzes studies to interpret healthcare data.

Education/Training: Master's/PhD (gl) in biostatistics (gl).

Salary Range: $90,000–$140,000+.

Shortage Indicator: Strong with data-driven medicine (gl).

Pathways & Notes: Roles in research (gl), pharma (gl), and public health (gl).

Cost-of-Living Lens: Industry roles can offset high metro COL (gl).

Quote: "Numbers tell the story of care."

Here's My Take: For math minds who want numbers to drive outcomes.

75. Epidemiologist

Description: Studies patterns of disease, outbreaks (gl), and prevention (gl) strategies.

Education/Training: Master's/PhD (gl) in epidemiology (gl) or public health (gl).

Salary Range: $80,000–$120,000+.

Shortage Indicator: Steady long term.

Pathways & Notes: Government, global health (gl), and research (gl).

Cost-of-Living Lens: Federal roles offer stability and benefits over base pay.

Quote: "Patterns reveal prevention (gl)."

Here's My Take: Ideal for investigators (gl) who want to protect populations (gl), not just individuals.

86. Cardiologist

Description: Diagnoses and treats heart conditions; cath lab (gl) procedures, imaging (gl), and prevention (gl).

Education/Training: MD (gl) or DO (gl) + residency (gl) + cardiology (gl) fellowship (gl).

Salary Range: $350,000–$600,000+.

Shortage Indicator: Strong.

Pathways & Notes: Interventional (gl) and electrophysiology (gl) subfields (gl).

Cost-of-Living Lens: Call stipends (gl) can significantly impact earnings.

Quote: "Every beat tells a story."

Here's My Take: Perfect for physicians who love both acute saves and long-term relationships.

87. Oncologist (Medical)

Description: Treats cancer (gl) through chemotherapy (gl), immunotherapy (gl), and targeted therapies (gl).

Education/Training: MD (gl) or DO (gl) + residency (gl) + oncology (gl) fellowship (gl).

Salary Range: $320,000–$550,000+.

Shortage Indicator: Strong; cancer incidence (gl) rising.

Pathways & Notes: Clinical trials (gl), palliative (gl) care, and research (gl).

Cost-of-Living Lens: Academic roles may pay less but bring research (gl) prestige (gl).

Quote: "Hope is the most powerful therapy."

Here's My Take: A calling for physicians balancing science and compassion through long battles.

88. Hematologist

Description: Diagnoses and treats blood disorders (gl), including anemia (gl), clotting (gl), and leukemia (gl).

Education/Training: MD (gl) or DO (gl) + fellowship (gl) in hematology (gl) and oncology (gl).

Salary Range: $300,000–$500,000+.

Shortage Indicator: Growing demand.

Pathways & Notes: Often combined with oncology (gl).

Cost-of-Living Lens: Private practice (gl) often pays more than academia.

Quote: "The story of health is in the blood."

Here's My Take: For physicians who want complexity (gl) and science-driven medicine.

89. Gastroenterologist

Description: Manages digestive system disorders; endoscopy (gl), colonoscopy (gl), and advanced procedures.

Education/Training: MD (gl) or DO (gl) + residency (gl) + fellowship (gl).

Salary Range: $350,000–$600,000+.

Shortage Indicator: High demand nationwide.

Pathways & Notes: ERCP (gl) and EUS (gl) training.

Cost-of-Living Lens: Procedure-heavy specialties (gl) often yield higher comp.

Quote: "The gut is the second brain."

Here's My Take: For doctors who value procedural skill and prevention (gl) impact.

90. Pulmonologist

Description: Treats respiratory (gl) diseases and manages asthma (gl), COPD (gl), interstitial (gl) lung disease (gl), and ICU (gl) consults (gl).

Education/Training: MD (gl) or DO (gl) + fellowship (gl).

Salary Range: $300,000–$475,000+.

Shortage Indicator: Strong.

Pathways & Notes: Overlaps with critical care (gl) and sleep medicine (gl).

Cost-of-Living Lens: Academic vs. private pay can differ significantly.

Quote: "Every breath is precious."

Here's My Take: For those who want chronic disease management with ICU (gl) acuity (gl).

91. Nephrologist

Description: Manages kidney disease (gl), dialysis (gl), hypertension (gl), and transplant (gl) care.

Education/Training: MD (gl) or DO (gl) + nephrology (gl) fellowship (gl).

Salary Range: $280,000–$400,000+.

Shortage Indicator: Strong with CKD (gl) prevalence (gl).

Pathways & Notes: Roles in dialysis (gl) companies and academic centers.

Cost-of-Living Lens: Regions with high ESRD (gl) rates may carry heavier workload (gl).

Quote: "Kidneys quietly run the show."

Here's My Take: For meticulous physicians who value continuity (gl) and lifesaving impact.

92. Endocrinologist

Description: Specializes (gl) in hormonal (gl) and metabolic (gl) disorders (gl), including diabetes (gl), thyroid (gl), and adrenal (gl) conditions.

Education/Training: MD (gl) or DO (gl) + fellowship (gl).

Salary Range: $250,000–$350,000+.

Shortage Indicator: Growing with diabetes (gl) prevalence (gl).

Pathways & Notes: Roles in clinics, research (gl), and academic medicine.

Cost-of-Living Lens: Lower-earning specialty (gl) but stable lifestyle.

Quote: "Hormones whisper; endocrinologists listen."

Here's My Take: For continuity (gl)-focused physicians who value long-term relationships.

93. Infectious Disease Physician

Description: Manages infections (gl), antibiotics (gl), HIV (gl), tropical diseases (gl), and stewardship (gl) programs.

Education/Training: MD (gl) or DO (gl) + ID (gl) fellowship (gl).

Salary Range: $220,000–$320,000+.

Shortage Indicator: High need; pipeline (gl) issues persist.

Pathways & Notes: Stewardship (gl) leadership, academic research (gl), and global health (gl).

Cost-of-Living Lens: Mission-driven work can mean trade-offs.

Quote: "Germs never sleep, and neither do we."

Here's My Take: For those driven by science and patient safety (gl).

94. Rheumatologist

Description: Diagnoses and treats autoimmune (gl) and musculoskeletal (gl) disorders (gl).

Education/Training: MD (gl) or DO (gl) + fellowship (gl).

Salary Range: $250,000–$350,000+.

Shortage Indicator: Severe shortage nationwide.

Pathways & Notes: Outpatient (gl)-focused; research (gl) and teaching opportunities.

Cost-of-Living Lens: Demand supports negotiation (gl).

Quote: "When the immune system misfires, clarity heals."

Here's My Take: Great for physicians who love detective work and chronic care.

95. Dermatologist

Description: Manages skin, hair, and nail diseases; procedural (gl) and cosmetic (gl) dermatology (gl).

Education/Training: MD (gl) or DO (gl) + dermatology (gl) residency (gl).

Salary Range: $300,000–$500,000+.

Shortage Indicator: Strong; very competitive residency (gl).

Pathways & Notes: Derm surgery (gl) and cosmetic subspecialties (gl).

Cost-of-Living Lens: High private practice (gl) potential.

Quote: "Skin health is whole health."

Here's My Take: For detail-driven physicians who want strong demand with lifestyle balance.

96. Allergist / Immunologist

Description: Treats allergies (gl), asthma (gl), and immune system disorders (gl).

Education/Training: MD (gl) or DO (gl) + fellowship (gl).

Salary Range: $250,000–$380,000+.

Shortage Indicator: Strong.

Pathways & Notes: Private practice (gl), academic medicine, or research (gl).

Cost-of-Living Lens: Outpatient (gl)-focused; flexible scheduling.

Quote: "When the body overreacts, clarity calms."

Here's My Take: For physicians who enjoy prevention (gl), diagnostics (gl), and quality-of-life wins.

97. Ophthalmologist

Description: Provides eye care and surgery (gl), including cataracts (gl), glaucoma (gl), and retina (gl) care.

Education/Training: MD (gl) or DO (gl) + ophthalmology (gl) residency (gl); fellowships (gl) optional.

Salary Range: $300,000–$500,000+.

Shortage Indicator: Moderate but stable.

Pathways & Notes: Retina (gl), cornea (gl), and oculoplastics (gl) subspecialties (gl).

Cost-of-Living Lens: Private practice (gl) can offer autonomy (gl) and strong earnings.

Quote: "Vision is the window to independence."

Here's My Take: For those who love precision and restoring sight.

98. Optometrist (OD)

Description: Provides vision exams, prescribes lenses, and diagnoses common eye conditions.

Education/Training: Doctor of Optometry (OD) (gl).

Salary Range: $115,000–$160,000+.

Shortage Indicator: Stable, especially in underserved (gl) regions.

Pathways & Notes: Ownership (gl) models are common.

Cost-of-Living Lens: Independent practice (gl) in rural (gl) areas may yield higher income.

Quote: "Clarity changes lives."

Here's My Take: Strong continuity (gl) care with lifestyle balance.

99. Audiologist

Description: Evaluates and treats hearing and balance disorders (gl); fits hearing aids (gl) and cochlear implants (gl).

Education/Training: Doctor of Audiology (AuD) (gl).

Salary Range: $85,000–$120,000+.

Shortage Indicator: Growing with aging population.

Pathways & Notes: Roles in ENT (gl), private practice (gl), and industry.

Cost-of-Living Lens: Industry and device roles may pay higher.

Quote: "Hearing connects us to life."

Here's My Take: A caring career restoring the joy of sound.

100. Dentist (General)

Description: Provides oral (gl) healthcare, preventive services, and restorative (gl) dental care.

Education/Training: DDS (gl) or DMD (gl); licensure (gl).

Salary Range: $150,000–$220,000+.

Shortage Indicator: Moderate overall; rural underserved (gl) areas have high demand.

Pathways & Notes: Oral surgery (gl), ortho (gl), and prosthodontics (gl) specialties (gl).

Cost-of-Living Lens: Private practice (gl) requires business acumen (gl).

Quote: "Smiles change confidence—and health."

Here's My Take: For those who love precision work, prevention (gl), and visible patient impact.

101. Oral and Maxillofacial Surgeon

Description: Performs surgery (gl) on face, jaw, and mouth—wisdom teeth, trauma (gl), implants (gl), pathology (gl).

Education/Training: DDS (gl)/DMD (gl) + 4–6 yr surgical residency (gl); board certification (gl).

Salary Range: $300,000–$600,000+.

Shortage Indicator: Specialized (gl) demand; fewer programs = higher need.

Pathways & Notes: Can subspecialize (gl) in cosmetic (gl) or craniofacial (gl) surgery (gl).

Cost-of-Living Lens: Private practice (gl) lucrative; malpractice (gl) premiums (gl) high in some states.

Quote: "Function and form restored in one cut."

Here's My Take: For those with surgical precision and artistic eye—it's surgery (gl) that blends utility with aesthetics (gl).

102. Orthodontist

Description: Specializes (gl) in alignment (gl) of teeth and jaws using braces (gl), aligners (gl), appliances (gl).

Education/Training: DDS (gl)/DMD (gl) + orthodontics (gl) residency (gl).

Salary Range: $250,000–$450,000+.

Shortage Indicator: Stable but competitive.

Pathways & Notes: Strong opportunities in private practice (gl) ownership (gl).

Cost-of-Living Lens: Urban saturation (gl) lowers rates; suburban/rural = higher returns.

Quote: "Straight teeth, confident smiles."

Here's My Take: For meticulous professionals who want visible, long-term results.

103. Periodontist

Description: Manages gum disease (gl), implants (gl), oral inflammation (gl).

Education/Training: DDS (gl)/DMD (gl) + periodontics (gl) residency (gl).

Salary Range: $220,000–$400,000+.

Shortage Indicator: Steady need with rising implant (gl) demand.

Pathways & Notes: Practices combine clinical care with surgery (gl).

Cost-of-Living Lens: High implant (gl) volume = higher income.

Quote: "Healthy gums anchor healthy lives."

Here's My Take: A specialty (gl) for those who value detail and prevention (gl) but enjoy procedures too.

104. Prosthodontist

Description: Restores and replaces teeth with prosthetics (gl), crowns (gl), bridges (gl), dentures (gl).

Education/Training: DDS (gl)/DMD (gl) + prosthodontics (gl) residency (gl).

Salary Range: $210,000–$350,000+.

Shortage Indicator: Niche (gl) specialty (gl) but high value.

Pathways & Notes: Close collaboration (gl) with oral surgery (gl) and oncology (gl).

Cost-of-Living Lens: Private practice (gl) margins strong with high-end cosmetic (gl) cases.

Quote: "Restoring smiles, restoring lives."

Here's My Take: For perfectionists who love artistry as much as anatomy (gl).

105. Dental Hygienist

Description: Provides cleanings, preventive (gl) care, and patient education.

Education/Training: Associate's (gl) or Bachelor's (gl) in Dental Hygiene; state licensure (gl).

Salary Range: $70,000–$100,000+.

Shortage Indicator: High; strong demand in most states.

Pathways & Notes: Flexible part-time options; bridge to dentistry (gl) possible.

Cost-of-Living Lens: Pay often tied to dental practice (gl) profitability (gl).

Quote: "Prevention (gl) starts in the chair."

Here's My Take: Great for those who want direct patient contact and lifestyle balance.

106. Dental Assistant

Description: Supports dentists in procedures, sterilization (gl), patient care, and scheduling.

Education/Training: Certificate (gl)/diploma (gl); DANB (gl) certification (gl) optional.

Salary Range: $40,000–$55,000+.

Shortage Indicator: Steady; critical to dental practice (gl) flow.

Pathways & Notes: Stepping stone to hygienist (gl) or dentist.

Cost-of-Living Lens: Benefits vary widely by office size.

Quote: "Every smile needs a strong assist."

Here's My Take: Perfect entry point for those exploring dental careers.

107. Chiropractor

Description: Provides spinal (gl) and musculoskeletal (gl) adjustments (gl), holistic (gl) pain management (gl).

Education/Training: Doctor of Chiropractic (DC) (gl).

Salary Range: $70,000–$120,000+.

Shortage Indicator: Stable; variable by region.

Pathways & Notes: Practice (gl) ownership (gl) common; integrative (gl) health collaborations (gl) growing.

Cost-of-Living Lens: Independent practice (gl) requires business skills to thrive.

Quote: "Alignment (gl) brings relief."

Here's My Take: A fit for hands-on healers with entrepreneurial spirit.

108. Podiatrist

Description: Treats foot, ankle, and lower-extremity (gl) conditions surgically and nonsurgically (gl).

Education/Training: Doctor of Podiatric Medicine (DPM) (gl) + residency (gl).

Salary Range: $150,000–$250,000+.

Shortage Indicator: Steady; demand rises with diabetes (gl) prevalence (gl).

Pathways & Notes: Subspecialties (gl) in sports (gl), wound care (gl), surgery (gl).

Cost-of-Living Lens: Outpatient (gl) and surgical practices (gl) lucrative in high-diabetes (gl) regions.

Quote: "Care begins from the ground up."

Here's My Take: For clinicians who like a surgical scope without full med school residency (gl) length.

109. Physician (Hospitalist)

Description: Provides general inpatient (gl) care—diagnosis (gl), management, coordination (gl).

Education/Training: MD (gl)/DO (gl) + residency (gl) (IM (gl), FP (gl), peds (gl)).

Salary Range: $250,000–$325,000+.

Shortage Indicator: Strong; hospital medicine (gl) exploded in last two decades.

Pathways & Notes: Roles in academic, community, nocturnist (gl), leadership.

Cost-of-Living Lens: Nocturnist (gl) premiums (gl) boost earnings.

Quote: "Inpatients (gl) need one clear captain."

Here's My Take: For physicians who thrive on variety, teamwork, and acute care.

110. Intensivist (Critical Care Physician)

Description: Manages ICU (gl) patients requiring advanced monitoring (gl) and life support (gl).

Education/Training: MD (gl)/DO (gl) + fellowship (gl) in critical care (gl).

Salary Range: $300,000–$500,000+.

Shortage Indicator: Strong, especially post-COVID.

Pathways & Notes: Specialties (gl) include surgical critical care (gl), neuro ICU (gl).

Cost-of-Living Lens: Demanding call schedules often offset by comp.

Quote: "Every detail can be life or death."

Here's My Take: For meticulous physicians who want to be at medicine's front lines.

111. Neonatologist

Description: Cares for critically ill newborns in NICU (gl) settings.

Education/Training: MD (gl)/DO (gl) + pediatrics (gl) + neonatology (gl) fellowship (gl).

Salary Range: $300,000–$450,000+.

Shortage Indicator: High; specialized (gl) demand.

Pathways & Notes: Academic centers dominate; leadership in NICU (gl) programs possible.

Cost-of-Living Lens: Large academic centers pay less but offer prestige (gl).

Quote: "The tiniest patients deserve the greatest care."

Here's My Take: For those with gentle hands, sharp minds, and endless patience.

112. Pediatrician (General)

Description: Provides preventive (gl) and acute care for infants, children, adolescents.

Education/Training: MD (gl)/DO (gl) + pediatrics (gl) residency (gl).

Salary Range: $190,000–$260,000+.

Shortage Indicator: Steady; shortages worse in rural (gl) areas.

Pathways & Notes: Subspecialize (gl) in neonatology (gl), adolescent (gl), developmental (gl) pediatrics (gl).

Cost-of-Living Lens: Lower pay vs adult specialties (gl), but lifestyle balance strong.

Quote: "Children aren't little adults—they're their own specialty (gl)."

Here's My Take: For physicians who love growth milestones (gl) and family-centered care.

113. Pediatric Subspecialist

Description: Focuses on complex conditions in children within a subspecialty (gl).

Education/Training: MD (gl)/DO (gl) + peds (gl) residency (gl) + fellowship (gl).

Salary Range: $210,000–$350,000+.

Shortage Indicator: Significant in many subspecialties (gl).

Pathways & Notes: Academic medicine, research (gl), advocacy (gl) common.

Cost-of-Living Lens: Subspecialty (gl) compensation lags adult equivalents.

Quote: "Children deserve specialized (gl) champions."

Here's My Take: For pediatricians (gl) drawn to complexity (gl) and advocacy (gl).

114. Geriatrician

Description: Provides comprehensive (gl) care for older adults, focusing on function (gl), polypharmacy (gl), and quality of life.

Education/Training: MD (gl)/DO (gl) + residency (gl) + geriatrics (gl) fellowship (gl).

Salary Range: $200,000–$280,000+.

Shortage Indicator: Severe shortage as population ages.

Pathways & Notes: Roles in outpatient (gl), nursing homes, academic centers.

Cost-of-Living Lens: Mission-driven incentives (gl) help offset lower base.

Quote: "Aging with dignity requires guides."

Here's My Take: For patient-centered physicians who value continuity (gl) and holistic (gl) care.

115. Obstetrician-Gynecologist (OB/GYN)

Description: Manages women's reproductive (gl) health, pregnancy, surgery (gl), deliveries.

Education/Training: MD (gl)/DO (gl) + OB/GYN (gl) residency (gl).

Salary Range: $280,000–$400,000+.

Shortage Indicator: Strong, especially rural (gl).

Pathways & Notes: Subspecialize (gl) in MFM (gl), REI (gl), GYN oncology (gl), urogynecology (gl).

Cost-of-Living Lens: Call burden (gl) can be intense; rural jobs pay premiums (gl).

Quote: "Caring for women through every chapter."

Here's My Take: For physicians who want procedural (gl) variety and lifelong patient relationships.

116. Maternal-Fetal Medicine Specialist (MFM)

Description: Manages high-risk pregnancies and fetal (gl) complications (gl).

Education/Training: MD (gl)/DO (gl) + OB/GYN (gl) + MFM (gl) fellowship (gl).

Salary Range: $350,000–$550,000+.

Shortage Indicator: Severe shortage nationwide.

Pathways & Notes: Roles in tertiary (gl) centers, academic medicine.

Cost-of-Living Lens: High COL (gl) metros see strong demand and packages.

Quote: "Guiding mothers and babies through complex journeys."

Here's My Take: For physicians drawn to complexity (gl) and advocacy (gl) at life's beginning.

117. Reproductive Endocrinologist (REI)

Description: Specializes (gl) in infertility (gl), IVF (gl), hormonal (gl) reproductive (gl) disorders (gl).

Education/Training: MD (gl)/DO (gl) + OB/GYN (gl) + REI (gl) fellowship (gl).

Salary Range: $300,000-$500,000+.

Shortage Indicator: Growing demand with advances in IVF (gl).

Pathways & Notes: Often combine clinical practice (gl) with lab direction.

Cost-of-Living Lens: Private practices (gl) lucrative in affluent (gl) areas.

Quote: "Helping families begin."

Here's My Take: A fit for physicians with patience and empathy for long journeys.

118. Gynecologic Oncologist

Description: Manages cancers (gl) of reproductive (gl) organs with surgery (gl), chemo (gl), research (gl).

Education/Training: MD (gl)/DO (gl) + OB/GYN (gl) + fellowship (gl).

Salary Range: $350,000-$550,000+.

Shortage Indicator: Strong; fellowship (gl) bottlenecks (gl).

Pathways & Notes: Academic centers dominate; research (gl) opportunities.

Cost-of-Living Lens: Salaries vary widely by institution (gl).

Quote: "Fighting cancers with skill and compassion."

Here's My Take: For surgeons driven by advocacy (gl) and complex care.

119. Urologist

Description: Treats urinary tract (gl) and male reproductive (gl) conditions; surgery (gl) + medical care.

Education/Training: MD (gl)/DO (gl) + urology (gl) residency (gl).

Salary Range: $325,000–$500,000+.

Shortage Indicator: Strong, particularly rural (gl).

Pathways & Notes: Robotics (gl) and oncology (gl) subfields (gl) strong.

Cost-of-Living Lens: Call and procedural (gl) load impact income significantly.

Quote: "Function and dignity restored."

Here's My Take: For physicians who enjoy procedural (gl) variety and tech-driven care.

120. Plastic Surgeon

Description: Restores or enhances function and appearance through surgical procedures.

Education/Training: MD (gl)/DO (gl) + plastic surgery (gl) residency (gl).

Salary Range: $350,000–$650,000+.

Shortage Indicator: Steady; competitive training.

Pathways & Notes: Subspecialties (gl) in hand (gl), craniofacial (gl), cosmetic (gl).

Cost-of-Living Lens: Private cosmetic (gl) practices most lucrative.

Quote: "Reconstruction (gl) meets artistry."

Here's My Take: For creative surgeons who blend function with form.

121. Thoracic Surgeon

Description: Performs surgeries (gl) on lungs, esophagus (gl), and chest organs.

Education/Training: MD (gl)/DO (gl) + 6–8 yr residency (gl)/fellowship (gl).

Salary Range: $400,000–$650,000+.

Shortage Indicator: Strong; long training pipeline (gl).

Pathways & Notes: Lung transplants (gl), oncology (gl) roles.

Cost-of-Living Lens: Academic salaries lower but research (gl) prestige (gl) high.

Quote: "Inside the chest lies life's rhythm."

Here's My Take: For elite surgeons who value technical mastery and complexity (gl).

122. Vascular Surgeon

Description: Treats arterial (gl) and venous (gl) disease with surgery (gl), stents (gl), grafts (gl).

Education/Training: MD (gl)/DO (gl) + fellowship (gl).

Salary Range: $350,000–$600,000+.

Shortage Indicator: High demand nationwide.

Pathways & Notes: Hybrid OR (gl) and endovascular (gl) procedures.

Cost-of-Living Lens: Call pay can be substantial.

Quote: "Flow is life."

Here's My Take: For physicians who thrive on precision and lifesaving interventions (gl).

123. Colorectal Surgeon

Description: Manages diseases of the colon, rectum (gl), and anus (gl) surgically and medically.

Education/Training: MD (gl)/DO (gl) + general surgery (gl) + fellowship (gl).

Salary Range: $325,000–$500,000+.

Shortage Indicator: Moderate but growing with colorectal cancer (gl) screening (gl).

Pathways & Notes: Academic centers emphasize research (gl); private practice (gl) procedural (gl).

Cost-of-Living Lens: Call-heavy role but compensated well.

Quote: "Every gut has a guardian."

Here's My Take: For surgeons who want impactful, technical, and continuity (gl)-rich work.

124. Otolaryngologist (ENT)

Description: Treats ear, nose, throat, and related head/neck conditions; surgical and medical.

Education/Training: MD (gl)/DO (gl) + ENT (gl) residency (gl).

Salary Range: $300,000–$500,000+.

Shortage Indicator: Steady but competitive.

Pathways & Notes: Subspecialize (gl) in peds (gl) ENT (gl), head & neck oncology (gl), facial plastics (gl).

Cost-of-Living Lens: Private practice (gl) lucrative; academic less so.

Quote: "Hearing, breathing, speaking—all ENT (gl) territory."

Here's My Take: A specialty (gl) for those who like variety and surgical finesse.

125. Emergency Medicine Physician

Description: Provides acute diagnosis (gl) and treatment in emergency departments (gl).

Education/Training: MD (gl)/DO (gl) + EM (gl) residency (gl); board certification (gl).

Salary Range: $280,000–$400,000+.

Shortage Indicator: Strong demand despite burnout (gl) and staffing shortages.

Pathways & Notes: Subspecialize (gl) in toxicology (gl), ultrasound (gl), critical care (gl).

Cost-of-Living Lens: Pay higher in rural (gl) and high-volume EDs (gl).

Quote: "Prepared for anything, anytime."

Here's My Take: For physicians who thrive on adrenaline (gl), pace, and quick decision-making.

126. Trauma Surgeon

Description: Provides immediate surgical interventions (gl) for life-threatening injuries.

Education/Training: MD (gl)/DO (gl) + general surgery (gl) + trauma (gl)/critical care (gl) fellowship (gl).

Salary Range: $400,000–$650,000+.

Shortage Indicator: Strong, especially in Level I (gl) and II (gl) trauma centers (gl).

Pathways & Notes: Roles overlap with critical care (gl) and academic leadership.

Cost-of-Living Lens: Call pay and trauma (gl) stipends (gl) often significant.

Quote: "When seconds decide survival, trauma surgeons step in."

Here's My Take: For decisive, adrenaline-ready physicians who thrive on unpredictability.

127. Emergency Medical Director

Description: Leads ED (gl) operations, staffing, quality, and patient flow.

Education/Training: MD (gl)/DO (gl) (EM (gl) board-certified (gl)); leadership experience.

Salary Range: $300,000–$450,000+.

Shortage Indicator: Moderate; leadership pipeline (gl) limited.

Pathways & Notes: Moves into hospital CMO (gl) or executive (gl) leadership possible.

Cost-of-Living Lens: High-volume urban EDs (gl) pay more but come with heavier stress.

Quote: "Leadership brings order to the chaos."

Here's My Take: A great match for physicians who balance clinical chops with administrative strategy.

128. Critical Care Transport Paramedic (CCT-P)

Description: Provides advanced prehospital (gl) and interfacility (gl) transport for critically ill patients.

Education/Training: Paramedic (gl) + critical care transport (gl) certification (gl) (FP-C (gl), CCP-C (gl)).

Salary Range: $60,000–$90,000+.

Shortage Indicator: High; specialized (gl) and physically demanding.

Pathways & Notes: Steps toward flight (gl) or leadership roles.

Cost-of-Living Lens: Hazard (gl) and overtime pay add substantially.

Quote: "Stability on the move saves lives."

Here's My Take: For medics who crave autonomy, intensity, and teamwork at altitude (gl) or highway speeds.

129. Flight Paramedic

Description: Provides advanced prehospital (gl) care in helicopters/fixed-wing aircraft.

Education/Training: Paramedic (gl); FP-C (gl) certification (gl) preferred; years of field experience.

Salary Range: $70,000–$100,000+.

Shortage Indicator: Specialized (gl) demand; competitive entry.

Pathways & Notes: Bridges into education, leadership, or ED (gl) roles.

Cost-of-Living Lens: Rural (gl) programs pay premiums (gl) to attract talent.

Quote: "Critical care at 5,000 feet."

Here's My Take: For those who thrive on adrenaline (gl) and complex saves in extreme settings.

130. Occupational Therapist Assistant (COTA)

Description: Supports OTs (gl) in restoring patient function (gl) and independence.

Education/Training: Associate's (gl) OTA (gl) program; licensure (gl) required.

Salary Range: $52,000–$70,000+.

Shortage Indicator: Steady demand in rehab (gl), SNF (gl), home health (gl).

Pathways & Notes: Ladders into OT (gl) with additional schooling.

Cost-of-Living Lens: Pay often stronger in hospitals vs schools.

Quote: "Small wins restore big independence."

Here's My Take: A great role for hands-on caregivers who like creativity and function (gl).

131. Physical Therapist Assistant (PTA)

Description: Works under PT (gl) to deliver exercises, mobility training, rehab (gl) care.

Education/Training: Associate's (gl) PTA (gl) program; state licensure (gl).

Salary Range: $55,000–$75,000+.

Shortage Indicator: Strong in SNF (gl) and outpatient (gl) rehab (gl).

Pathways & Notes: Some bridge to DPT (gl) with further education.

Cost-of-Living Lens: Rural (gl) demand = higher hiring bonuses.

Quote: "Helping patients step forward again."

Here's My Take: For those who like coaching and motivating patients daily.

132. Speech-Language Pathology Assistant (SLPA)

Description: Provides support for speech therapy (gl) under SLP (gl) supervision (gl).

Education/Training: Associate's (gl)/Bachelor's (gl) + SLPA (gl) certificate (gl) (state-specific).

Salary Range: $45,000–$65,000+.

Shortage Indicator: Strong in schools and peds (gl) clinics.

Pathways & Notes: Often bridge to full SLP (gl) roles.

Cost-of-Living Lens: School contracts (gl) balance lower pay with lifestyle perks.

Quote: "Every sound practiced is progress."

Here's My Take: A strong entry point into allied health (gl) for communicators at heart.

133. Cytotechnologist

Description: Examines cells under microscopes (gl) to detect cancer (gl) and disease.

Education/Training: Bachelor's (gl) in cytotechnology (gl) or MLS (gl) + ASCP (gl) certification (gl).

Salary Range: $70,000–$100,000+.

Shortage Indicator: High, with lab workforce shortages.

Pathways & Notes: Roles in cancer (gl) centers, pathology (gl) labs.

Cost-of-Living Lens: Salaries vary widely by region and system size.

Quote: "Cancer often whispers first through a cell."

Here's My Take: For microscope (gl) enthusiasts who want early detection impact.

134. Histotechnologist

Description: Prepares tissue samples for microscopic (gl) analysis and diagnosis (gl).

Education/Training: Bachelor's (gl)/Associate's (gl) in histotechnology (gl); ASCP (gl) certification (gl).

Salary Range: $55,000–$78,000+.

Shortage Indicator: Persistent shortage in pathology (gl) labs.

Pathways & Notes: Supervisor (gl) or lead histology (gl) roles.

Cost-of-Living Lens: Academic centers pay less but offer learning exposure.

Quote: "Every slice of tissue tells a story."

Here's My Take: Perfect for detail-oriented lab pros who like precision behind the scenes.

135. Cytogenetic Technologist

Description: Analyzes chromosomes (gl) for genetic (gl) disorders (gl), cancers (gl), abnormalities (gl).

Education/Training: Bachelor's (gl) in cytogenetics (gl) or MLS (gl); ASCP (gl) certification (gl).

Salary Range: $72,000–$105,000+.

Shortage Indicator: Strong, with demand in research (gl) and oncology (gl) labs.

Pathways & Notes: Roles in genetics (gl) labs, academic centers.

Cost-of-Living Lens: Salaries higher in private biotech (gl) than academic labs.

Quote: "Chromosomes (gl) are the blueprint (gl) of health."

Here's My Take: For science-minded professionals fascinated by genetics (gl).

136. Nuclear Medicine Technologist

Description: Performs diagnostic imaging (gl) with radioactive (gl) tracers (gl) (PET (gl), SPECT (gl)).

Education/Training: Associate's (gl)/Bachelor's (gl); ARRT(N) (gl) or NMTCB (gl) credential (gl).

Salary Range: $72,000-$110,000+.

Shortage Indicator: Moderate but stable; specialized (gl) demand.

Pathways & Notes: Bridges into PET/CT (gl) or research (gl) roles.

Cost-of-Living Lens: Cross-credentialing (gl) boosts pay significantly.

Quote: "Radiotracers (gl) reveal hidden truths."

Here's My Take: For techs who love imaging (gl) and advanced physics (gl) in medicine.

137. Radiation Therapist

Description: Delivers radiation (gl) treatments to cancer (gl) patients with precision.

Education/Training: Associate's (gl)/Bachelor's (gl) in radiation therapy (gl); ARRT (gl) credential (gl).

Salary Range: $78,000-$115,000+.

Shortage Indicator: High demand tied to oncology (gl) volume.

Pathways & Notes: Roles in cancer (gl) centers, research (gl), dosimetry (gl).

Cost-of-Living Lens: Urban cancer (gl) centers pay more but workloads heavy.

Quote: "Precision beams, targeted healing."

Here's My Take: For compassionate techs who want hands-on roles in oncology (gl).

138. Dosimetrist

Description: Plans radiation therapy (gl) treatments, calculating doses (gl) and targeting tumors (gl).

Education/Training: Bachelor's (gl) in dosimetry (gl) or radiation science (gl); CMD (gl) certification (gl).

Salary Range: $95,000–$135,000+.

Shortage Indicator: Strong, with limited training programs.

Pathways & Notes: Often promoted from radiation therapist (gl) role.

Cost-of-Living Lens: Salaries higher in oncology (gl) specialty (gl) centers.

Quote: "Math meets medicine to fight cancer."

Here's My Take: For analytical professionals who like high-impact behind-the-scenes work.

139. Medical Physicist

Description: Ensures accuracy and safety of radiation (gl) treatments; calibrates (gl) and maintains radiation (gl) equipment.

Education/Training: Master's (gl)/PhD (gl) in medical physics (gl); board certification (gl) (ABR (gl)).

Salary Range: $140,000–$200,000+.

Shortage Indicator: Strong in oncology (gl) centers.

Pathways & Notes: Research (gl), teaching, leadership roles available.

Cost-of-Living Lens: Salaries scale with experience and institution (gl) size.

Quote: "Physics keeps radiation (gl) safe and effective."

Here's My Take: Best for math/science experts who want direct patient impact without bedside care.

140. Perfusion Technologist (Entry-Level)

Description: Assists perfusionists (gl) in cardiac surgery (gl) support and ECMO (gl) circuits (gl).

Education/Training: Bachelor's (gl) in science; training program entry.

Salary Range: $55,000–$75,000+.

Shortage Indicator: Strong due to limited pipeline (gl).

Pathways & Notes: Ladder to perfusionist (gl) (CCP (gl) credential (gl)).

Cost-of-Living Lens: Hospitals pay more than research (gl) centers.

Quote: "Circulation (gl) support starts here."

Here's My Take: A rare entry lane for those fascinated by cardiac surgery (gl) technology.

141. Transplant Coordinator (RN)

Description: Coordinates organ donation, recipient evaluation (gl), and post-transplant care.

Education/Training: RN (gl); transplant training/certification (gl).

Salary Range: $85,000–$125,000+.

Shortage Indicator: Growing with transplant volume increases.

Pathways & Notes: Highly specialized (gl); strong continuity (gl) of care.

Cost-of-Living Lens: Large academic centers lead compensation.

Quote: "Every match is a second chance."

Here's My Take: For nurses who thrive on detail, logistics (gl), and profound human stories.

142. Organ Procurement Coordinator

Description: Facilitates organ recovery and donation logistics (gl); interfaces with families and surgical teams.

Education/Training: RN (gl) or healthcare degree; OPO (gl) training.

Salary Range: $80,000–$115,000+.

Shortage Indicator: Strong, with high emotional demands.

Pathways & Notes: Often tied to nonprofit (gl) OPOs (gl); leadership possible.

Cost-of-Living Lens: Salaries vary but mission is priceless.

Quote: "Donation turns loss into legacy."

Here's My Take: For resilient professionals who want purpose-driven work.

143. Clinical Geneticist (MD/DO)

Description: Physician specializing (gl) in diagnosing genetic (gl) disorders (gl), counseling (gl), and treatment.

Education/Training: MD (gl)/DO (gl) + genetics (gl) fellowship (gl).

Salary Range: $180,000–$260,000+.

Shortage Indicator: Severe; very few trained annually.

Pathways & Notes: Roles in pediatrics (gl), oncology (gl), prenatal (gl) care.

Cost-of-Living Lens: Academic centers dominate; salaries modest vs other specialties (gl).

Quote: "Genes guide, but clinicians interpret."

Here's My Take: For science-driven physicians who want to decode rare diseases (gl).

144. Pathologist

Description: Diagnoses diseases through lab analysis of tissue, blood, and fluids.

Education/Training: MD (gl)/DO (gl) + pathology (gl) residency (gl).

Salary Range: $250,000–$400,000+.

Shortage Indicator: Strong, especially in subspecialties (gl).

Pathways & Notes: Options in forensics (gl), molecular (gl), transfusion medicine (gl).

Cost-of-Living Lens: Academic vs private income gap can be wide.

Quote: "Diagnosis (gl) begins at the microscope (gl)."

Here's My Take: Best for physicians who like detective work without daily patient care.

145. Forensic Pathologist

Description: Investigates causes of death via autopsies (gl) and lab studies.

Education/Training: MD (gl)/DO (gl) + pathology (gl) + forensic (gl) fellowship (gl).

Salary Range: $200,000–$300,000+.

Shortage Indicator: National shortage; many ME (gl) offices understaffed.

Pathways & Notes: Government roles often come with pensions (gl).

Cost-of-Living Lens: Public roles pay less but carry stability.

Quote: "Every life leaves evidence."

Here's My Take: For those with resilience and curiosity who want to serve justice.

146. Medical Examiner (ME)

Description: Physician overseeing death investigations (gl) and legal determinations (gl).

Education/Training: MD (gl)/DO (gl); board-certified (gl) in forensic pathology (gl).

Salary Range: $220,000–$325,000+.

Shortage Indicator: Severe shortage nationally.

Pathways & Notes: Public health (gl) and legal collaboration (gl) essential.

Cost-of-Living Lens: Salaries lower but mission is profound.

Quote: "Speaking for the silent."

Here's My Take: For physicians who value truth and service to families and justice.

147. Coroner

Description: Elected or appointed official determining causes of death (often non-physician).

Education/Training: Varies by jurisdiction (gl); may be law enforcement (gl), RN (gl), or physician.

Salary Range: $50,000–$110,000+.

Shortage Indicator: Variable; role shrinking where MEs (gl) replace coroners.

Pathways & Notes: Political and legal connections (gl) essential.

Cost-of-Living Lens: Salaries lower; civic service (gl) aspect.

Quote: "Accountability starts at death's door."

Here's My Take: For civic-minded leaders with resilience and integrity.

148. Occupational Therapist (Hand Therapy Specialty)

Description: Restores function (gl) for hand injuries, burns (gl), post-surgical recovery.

Education/Training: OTR/L (gl) + CHT (gl) certification (gl).

Salary Range: $85,000–$115,000+.

Shortage Indicator: High; niche (gl) specialty (gl).

Pathways & Notes: Strong demand in ortho (gl) and plastics (gl) rehab (gl).

Cost-of-Living Lens: Urban trauma (gl) centers offer highest pay.

Quote: "Hands are life's tools—restored through therapy (gl)."

Here's My Take: For creative OTs (gl) who love fine motor function (gl) and surgical collaboration (gl).

149. Certified Diabetes Educator (CDE)

Description: Provides education, coaching, and management for patients with diabetes (gl).

Education/Training: RN (gl), RD (gl), PharmD (gl), or other health professional + CDCES (gl) credential (gl).

Salary Range: $70,000–$95,000+.

Shortage Indicator: Strong with rising diabetes (gl) prevalence (gl).

Pathways & Notes: Hospital, outpatient (gl), community roles.

Cost-of-Living Lens: Salaries modest, but mission impact high.

Quote: "Knowledge is insulin (gl) for the mind."

Here's My Take: For educators who want to empower patients toward lifelong management.

150. Registered Dietitian Nutritionist (RDN)

Description: Provides medical nutrition therapy (gl), counseling (gl), and dietary planning.

Education/Training: Bachelor's (gl) + dietetic internship (gl); RDN (gl) credential (gl); Master's (gl) soon required.

Salary Range: $65,000–$95,000+.

Shortage Indicator: Strong in hospitals, outpatient (gl), community health (gl).

Pathways & Notes: Specialty (gl) certs (gl) (CNSC (gl), CDE (gl)) expand roles.

Cost-of-Living Lens: Salaries modest, but broad settings to choose from.

Quote: "Food is medicine when guided by science."

Here's My Take: For those passionate about blending science, prevention (gl), and daily life habits.

151. Nutrition Support Specialist (CNSC)

Description: Provides advanced expertise in parenteral (gl) and enteral (gl) nutrition for critically ill patients.

Education/Training: RN (gl), RDN (gl), PharmD (gl), or MD (gl) with Certified Nutrition Support Clinician (gl) credential (gl).

Salary Range: $78,000–$110,000+.

Shortage Indicator: Moderate but growing as ICU (gl) acuity (gl) rises.

Pathways & Notes: Roles in hospitals, ICUs (gl), and outpatient (gl) programs.

Cost-of-Living Lens: Urban centers and academic ICUs (gl) pay premiums (gl).

Quote: "Feeding critically ill patients is precision medicine too."

Here's My Take: A niche (gl) but vital role for detail-driven clinicians who want measurable impact.

152. Public Health Nurse

Description: Provides community outreach, screenings (gl), education, and disease prevention (gl) programs.

Education/Training: BSN (gl); MPH (gl) beneficial for leadership roles.

Salary Range: $70,000–$100,000+.

Shortage Indicator: Strong in underserved communities.

Pathways & Notes: Bridges into policy (gl), epidemiology (gl), or school health.

Cost-of-Living Lens: Government pay stable but rarely high; benefits offset base.

Quote: "Prevention begins where people live."

Here's My Take: Best for nurses who want to change population health (gl), not just patient health.

153. Community Health Worker (CHW)

Description: Provides frontline outreach, health education, and navigation (gl) for underserved populations.

Education/Training: High school diploma + CHW (gl) training/certification (gl).

Salary Range: $42,000–$58,000+.

Shortage Indicator: High demand in value-based care (gl) models.

Pathways & Notes: Entry role leading to nursing, social work (gl), public health (gl).

Cost-of-Living Lens: Modest salaries but mission-driven benefits high.

Quote: "Trust is the bridge to care."

Here's My Take: Perfect for connectors who know their communities and want to improve access.

154. Epidemiology Field Officer

Description: Investigates outbreaks (gl), collects data, supports disease prevention (gl) in the field.

Education/Training: MPH (gl) or related; CDC (gl) Epidemic Intelligence Service (gl) pathway possible.

Salary Range: $72,000–$105,000+.

Shortage Indicator: Strong with public health (gl) crises (gl).

Pathways & Notes: Roles in global health (gl), CDC (gl), WHO (gl).

Cost-of-Living Lens: Federal jobs offer stability, not high pay.

Quote: "Tracking diseases requires boots on the ground."

Here's My Take: For adventurous investigators who want to be on the frontlines of prevention (gl).

155. School Nurse

Description: Provides health care, screenings (gl), and emergency response in schools.

Education/Training: RN (gl); BSN (gl) preferred; school nurse credential (gl) in some states.

Salary Range: $58,000–$75,000+.

Shortage Indicator: Widespread shortage nationwide.

Pathways & Notes: Ladders into public health (gl) or pediatric (gl) specialties (gl).

Cost-of-Living Lens: Pay modest, summers often off; benefits strong in public systems.

Quote: "Every child deserves health support at school."

Here's My Take: Ideal for nurses who value continuity (gl) and advocacy (gl) for kids.

156. Occupational Health Nurse

Description: Promotes workplace safety, injury prevention (gl), and employee wellness.

Education/Training: RN (gl)/BSN (gl); COHN (gl) certification (gl) optional.

Salary Range: $75,000–$105,000+.

Shortage Indicator: Stable, strong in manufacturing and corporate settings.

Pathways & Notes: Moves into safety officer (gl) or HR (gl)/benefits leadership.

Cost-of-Living Lens: Corporate pay often higher than hospital-based roles.

Quote: "Healthier workers build healthier companies."

Here's My Take: For nurses who like blending clinical care with prevention (gl) and strategy.

157. Infection Preventionist

Description: Monitors, educates, and manages infection control (gl) programs in hospitals.

Education/Training: RN (gl), MT (gl), MPH (gl); CIC (gl) credential (gl) preferred.

Salary Range: $78,000–$115,000+.

Shortage Indicator: Very high demand post-COVID (gl).

Pathways & Notes: Steps into quality (gl), risk (gl), or public health (gl) leadership.

Cost-of-Living Lens: Large health systems pay more; travel IPs (gl) exist.

Quote: "Every infection prevented is a life protected."

Here's My Take: For clinicians who love data, surveillance (gl), and systems improvement.

158. Industrial Hygienist

Description: Identifies and controls workplace environmental hazards (gl) (chemical (gl), physical (gl), biological (gl)).

Education/Training: Bachelor's (gl)/Master's (gl) in industrial hygiene (gl), safety, or public health (gl); CIH (gl) credential (gl).

Salary Range: $75,000–$110,000+.

Shortage Indicator: Growing with occupational safety regulations (gl).

Pathways & Notes: Government, private industry, consulting.

Cost-of-Living Lens: Industry roles more lucrative than public sector.

Quote: "Invisible hazards need visible solutions."

Here's My Take: For science-minded professionals who want to protect health at work.

159. Health Educator

Description: Designs and delivers programs to promote wellness and prevention (gl).

Education/Training: Bachelor's (gl)/Master's (gl) in public health (gl)/education; CHES (gl) credential (gl).

Salary Range: $55,000–$78,000+.

Shortage Indicator: Moderate but expanding with value-based care (gl).

Pathways & Notes: Roles in hospitals, schools, nonprofits (gl).

Cost-of-Living Lens: Salaries modest; grants (gl) fund many positions.

Quote: "Knowledge saves lives."

Here's My Take: Perfect for teachers at heart who want to prevent illness instead of treating it.

160. Wellness Coach (Health Coach)

Description: Supports lifestyle change, nutrition, exercise, and stress management (gl).

Education/Training: Certificate (gl) programs; NBHWC (gl) credential (gl) rising in recognition (gl).

Salary Range: $48,000–$72,000+.

Shortage Indicator: Growing demand in corporate and concierge medicine (gl).

Pathways & Notes: Flexible self-employment (gl) and telehealth (gl) roles.

Cost-of-Living Lens: Private pay clients increase income potential.

Quote: "Coaching unlocks healthier habits."

Here's My Take: For motivators who thrive on accountability partnerships.

161. Genomics Data Analyst

Description: Interprets genomic (gl) datasets (gl) for research (gl), precision medicine (gl), and diagnostics (gl).

Education/Training: Bachelor's (gl)/Master's (gl) in bioinformatics (gl); strong coding (gl) skills.

Salary Range: $82,000–$120,000+.

Shortage Indicator: Very high with precision medicine (gl) expansion.

Pathways & Notes: Pharma (gl), academic, and biotech (gl) roles abundant.

Cost-of-Living Lens: Remote opportunities expanding.

Quote: "Big data makes personal medicine possible."

Here's My Take: For data-savvy pros who want to connect genes (gl) to cures.

162. Clinical Informaticist

Description: Optimizes EHRs (gl) and digital tools for better clinical workflows (gl).

Education/Training: RN (gl), PharmD (gl), MD (gl), or IT (gl) background; board certification (gl) in informatics (gl).

Salary Range: $95,000–$140,000+.

Shortage Indicator: Strong with ongoing digital health push.

Pathways & Notes: Leads to CNIO (gl), CMIO (gl), or CIO (gl) roles.

Cost-of-Living Lens: Epic (gl)/Cerner (gl) certifications (gl) boost pay.

Quote: "Technology should serve patients, not slow them."

Here's My Take: Perfect for clinicians who want to fix the systems we all complain about.

163. Telehealth Coordinator

Description: Implements and manages telemedicine (gl) programs, workflows (gl), and compliance (gl).

Education/Training: Health admin (gl), nursing, or IT (gl) background; certificate (gl) programs emerging.

Salary Range: $65,000–$95,000+.

Shortage Indicator: Growing rapidly with virtual care expansion.

Pathways & Notes: Roles in hospitals, startups (gl), and private groups.

Cost-of-Living Lens: Hybrid/remote pay models common.

Quote: "Virtual care needs real coordination."

Here's My Take: For problem-solvers who like to build new systems of access.

164. Healthcare Data Scientist

Description: Uses AI (gl), statistics (gl), and predictive (gl) models to improve patient outcomes.

Education/Training: Master's (gl)/PhD (gl) in data science (gl)/health informatics (gl).

Salary Range: $110,000–$160,000+.

Shortage Indicator: Extremely strong; top growth field.

Pathways & Notes: Pharma (gl), health systems, startups (gl) all hiring.

Cost-of-Living Lens: Tech salaries higher than clinical equivalents.

Quote: "Data is medicine's new stethoscope."

Here's My Take: For coders (gl) who want to shape the future of health, not just apps.

165. Medical Science Liaison (MSL)

Description: Connects pharmaceutical (gl) companies with clinicians, sharing scientific evidence (gl).

Education/Training: PharmD (gl), PhD (gl), MD (gl); strong communication skills.

Salary Range: $125,000–$180,000+.

Shortage Indicator: Competitive but strong demand in pharma (gl).

Pathways & Notes: Step into medical affairs (gl) or industry leadership.

Cost-of-Living Lens: Travel-heavy but lucrative.

Quote: "Science needs translators too."

Here's My Take: Best for extroverted scientists who want to leave the lab but stay close to discovery.

166. Pharmaceutical Sales Representative

Description: Markets and educates clinicians about medications and therapies.

Education/Training: Bachelor's (gl) degree; sales training; clinical background a plus.

Salary Range: $80,000–$130,000+ with commission (gl).

Shortage Indicator: Stable but shifting with digital marketing (gl).

Pathways & Notes: Ladders into account manager (gl) or marketing director roles.

Cost-of-Living Lens: Commission-driven; urban markets more competitive.

Quote: "Knowledge drives prescribing confidence."

Here's My Take: A fit for persuasive, people-oriented professionals with resilience.

167. Health Economist

Description: Analyzes healthcare costs, outcomes, and value-based (gl) models.

Education/Training: Master's (gl)/PhD (gl) in economics (gl), public health (gl), or health policy (gl).

Salary Range: $95,000–$150,000+.

Shortage Indicator: Growing with policy reforms and cost scrutiny.

Pathways & Notes: Academia, consulting, payer (gl), government roles.

Cost-of-Living Lens: Policy roles less lucrative than industry.

Quote: "Numbers guide policy and practice."

Here's My Take: For math and policy minds who want to shape system-level change.

168. Health Policy Analyst

Description: Evaluates and recommends healthcare legislation (gl), programs, and reforms.

Education/Training: Master's (gl) in public policy (gl), public health (gl), or law.

Salary Range: $70,000–$110,000+.

Shortage Indicator: Stable but competitive in government.

Pathways & Notes: Progression into advocacy (gl), consulting, or leadership.

Cost-of-Living Lens: Federal pay scales (gl) standardized; industry consulting pays more.

Quote: "Policy is the hidden hand of healthcare."

Here's My Take: Best for those who like the big picture and influencing systems.

169. Healthcare Lobbyist

Description: Advocates for healthcare organizations or industries to influence legislation (gl).

Education/Training: Background in law, policy (gl), or health admin (gl).

Salary Range: $95,000–$160,000+.

Shortage Indicator: Competitive; demand strong around major reforms.

Pathways & Notes: Consulting firms, trade associations (gl), private industry.

Cost-of-Living Lens: DC (gl) and state capitals dominate opportunities.

Quote: "Behind every policy is someone advocating."

Here's My Take: For persuasive professionals who want to influence the direction of healthcare.

170. Hospital Administrator

Description: Manages hospital operations, budgets, staffing, and compliance (gl).

Education/Training: MHA (gl), MBA (gl), MPH (gl); leadership experience required.

Salary Range: $150,000–$350,000+.

Shortage Indicator: Strong, especially in rural (gl) or struggling hospitals.

Pathways & Notes: Routes to CEO (gl), COO (gl) roles.

Cost-of-Living Lens: Salaries tied to system size; rural (gl) = broader authority.

Quote: "Hospitals run on leadership, not luck."

Here's My Take: For vision-driven leaders who thrive on complexity and coordination.

171. Clinic Manager

Description: Oversees daily operations of outpatient (gl) practices and clinics.

Education/Training: Bachelor's (gl)/Master's (gl) in health admin (gl) or related.

Salary Range: $80,000–$120,000+.

Shortage Indicator: Strong with outpatient (gl) growth.

Pathways & Notes: Steps toward hospital administration.

Cost-of-Living Lens: Salaries modest but balanced with manageable scope.

Quote: "Every clinic needs a steady hand."

Here's My Take: A great fit for organizers who want impact at the local level.

172. Health System CEO

Description: Sets vision, strategy, and culture for multi-hospital systems.

Education/Training: MHA (gl), MBA (gl), MD (gl)/DO (gl)/RN (gl) with leadership background.

Salary Range: $500,000–$1.5M+.

Shortage Indicator: Competitive; boards (gl) seek proven turnarounds (gl).

Pathways & Notes: Top executive (gl) role in healthcare.

Cost-of-Living Lens: Comp packages heavy on incentives (gl) and bonuses.

Quote: "The culture of a system flows from the top."

Here's My Take: For big-picture leaders who thrive under scrutiny and responsibility.

173. Chief Nursing Officer (CNO)

Description: Directs nursing practice, quality, staffing, and Magnet® alignment.

Education/Training: RN (gl) + MSN (gl)/DNP (gl); leadership experience.

Salary Range: $200,000–$350,000+.

Shortage Indicator: Strong; pipeline (gl) limited.

Pathways & Notes: Key to executive (gl) team; Magnet® hospitals emphasize CNO leadership.

Cost-of-Living Lens: Salaries higher in large systems.

Quote: "Nursing leadership is culture leadership."

Here's My Take: For nurses who want to shape the practice of thousands.

174. Chief Medical Officer (CMO)

Description: Leads clinical quality (gl), safety (gl), and medical staff affairs.

Education/Training: MD (gl)/DO (gl) + leadership training (gl) (CPE (gl), MBA (gl)).

Salary Range: $280,000–$500,000+.

Shortage Indicator: Strong across systems.

Pathways & Notes: Bridges to CEO (gl) or system leadership.

Cost-of-Living Lens: Salaries scale with hospital size and complexity.

Quote: "Standards plus empathy equals adoption."

Here's My Take: Best for physicians who want to move from bedside to boardroom impact.

175. Chief Information Officer (CIO, Healthcare)

Description: Directs IT (gl) strategy, cybersecurity (gl), and digital transformation (gl) in healthcare.

Education/Training: IT (gl)/health informatics (gl) background; MBA (gl)/MHA (gl) helpful.

Salary Range: $200,000–$350,000+.

Shortage Indicator: Strong, especially with cybersecurity (gl) threats.

Pathways & Notes: Leads digital health initiatives (gl) and AI (gl) adoption.

Cost-of-Living Lens: Salaries competitive with tech but often lower than private sector.

Quote: "Digital strategy is clinical strategy now."

Here's My Take: For visionary tech leaders who want to steer healthcare's future.

176. Chief Financial Officer (CFO, Healthcare)

Description: Oversees financial health of hospitals or systems—budgets, revenue cycles (gl), capital planning (gl).

Education/Training: CPA (gl), MBA (gl), or MHA (gl); healthcare finance expertise critical.

Salary Range: $250,000–$500,000+.

Shortage Indicator: Moderate; high demand for turnaround (gl) specialists.

Pathways & Notes: Bridges into CEO (gl)/COO (gl) or consulting.

Cost-of-Living Lens: Compensation scales dramatically with system size.

Quote: "Numbers tell the story of mission sustainability (gl)."

Here's My Take: For finance-minded leaders who want to balance dollars with dignity in care.

177. Chief Operating Officer (COO, Healthcare)

Description: Manages daily hospital operations—clinical services, facilities, efficiency.

Education/Training: MHA (gl), MBA (gl), or clinical degree + leadership.

Salary Range: $250,000–$450,000+.

Shortage Indicator: Strong in complex systems.

Pathways & Notes: Often the next step to CEO (gl).

Cost-of-Living Lens: Scale of operations = scale of pay.

Quote: "Operations are where strategy meets reality."

Here's My Take: A fit for problem-solvers who love orchestrating moving parts.

178. Chief Human Resources Officer (CHRO, Healthcare)

Description: Leads workforce strategy, recruitment (gl), retention (gl), culture, benefits.

Education/Training: HR (gl) degree or MBA (gl); SHRM-SCP (gl) certification (gl) helpful.

Salary Range: $180,000–$325,000+.

Shortage Indicator: Strong with ongoing staffing crises (gl).

Pathways & Notes: Expanding role in employee engagement (gl) and DEI (gl).

Cost-of-Living Lens: Large systems offer richer comp packages.

Quote: "Culture is built through people practices."

Here's My Take: For leaders who believe retention (gl) and alignment are the real bottom line.

179. Chief Diversity & Inclusion Officer (CDIO)

Description: Develops strategies for equity (gl), diversity (gl), and inclusion (gl) in healthcare organizations.

Education/Training: Master's (gl) in HR (gl), public policy (gl), or related; diversity leadership experience.

Salary Range: $150,000–$250,000+.

Shortage Indicator: Growing with equity (gl) imperatives (gl).

Pathways & Notes: Integrates with HR (gl), patient experience (gl), community engagement (gl).

Cost-of-Living Lens: Compensation varies by system size and mission focus.

Quote: "Inclusion (gl) is the foundation of trust in care."

Here's My Take: For values-driven leaders who want culture change to last.

180. Chief Quality Officer (CQO)

Description: Directs quality, safety, accreditation (gl), and outcomes improvement.

Education/Training: MD (gl)/DO (gl), RN (gl), or admin background + quality certifications (gl) (CQM (gl), Lean Six Sigma (gl)).

Salary Range: $200,000–$325,000+.

Shortage Indicator: High with pay-for-performance (gl) metrics (gl).

Pathways & Notes: Roles integrate with patient safety, compliance (gl), and regulatory bodies (gl).

Cost-of-Living Lens: Salaries scale with system size and accreditation (gl) status.

Quote: "Quality is not a department—it's the way we work."

Here's My Take: For system-thinkers who want to hardwire safety and alignment.

181. Chief Innovation Officer

Description: Drives digital health, AI (gl), new models of care, and strategic transformation (gl).

Education/Training: MBA (gl), MPH (gl), MD (gl), or IT (gl) background with innovation track record.

Salary Range: $190,000–$325,000+.

Shortage Indicator: Emerging, competitive roles.

Pathways & Notes: Often hybrid of strategy and tech; ties to venture (gl) arms.

Cost-of-Living Lens: Large systems or urban innovation hubs (gl) pay most.

Quote: "Tomorrow's care requires today's imagination."

Here's My Take: For bold leaders who want to push healthcare into the future.

182. Chief Experience Officer (CXO, Healthcare)

Description: Leads patient, family, and employee experience strategies.

Education/Training: Master's (gl) in health admin (gl), communications (gl), or clinical background; CPXP (gl) credential (gl).

Salary Range: $150,000–$275,000+.

Shortage Indicator: Growing with value-based care (gl) and patient-centered (gl) metrics (gl).

Pathways & Notes: Collaborates closely with CNO (gl), CMO (gl), HR (gl).

Cost-of-Living Lens: Larger systems pay higher; nonprofits (gl) focus on mission over money.

Quote: "Experience is the outcome patients remember."

Here's My Take: For empathetic leaders who believe culture is as critical as care.

183. Chief Strategy Officer (CSO, Healthcare)

Description: Shapes long-term organizational growth, partnerships (gl), and market positioning (gl).

Education/Training: MBA (gl)/MHA (gl); consulting or strategy background.

Salary Range: $200,000–$350,000+.

Shortage Indicator: Competitive but key role in system growth.

Pathways & Notes: Bridges into CEO (gl) succession (gl) paths.

Cost-of-Living Lens: Larger markets = higher base and bonus packages.

Quote: "Strategy is tomorrow's playbook for care."

Here's My Take: For vision-driven planners who want to shape the chessboard of healthcare.

184. Chief Population Health Officer

Description: Directs population health (gl), chronic disease management (gl), community wellness.

Education/Training: MD (gl), RN (gl), or MPH (gl); background in value-based care (gl).

Salary Range: $180,000–$300,000+.

Shortage Indicator: High as systems shift to risk-based (gl) contracts (gl).

Pathways & Notes: Key roles in ACOs (gl) and integrated delivery systems (gl).

Cost-of-Living Lens: Salaries tied to risk-sharing (gl) arrangements.

Quote: "Population health (gl) is the bridge from care to community."

Here's My Take: For leaders passionate about shifting focus from sick care to health.

185. Chief Patient Safety Officer (CPSO)

Description: Oversees system-wide patient safety programs, root cause analyses (gl), and safety culture.

Education/Training: MD (gl), RN (gl), PharmD (gl), or admin + safety training (gl) (CPPS (gl) credential (gl)).

Salary Range: $180,000–$300,000+.

Shortage Indicator: High, tied to regulatory (gl) and liability (gl) pressures.

Pathways & Notes: Works closely with CQO (gl) and risk management.

Cost-of-Living Lens: Academic systems offer influence; private pay higher.

Quote: "Every patient deserves a harm-free journey."

Here's My Take: For leaders who want to prevent errors and protect lives.

Reaching the end of the Field of 185 isn't about checking boxes — it's about expanding your horizon. By now, you've seen that healthcare is more than a job market. It's an ecosystem (gl): part science, part service, part calling.

Maybe you've already spotted your match. Maybe you've circled three or four possibilities you never considered. Or maybe you've realized your current role is only half-aligned (gl), and there's a pivot (gl) waiting to happen. That's good news. Alignment isn't about getting it right once — it's about recalibrating (gl) as you grow.

Here's what I know after decades in healthcare recruitment (gl): there's a place for you. Whether you're drawn to adrenaline or analysis, compassion or compliance (gl), leadership or lab work — the right role doesn't just pay the bills, it fuels your purpose.

So take this Field of 185 with you. Highlight it. Dog-ear it. Argue with it. Most importantly, let it challenge you to stop settling for misalignment (gl). Healthcare needs you at your best, and you deserve a role where that best can shine.

Stay aligned. Stay curious. And always, StaySm:)in'!

Chapter 55
85 Careers of the Future

The Hub of Healing

If you've ever wondered where healthcare is headed, look closer.

It isn't waiting in a distant tomorrow — it's already here, quietly unfolding in hospital basements, biotech labs, and home devices that listen before they alert.

The future of care doesn't wait for permission.

It learns. It adapts. It predicts. It personalizes — faster than any textbook can keep up.

But here's the truth that matters most:

Technology will never replace healthcare professionals.

It will reveal what makes them irreplaceable.

Each role you're about to meet represents one heartbeat of that transformation — where artificial intelligence meets human ethics, where data meets dignity, and where science meets soul.

This is what happens when alignment becomes innovation.

The Precision Pavilion

Data, Diagnostics, and Personalized Medicine

Welcome to healthcare's predictive core — where algorithms learn empathy, genomes become guides, and data shapes destiny.

The Precision Pavilion belongs to the healers who translate complexity into clarity.

They make medicine not just faster, but smarter, safer, and uniquely human.

Corridor 1 The Algorithmic Diagnostic Wing

AI, Predictive Medicine, and Next-Gen Discovery

1. AI Imaging Liaison

Pathway: Radiologic Technologist or Imaging Specialist cross-trained in AI analytics and machine-learning interpretation.

Mason's Take: You're the interpreter between radiologists and algorithms — part human translator, part digital detective. You'll ensure that every AI decision is traceable, transparent, and trustworthy. Machines can see the pixels, but you'll see the person. The future of diagnostics depends on people who can make sense of what the code can't explain.

2. Predictive Care Coordinator

Pathway: RN, data analyst, or population-health professional with certification in predictive modeling and clinical forecasting.

Mason's Take: You're the weather forecaster of wellness. Your dashboards don't just show risk — they reveal possibility. You'll catch problems before they storm, and you'll turn prevention into poetry. Behind every metric is a life, and you'll treat each one like the miracle it already is.

3. Genomic Data Navigator

Pathway: RN, Medical Laboratory Scientist, or health-informatics specialist with training in genomics or bioinformatics.

Mason's Take: You're half detective, half DNA decoder. You'll translate genetic reports into personalized treatment plans that patients can actually understand. Precision medicine may speak in base pairs, but you'll make it sound like hope. Every gene you interpret is another thread in the story of what's possible.

4. Digital Twin Engineer

Pathway: Biomedical Engineer or Data Scientist trained in simulation modeling, physiology, and AI.

Mason's Take: You build virtual replicas of patients, organs, and even entire hospitals — so teams can test treatments before they touch skin. You'll prevent harm, accelerate discovery, and design healing like an architect designs light. This is empathy through engineering — every model a rehearsal for saving a life.

5. Clinical Algorithm Auditor

Pathway: Clinician, Data Scientist, or Ethicist with specialization in AI governance and bias detection.

Mason's Take: You're the conscience behind the code. Algorithms may be powerful, but they need watchdogs with wisdom. You'll test every output for fairness, accuracy, and humanity. The future depends on your refusal to let efficiency eclipse ethics.

6. Precision Pharmacogenomics Specialist

Pathway: Pharmacist, Genetic Counselor, or Laboratory Scientist with pharmacogenomics certification.

Mason's Take: You're the matchmaker of meds and molecules. No more one-size-fits-all — you'll tailor therapies to each patient's genes. Adverse reactions will drop; outcomes will rise. You're not dispensing drugs; you're delivering precision.

7. AI-Augmented Pathologist

Pathway: Pathologist or Laboratory Director with training in AI image-recognition and molecular diagnostics.

Mason's Take: You'll work side-by-side with algorithms that never sleep, amplifying your accuracy without replacing your intuition. The microscope of the future will listen, learn, and label — but it will still need your judgment. In this role, you'll prove that humanity is the best validation protocol.

8. Remote Robotics Surgeon

Pathway: Surgeon or Procedural Specialist certified in tele-robotic and haptic-surgery systems.

Mason's Take: You'll operate across continents, guided by fiber optics and feedback sensors so precise they feel like touch. Your OR may be miles away, but your focus won't flinch. You'll make "distance" irrelevant — and turn global access into reality.

9. Predictive Population Analyst

Pathway: Epidemiologist or Biostatistician with AI-driven predictive-modeling and behavioral-data expertise.

Mason's Take: You're the oracle of outcomes — identifying health crises before they happen. You'll track trends, social patterns, and unseen risks that shape public health. You'll turn raw data into resilience. This is epidemiology evolved.

10. Synthetic Biology Designer

Pathway: Biotechnologist, Cellular Engineer, or Bioinformatics Specialist with synthetic-genomics training.

Mason's Take: You'll design life itself — engineering cells to fight disease, grow organs, and repair tissue from within. It sounds futuristic, but it's already unfolding. Alignment here means remembering that every discovery carries a heartbeat. You're not just editing genes; you're rewriting the language of healing.

Corridor 2 · The Virtual Continuum

Hybrid Care, Hospital-at-Home, and Telepresence Medicine

11. Hospital-at-Home Systems Architect

Pathway: Healthcare administrator or clinical operations specialist with training in virtual acute-care delivery and IoT integration.

Mason's Take: You're designing hospitals without walls. You'll choreograph nurses, sensors, and satellite logistics so seamlessly that patients heal from home with ICU-level oversight. You're building the blueprint for comfort-driven, data-anchored care. When patients say, "I never thought this was possible," you'll smile — because you made it so.

12. Tele-Surgical Operations Coordinator

Pathway: Perioperative RN or biomedical engineer with certification in tele-robotic workflow management.

Mason's Take: You're the air-traffic controller of remote surgery. You'll synchronize cameras, consoles, and cross-continental teams. Precision is your poetry. If your calm can steady a surgeon's hand three time zones away, you've mastered the new art of presence.

13. Virtual ICU Nurse (Advanced Tele-Critical Care RN)

Pathway: ICU nurse with tele-critical care and AI-monitoring credentials.

Mason's Take: You'll save lives through screens — reading micro-movements, waveform whispers, and patient patterns that machines can't interpret alone. You'll prove that compassion carries bandwidth. Even in slippers, you'll be standing guard.

14. Home-Based Infusion Technologist

Pathway: Infusion RN or clinical technician certified in smart-pump and remote medication-monitoring systems.

Mason's Take: You turn living rooms into micro-clinics. Your briefcase hums with technology and trust. You'll bring calm to chaos, safety to syringes, and precision to every drip. Remember: in your hands, comfort is clinical.

15. Bio-Wearable Integration Specialist

Pathway: Biomedical engineer or digital-health technologist trained in sensor design and human-factors engineering.

Mason's Take: You're merging skin and circuitry. From glucose tattoos to cardiac patches, you'll make devices disappear into daily life. Study anatomy and empathy equally — both determine the fit. You'll help people live monitored without feeling monitored.

16. Virtual Rehabilitation Coach

Pathway: Physical or occupational therapist with VR/AR rehabilitation certification.

Mason's Take: You'll transform therapy from repetition to revelation. Patients will box with avatars, climb digital mountains, and regain mobility through motion-tracking miracles. You'll gamify grit — and healing will feel like winning again.

17. Remote Patient Experience Designer

Pathway: Healthcare UX designer or service-design specialist with training in clinical workflow and human-computer interaction.

Mason's Take: You'll make telehealth feel like care, not customer service. Every pixel and pause will carry purpose. You'll build digital empathy into buttons and timing. If you can make a patient feel seen through a screen, you've already healed something.

18. Health Drone Logistics Pilot

Pathway: Licensed UAV operator with medical supply-chain and FAA Part 107 certification.

Mason's Take: You're the new courier of compassion — delivering blood, vaccines, and hope to places roads can't reach. You'll chart flight paths between innovation and impact. Keep your eyes skyward and your purpose grounded.

19. Ambient Home Sensor Analyst

Pathway: Health informatics or biomedical data specialist trained in ambient AI and predictive alert systems.

Mason's Take: You'll turn ordinary homes into silent safety nets. Your algorithms will hear the coughs, stumbles, and silences that signal distress. Privacy and protection will be your balancing act. You'll guard dignity with data.

20. Cross-Reality Medical Interpreter

Pathway: Certified medical interpreter trained in AR/VR environments and speech-to-avatar translation.

Mason's Take: You'll make language barriers vanish — even inside holographic hospitals. You'll ensure that every patient, regardless of tongue or tech, is truly understood. This isn't translation; it's transformation.

Corridor 3 · The Bio-Innovation Bay

Genomics, Regeneration, and Living Technology

21. Regenerative Tissue Engineer

Pathway: Biomedical engineer or cellular biologist with specialization in regenerative medicine and 3-D bioprinting.

Mason's Take: You're sculpting the raw material of life. You'll grow cartilage, skin, and organs from stem-cell blueprints. Every new tissue you build rewrites the definition of recovery. You're not fixing what's broken — you're creating what's never existed before.

22. Neuro-Interface Clinician

Pathway: Neurologist, RN, or biomedical engineer trained in brain-computer interface (BCI) technology.

Mason's Take: You translate thought into motion. You'll help paralyzed patients move robotic limbs just by imagining it. Keep your curiosity electric and your ethics grounded — because you're literally rewiring what it means to be human.

23. Cellular Immunotherapy Coordinator

Pathway: Oncology nurse or lab technologist with certification in cell-therapy operations (CAR-T, NK, TIL platforms).

Mason's Take: You're the project manager of miracles. You'll shepherd living medicines from freezer to vein. You'll comfort families and coordinate scientists — a bridge between lab coats and love. When remission happens, you'll know you helped design it.

24. Bio-Ink Developer

Pathway: Materials scientist or chemical engineer specializing in biopolymers and organ-printing substrates.

Mason's Take: You're inventing the ink that can save lives. Each droplet you refine becomes bone, vessel, or valve. The secret ingredient is patience — because perfection here prints in layers of hope.

25. Genetic Wellness Advisor

Pathway: Genetic counselor or preventive-health specialist with certification in consumer genomics and epigenetics.

Mason's Take: You'll decode not just disease risk, but possibility. You'll teach people how lifestyle can switch genes on or off. You're proof that knowledge isn't power — it's prevention.

26. Microbiome Restoration Scientist

Pathway: Microbiologist or gastroenterology researcher trained in microbiome sequencing and microbial therapeutics.

Mason's Take: You're curating the body's inner galaxy. Every culture you balance brings immune systems back into tune. You'll help people heal from the inside out — one microbial symphony at a time.

27. Biofabrication Operations Director

Pathway: Manufacturing or biomedical leader with experience in clean-room production and regulatory compliance for living materials.

Mason's Take: You run the factory of the future — where the product is living tissue. You'll blend engineering, ethics, and elegance. Alignment here means quality control with a conscience.

28. Neural Rehabilitation Programmer

Pathway: Physical therapist or neuroscientist cross-trained in neuro-prosthetic programming and adaptive AI.

Mason's Take: You teach computers compassion through motion. Every line of code helps neurons reconnect. You'll redefine recovery for patients once told "never again."

29. Epigenetic Therapy Designer

Pathway: Pharmacologist or molecular biologist specializing in gene-expression modulation and personalized oncology.

Mason's Take: You'll write prescriptions for possibility — drugs that switch genes back on for healing. You're the poet of proteins, editing disease at its source.

30. Cryobiology Conservation Specialist

Pathway: Laboratory scientist or biobank manager trained in cryogenic storage and cellular preservation.

Mason's Take: You're the guardian of tomorrow's cures. Inside your tanks sleep tissues that could save generations. Stewardship here is sacred.

Corridor 4 · The Wellness Wing

Prevention, Longevity, and Whole-Person Intelligence

31. Longevity Medicine Specialist

Pathway: Physician, NP, or PA trained in longevity medicine, metabolic science, and precision prevention.

Mason's Take: You'll replace fear of aging with fascination. You'll help patients extend not just their years, but their vitality. Longevity is alignment across time.

32. Digital Wellness Strategist

Pathway: Public-health professional or UX researcher trained in behavioral-health technology and data ethics.

Mason's Take: You'll design the apps that quietly teach better sleep, calmer minds, and longer lives. Every nudge you build becomes an act of care.

33. Emotional-AI Therapist

Pathway: Licensed therapist or psychologist certified in AI-enhanced cognitive and affective computing systems.

Mason's Take: You'll collaborate with empathetic machines — but keep the heart of therapy human. Insight will always beat algorithm.

34. Climate Health Strategist

Pathway: Environmental-health or public-policy professional trained in climate medicine and resilience design.

Mason's Take: You'll connect weather to wellness. Heat, smoke, and storms will become clinical variables. Prevention begins with the planet.

35. Sleep Architecture Specialist

Pathway: Respiratory therapist, sleep technologist, or neurophysiologist specializing in digital polysomnography and circadian analytics.

Mason's Take: You'll turn exhaustion into equilibrium. Sleep isn't lazy — it's clinical.

36. Wellness Data Scientist

Pathway: Data analyst or epidemiologist with expertise in wearable-sensor and real-time health analytics.

Mason's Take: You'll read the rhythm of wellbeing like a language. Numbers will become narratives of prevention.

37. Integrative Nutrition Technologist

Pathway: Dietitian or food-science professional trained in nutrigenomics and personalized diet algorithms.

Mason's Take: You'll make food as precise as medicine. Your menus will be powered by biology, not fads.

38. Corporate Resilience Director

Pathway: Organizational psychologist or HR leader trained in burnout prevention and trauma-informed leadership.

Mason's Take: You'll build cultures where people stay because they fit. Alignment will become a retention strategy.

39. Behavioral Design Engineer

Pathway: Cognitive scientist or behavioral economist specializing in digital nudging and habit formation.

Mason's Take: You'll design environments that make healthy choices automatic. Kindness will be coded into the system.

40. Community Longevity Coordinator

Pathway: Public-health worker or nurse leader with geroscience and social-wellness training.

Mason's Take: You'll turn neighborhoods into healing ecosystems. Connection will become clinical.

Corridor 5 · The Neuro-Frontier

Cognition, Neural Care, and the Science of Thoughtful Healing

41. Cognitive Enhancement Clinician

Pathway: Neurologist, NP, or psychologist trained in neuro-stimulation and cognitive-training ethics.

Mason's Take: You'll expand human potential without losing human values. Progress guided by principle.

42. Memory Restoration Engineer

Pathway: Biomedical engineer or neuroscientist specializing in neural-encoding and hippocampal prosthetics.

Mason's Take: You'll rebuild memories — and with them, identities. Every recollection will feel like a sunrise.

43. Digital Neuro-Therapist

Pathway: Licensed therapist using VR/AR cognitive rehabilitation and neurofeedback platforms.

Mason's Take: You'll turn therapy into immersive healing journeys. Experience will become medicine.

44. Neuro-Ethics Consultant

Pathway: Ethicist, attorney, or philosopher trained in neurotechnology governance and privacy law.

Mason's Take: You'll protect the mind as fiercely as medicine protects the body. Innovation must answer to conscience.

45. Brain-Computer Rehabilitation Coach

Pathway: PT or OT trained in BCI prosthetics and adaptive neuro-AI.

Mason's Take: You'll help patients move by thinking. Intent will become action again.

46. Consciousness Research Coordinator

Pathway: Research scientist or anesthesiologist studying neural correlates of awareness.

Mason's Take: You'll explore what it means to be awake, aware, and alive — with science and humility.

47. Neural Data Guardian

Pathway: Health-IT security or informatics specialist certified in neural-data protection.

Mason's Take: You'll guard the most personal data on Earth — thoughts. Privacy will become sacred again.

48. Sensory Restoration Specialist

Pathway: Audiologist, ophthalmic technologist, or biomedical engineer working in sensory neuroprosthetics.

Mason's Take: You'll bring sound to silence and light to darkness. Perception will be your canvas.

49. Neuro-AI Translator

Pathway: Data scientist or neurologist trained in explainable AI for brain diagnostics.

Mason's Take: You'll help machines understand minds — without forgetting the humans behind them.

50. Digital Empathy Designer

Pathway: UX designer or behavioral scientist specializing in human-AI emotional interaction.

Mason's Take: You'll teach technology how to care. Compassion will be your programming language.

Corridor 6 · The Diagnostic Frontier

AI Imaging, Wearables, and Precision Detection

This corridor hums with pattern recognition and pulse sensors.

Here, detection becomes prevention, and diagnostics become dialogue.

It's not about finding what's wrong — it's about finding it early enough to make it right.

The future belongs to the clinicians who can see clearly — through data, design, and discernment.

51. AI Imaging Validator

Pathway: Radiologic technologist or data scientist trained in algorithmic bias detection and medical image verification.

Mason's Take: You'll stand guard between machine predictions and human consequences. You'll question every pixel and pattern, because accuracy isn't enough — alignment is. You're the conscience behind the code that reads lives.

52. Multi-Modal Diagnostic Integrator

Pathway: Biomedical informatics specialist skilled in combining imaging, lab, and genomic data for predictive analytics.

Mason's Take: You'll connect the dots between scans, samples, and stories. You'll give clinicians a full picture, not just snapshots. You're the orchestra conductor of diagnostics — keeping complexity in harmony.

53. Smart Sensor Nurse

Pathway: Registered nurse or clinical technologist certified in wearable diagnostics and biosensor analytics.

Mason's Take: You'll listen to what patients can't feel yet — the subtle signals before symptoms start. You'll make "checkups" continuous. You'll help healthcare keep its promise: heal early, not react late.

54. Molecular Diagnostics Engineer

Pathway: Clinical laboratory scientist or biochemist trained in molecular assay design and automation.

Mason's Take: You'll shrink labs into portable systems. Your reagents and robotics will reveal truth faster than fear can spread. You're proof that precision can be mobile — and lifesaving.

55. Predictive Pathology Analyst

Pathway: Pathologist or data scientist specializing in digital pathology and AI histopathology.

Mason's Take: You'll turn microscopic slides into massive insight. Every stained cell tells a story, and you'll be fluent in its language. You'll help shift pathology from reaction to prevention.

56. Continuous Glucose Systems Coach

Pathway: Certified diabetes educator or nurse technologist trained in real-time glucose-monitoring platforms.

Mason's Take: You'll help patients see their biology in motion. Every data point becomes a decision, every meal a moment of agency. You're teaching people to become scientists of their own health.

57. Digital Biomarker Scientist

Pathway: Data scientist or biostatistician specializing in behavioral and physiological digital biomarkers.

Mason's Take: You'll turn motion, speech, and sleep into diagnostic signals. You'll detect risk in patterns most people never notice. You'll prove that wellness leaves footprints — and you know how to read them.

58. Nanodiagnostics Technician

Pathway: Laboratory technologist or nanomaterials scientist trained in nanoscale biosensing and molecular imaging.

Mason's Take: You'll work on the invisible frontier — detecting disease with sensors smaller than cells. You'll see illness before even microscopes can. Your precision will feel like prophecy.

59. Portable Lab Systems Specialist

Pathway: Biomedical engineer or clinical technologist trained in lab-on-a-chip and mobile diagnostics.

Mason's Take: You'll put laboratories into backpacks. In rural towns, disaster zones, and everywhere time matters, your work will deliver answers where hope once waited. You are mobility, in medicine form.

60. AI Radiology Workflow Architect

Pathway: Imaging administrator or software engineer experienced in radiology AI integration and workflow optimization.

Mason's Take: You'll choreograph humans and algorithms like a duet. You'll speed diagnosis without sacrificing discernment. Every streamlined scan can mean one more life spared from delay.

Corridor 7 · The Power Panel

Robotics, Automation, and Sustainable Systems

This corridor hums, glows, and occasionally whirs.

It's the domain of engineers with heart and clinicians with circuitry in their veins.

They build the exoskeletons, maintain the robotic arms, and design hospitals that heal both people and the planet.

Here, sustainability meets precision — and care runs on clean current.

61. Surgical Robotics Integration Specialist

Pathway: OR nurse, biomedical engineer, or technologist with certification in robotic-surgery systems integration.

Mason's Take: You'll be the bridge between surgeon and machine. You'll make every incision safer through synchronization and setup. The robot may move the scalpel — but you move the system.

62. Clinical Exoskeleton Technician

Pathway: Physical therapist, biomedical technologist, or prosthetics specialist trained in robotic mobility systems.

Mason's Take: You'll help people walk again — powered by exosuits that feel like science fiction until the moment someone stands up and smiles. Engineering becomes empathy, made mechanical.

63. Surgical Drone Operator

Pathway: Perioperative technologist or biomedical engineer certified in tele-robotic UAV systems.

Mason's Take: You'll extend a surgeon's capability across distance when speed is the difference between salvage and loss. When care must move fast, you'll be the connection that makes it possible.

64. Medical Robotics Maintenance Engineer

Pathway: Robotics or mechatronics engineer with healthcare-device compliance certification.

Mason's Take: You'll keep life-saving machines flawless. Behind every smooth case is your calibration, your standards, your quiet excellence. You may not wear scrubs, but you protect outcomes.

65. Sustainable Hospital Systems Designer

Pathway: Environmental engineer or healthcare architect trained in LEED, carbon-reduction, and smart-grid systems.

Mason's Take: You'll turn hospitals into ecosystems — resilient, efficient, and restorative. Every watt saved and every drop reused becomes an act of healing. Sustainability is the new sterility.

66. Energy Resilience Officer

Pathway: Facilities or energy manager with experience in renewable microgrids and critical-infrastructure protection.

Mason's Take: You'll keep life-support alive when the grid goes dark. You're the steady hand in every storm — powering the promise that hospitals never sleep.

67. Medical Device Cybersecurity Analyst

Pathway: IT security professional trained in healthcare-device protection and cybersecurity compliance.

Mason's Take: You'll defend patients from invisible danger — not viruses in bodies, but vulnerabilities in code. Your vigilance makes every monitor, pump, and alarm a little safer.

68. Automation Workflow Engineer

Pathway: Industrial engineer or clinical operations specialist trained in RPA and AI optimization.

Mason's Take: You'll replace burnout with breathing room by automating the noise. You'll give clinicians back their rarest resource — time — and make room for one more human conversation.

69. Smart Building Health Technologist

Pathway: Biomedical or facilities technologist specializing in IoT sensors, air-quality systems, and wellness architecture.

Mason's Take: You'll make walls breathe and rooms respond. Light, temperature, and sound will adjust to healing rhythms. You'll turn buildings into active partners in care.

70. Renewable Medical Materials Scientist

Pathway: Materials scientist or environmental chemist focused on biodegradable medical supplies and circular-economy design.

Mason's Take: You'll invent the next generation of gloves, gowns, and gear — sustainable, sterile, and smart. You'll leave no trace except better outcomes.

Corridor 8 · The Data Nexus

AI Governance, Ethics, and the Alignment of Digital Intelligence

This is the quiet hum beneath healthcare's heartbeat.

Here, accuracy meets empathy, and privacy becomes sacred.

The professionals in this corridor don't just manage information — they guard truth, transparency, and trust.

Every clean dataset is a story protected. Every algorithm reviewed is a life safeguarded.

71. Clinical AI Auditor

Pathway: Clinician, data scientist, or compliance professional trained in AI governance and bias mitigation.

Mason's Take: You'll keep algorithms honest. When a machine influences who gets care, you'll make sure the math matches morality. You're not anti-technology — you're pro-humanity.

72. Digital Ethics Officer

Pathway: Legal, ethics, or informatics professional with training in healthcare AI and data responsibility.

Mason's Take: You'll be the conscience of innovation. Every boundary you uphold protects trust before it breaks. Progress without principle isn't progress — it's risk.

73. Algorithmic Transparency Specialist

Pathway: Data analyst or policy strategist focused on explainable AI and model interpretability.

Mason's Take: You'll open the black box. You'll make complex systems understandable for patients, clinicians, and leaders. Clarity is care.

74. Clinical Language Model Trainer

Pathway: Linguist, data scientist, or clinician specializing in medical NLP model development and supervision.

Mason's Take: You'll teach machines to speak medicine responsibly. Every dataset is a reflection of real lives. Your job is to make sure AI doesn't just talk — it listens.

75. Health Data Privacy Architect

Pathway: Information-security engineer or health IT professional with HIPAA, ISO, and interoperability privacy specialization.

Mason's Take: You'll build digital vaults for the world's most personal information. Your systems will make invisible safety feel real. You'll design trust at scale.

Corridor 8 · The Data Nexus

AI Governance, Ethics, and the Alignment of Digital Intelligence

This is the quiet hum beneath healthcare's heartbeat.

Here, accuracy meets empathy, and privacy becomes sacred.

The professionals in this corridor don't just manage information — they guard truth, transparency, and trust.

Every clean dataset is a story protected. Every algorithm reviewed is a life safeguarded.

76. Synthetic Data Scientist

Pathway: Computational scientist or biostatistician trained in synthetic patient data generation and de-identification ethics.

Mason's Take: You'll make privacy compatible with progress. You'll create data that mimics reality — without revealing identity. You're the quiet genius behind safe innovation.

77. Human–AI Collaboration Designer

Pathway: UX researcher or behavioral scientist focused on clinician–AI workflow optimization.

Mason's Take: You'll choreograph the dance between human intuition and machine precision. You'll know exactly when the algorithm should lead — and when to step aside for empathy.

78. Digital Twin Health Analyst

Pathway: Data scientist or biomedical engineer skilled in patient-simulation modeling and predictive analytics.

Mason's Take: You'll create digital versions of real patients to test treatments, reduce risk, and personalize recovery. Every outcome you improve will echo twice — once in code, once in life.

79. Cyber Resilience Strategist

Pathway: IT security professional or systems engineer with expertise in critical-infrastructure protection for hospitals.

Mason's Take: You'll defend care from chaos. When ransomware hits or networks fail, you'll restore order in the dark. You're the shield that lets others keep saving lives.

80. Data Equity Officer

Pathway: Public-health or data-policy leader with training in equity analytics and inclusive algorithm design.

Mason's Take: You'll ensure healthcare data reflects everyone — not just the majority. You'll fix blind spots before they become bias. You'll turn inclusion into infrastructure.

Corridor 9 · The Leadership League

Alignment, Innovation, and the Future of Human-Centered Leadership

This corridor doesn't echo with footsteps — it resonates with purpose.

Here, leadership isn't a position; it's a practice.

These roles exist for the builders of culture, the architects of alignment, and the champions who measure success not in profits, but in pride, presence, and people.

81. Chief Alignment Officer

Pathway: Senior healthcare executive or nurse leader trained in organizational psychology, workforce engagement, and transformational leadership.

Mason's Take: You'll align the human pulse with the hospital pulse. You'll turn burnout into belonging and metrics into meaning. When others chase benchmarks, you'll build belief. You'll be the steward of purpose in motion.

82. Chief Empathy Architect

Pathway: Executive or organizational designer with expertise in emotional intelligence, experience strategy, and leadership science.

Mason's Take: You'll redesign leadership from the inside out. You'll hardwire compassion into culture and call it infrastructure. You'll remind every executive that ROI means Return on Integrity.

83. Director of Healthcare Storytelling

Pathway: Communications or patient-experience professional with background in narrative medicine, journalism, or digital media.

Mason's Take: You'll collect the stories that keep systems human. You'll translate data into dignity and outcomes into emotion. You'll make empathy memorable — and unforgettable.

84. Chief Wellbeing & Retention Officer

Pathway: HR or nursing leader trained in resilience strategy, trauma-informed leadership, and evidence-based engagement.

Mason's Take: You'll rewrite turnover trends with tenderness. You'll prove that retention isn't a metric — it's a relationship. Every thank-you note, every flexible schedule, every listening round will be a quiet revolution.

85. Chief Innovation & Alignment Strategist

Pathway: Healthcare administrator, clinician, or consultant specializing in organizational transformation and AI–human integration.

Mason's Take: You'll stand where systems meet souls. You'll integrate **SCRUB*fit*™**, **PACES™**, and **CARESET™** thinking into leadership DNA. You'll make alignment scalable — and the future sustainable.

Mason's Closing Reflection

Eighty-five roles.

Each one real, rising, and redefining what it means to work in healthcare.

Some heal with hands, others with hardware; some with words, others with code.

But all share one pulse — the alignment of purpose, possibility, and people.

The corridors of Hopewell aren't fiction.

They're blueprints.

They show what happens when design meets devotion, and when the next generation of healthcare leaders refuses to choose between heart and innovation.

Healthcare's future isn't waiting for permission — it's waiting for you.

Chapter 56

50 Healthcare
Side Hustles

50 Side Hustles to Test-Drive Your Future in Healthcare

Not everyone enters healthcare wearing scrubs or a white coat. Some start small — testing the waters before taking the leap. Sometimes that's the smartest path forward. That's where side hustles come in.

Think of these as test-drives — an opportunity to "dip your toes in the water," so to speak. These are flexible roles with low barriers to entry that give you a front-row seat to the rhythms, frustrations, and joys of healthcare. Some are patient-facing. Others happen quietly behind the scenes. A few orbit outside hospitals but still revolve around health and healing. The beauty of side hustles is that they're real work, real pay (or at least real experience), and real clues about whether a healthcare career is your calling — or simply a curiosity.

In the pages ahead, you'll find 50 side hustles that range from classic starter jobs like patient transport or medical scribing to creative gigs like health blogging or volunteering on a crisis hotline. Each profile explains what the role is, what alignment traits it tests, how much you can expect to earn (or save), and how it can springboard into a bigger career. And because I've lived long enough in this world to know that the smallest jobs can spark the biggest callings, you'll also get my personal take on why each hustle matters.

Let's begin — your first step into healthcare might be closer, simpler, and more rewarding than you ever imagined.

Part I — Front-Desk & First Impressions

1. Patient Care Representative

Description: Handles registration, verifies insurance, checks patients in, and serves as the first point of contact.

Alignment Preview: Great for multitaskers who can handle stress with a smile and calm anxious patients.

Pay / Perks: $15–22/hr; flexible shifts.

Springboard Potential: Patient advocacy, health-information management, or supervisory roles.

Mason's Take: Don't underestimate the first hello — alignment often begins with eye contact and a smile at the front desk. Your calm can shape the entire visit.

2. Telephone Operator / Call Center Scheduler

Description: Manages incoming calls, schedules appointments, and routes patients to the right departments.

Alignment Preview: Tests patience, clarity, and real-time problem-solving.

Pay / Perks: $14–20/hr; often remote or hybrid.

Springboard Potential: Scheduling coordinator, practice manager, or patient-navigation roles.

Mason's Take: If you can survive the switchboard at 4:59 p.m. on a Friday, you're tougher than half the doctors in the building. You'll also master communication — a skill that travels everywhere in healthcare.

3. Hospital Gift Shop Clerk

Description: Sells flowers, snacks, cards, and comfort items in the hospital gift shop.

Alignment Preview: Low-stress way to test hospital comfort while practicing empathy with patients' families.

Pay / Perks: $12–18/hr; sometimes volunteer.

Springboard Potential: Admissions, volunteer services, or hospitality roles.

Mason's Take: Healing sometimes starts with a balloon and a candy bar. You'll witness joy, grief, and gratitude — often in the same ten-minute window.

4. Medical Receptionist / Clinic Greeter

Description: Greets patients, manages paperwork, collects copays, and keeps the front office running.

Alignment Preview: Perfect for those who enjoy order, face-to-face interaction, and being the calm in the storm.

Pay / Perks: $15–22/hr.

Springboard Potential: Administrative leadership, practice management, or care coordination.

Mason's Take: The best receptionists aren't gatekeepers — they're guides. You'll learn to balance empathy with efficiency, a skill every leader needs.

Part II — Paperwork, Process & Precision

5. Medical Records Clerk / HIM Scanner

Description: Scans, organizes, and digitizes patient records, ensuring HIPAA compliance.

Alignment Preview: Tests attention to detail and respect for privacy.

Pay / Perks: $15–21/hr.

Springboard Potential: Coding, privacy officer, or health-information management paths.

Mason's Take: Every chart you scan could prevent a medical error. Precision here saves lives downstream.

6. Billing Assistant

Description: Processes claims, enters charges, and follows up on rejected insurance claims.

Alignment Preview: Ideal for detail-driven people who like paperwork puzzles.

Pay / Perks: $16–23/hr.

Springboard Potential: Coding certifications (CPC, CCS) and revenue-cycle careers.

Mason's Take: If you love sudoku, you'll love untangling insurance. You'll gain a crash course in how money flows through medicine — a lesson worth every keystroke.

7. Insurance Verification Coordinator

Description: Calls insurance companies, confirms coverage, and manages prior authorizations.

Alignment Preview: Great for rule-followers who can advocate firmly when needed.

Pay / Perks: $17–25/hr.

Springboard Potential: Insurance specialist, utilization review, or revenue-cycle management.

Mason's Take: You'll learn fast that "not medically necessary" can mean wildly different things. You're the translator between policy and people — stay persistent.

Part III — Hands-On Care Starters

8. Patient Transporter

Description: Moves patients between rooms, departments, and tests — always with safety and compassion.

Alignment Preview: Tests physical stamina, bedside manner, and empathy.

Pay / Perks: $13–20/hr; entry-level.

Springboard Potential: CNA or orderly roles.

Mason's Take: A smile and a steady hand on a stretcher can lower blood pressure faster than meds. You'll see humanity from hallway A to Z.

9. Medical Scribe

Description: Works beside providers to document patient visits in the EHR.

Alignment Preview: Tests focus, endurance, and curiosity about clinical reasoning.

Pay / Perks: $15–22/hr; flexible for students.

Springboard Potential: Med school, nursing, or PA programs.

Mason's Take: You'll learn more about real-world medicine in three months as a scribe than in a year of lectures. Observe everything — the best clinicians are constant learners.

10. Pharmacy Technician Trainee / Cashier

Description: Assists pharmacists with filling prescriptions, stocking, and ringing up meds; many employers train from scratch.

Alignment Preview: Tests accuracy, responsibility, and calm multitasking.

Pay / Perks: $15–20/hr to start; certification can raise this.

Springboard Potential: Certified Pharmacy Tech, hospital pharmacy, or retail lead roles.

Mason's Take: Pharmacy is half science, half empathy under pressure. You'll see that every pill bottle holds both chemistry and trust.

Part IV — Care at Home & in the Community

11. Phlebotomy Tech-in-Training

Description: Learns to draw blood for lab tests under supervision before certification.

Alignment Preview: Perfect for steady hands and calm voices.

Pay / Perks: $15–22/hr training; $20–28/hr certified.

Springboard Potential: Phlebotomist, Lab Tech, or PA/MD paths.

Mason's Take: If you can convince a terrified patient to roll up their sleeve, you've already mastered healthcare diplomacy. Precision earns trust — and trust is everything.

12. Certified Nursing Assistant (CNA) — Fast Track

Description: Provides hands-on care — vitals, hygiene, feeding, mobility — after a short course and exam.

Alignment Preview: Great for compassionate, physically active people comfortable with bedside realities.

Pay / Perks: $16–23/hr; training 4–12 weeks.

Springboard Potential: LPN, RN, or allied-health programs.

Mason's Take: Many careers begin here — with the simple act of helping someone out of bed with dignity. Every shift is a master class in humility and heart.

13. Central Sterile Tech (Instrument Processing)

Description: Cleans and sterilizes surgical instruments; sets up trays for ORs.

Alignment Preview: Ideal for detail-oriented introverts who like essential, behind-the-scenes work.

Pay / Perks: $17–25/hr; on-the-job training common.

Springboard Potential: Sterile Processing Supervisor, OR Tech, Surgical Assistant.

Mason's Take: No surgeon moves without you. Quiet precision makes miracles possible.

14. Companion Caregiver

Description: Provides non-medical support for seniors — conversation, errands, meal prep, and light home help.

Alignment Preview: Tests patience, empathy, and comfort with aging populations.

Pay / Perks: $13–18/hr; flexible schedules.

Springboard Potential: CNA, Home Health Aide, or gerontology-focused nursing.

Mason's Take: Sometimes the most powerful medicine is simply presence. If you can sit through silence and still connect, you're already a healer.

15. Home Health Aide (HHA)

Description: Assists patients with daily living tasks in their homes; requires short certification.

Alignment Preview: Ideal for those who want one-on-one care and flexibility.

Pay / Perks: $14–20/hr.

Springboard Potential: LPN/RN, hospice care, or case management.

Mason's Take: You're invited into someone's most private world — their home. Respect and trust mean everything here. Honor that and you'll change lives.

16. Non-Emergency Medical Transport (NEMT) Driver

Description: Transports patients to appointments, dialysis, or rehab safely and on time.

Alignment Preview: Perfect for people who like driving, being punctual, and offering reassuring conversation.

Pay / Perks: $14–22/hr; sometimes per-trip rates.

Springboard Potential: EMT training or healthcare logistics.

Mason's Take: You're not just a driver — you're the bridge to care. A ride that shows up on time can be the difference between stability and setback.

17. Crisis Hotline Volunteer

Description: Provides emotional support and resources via phone or chat for people in crisis; training provided.

Alignment Preview: Tests empathy, calm under pressure, and active listening.

Pay / Perks: Unpaid but invaluable experience; flexible remote shifts.

Springboard Potential: Social work, counseling, psychiatric nursing.

Mason's Take: You'll never forget the moment someone says, "Thank you for listening." You held space for a life — that's real impact.

18. CPR / First Aid Instructor (Red Cross or AHA)

Description: Teaches CPR, AED, and First Aid after a short instructor course.

Alignment Preview: Great for natural teachers who want to empower others with lifesaving skills.

Pay / Perks: $18–30/hr; often freelance or per class.

Springboard Potential: Training coordinator, EMS educator, or safety officer.

Mason's Take: Few side hustles let you say, "I gave someone skills that might save a life." This one does — and you'll walk away changed.

19. Peer Recovery Support Specialist

Description: Supports individuals recovering from substance use disorder; often based on lived experience plus certification.

Alignment Preview: Best for empathetic, nonjudgmental communicators with resilience and boundaries.

Pay / Perks: $16–22/hr; flexible.

Springboard Potential: Addiction counseling, psychiatric nursing, public health.

Mason's Take: Turning your scars into someone else's survival guide — that's purpose at its purest. Your empathy becomes medicine.

20. Doula-in-Training

Description: Provides non-medical labor support, education, and advocacy for birthing families.

Alignment Preview: Great for nurturing personalities and advocates for women's health and birth equity.

Pay / Perks: $300–800 per birth; often freelance.

Springboard Potential: Midwife, OB nurse, lactation consultant.

Mason's Take: If you believe birth is as much about support as science, this is your calling. You'll witness the moment life begins — and feel honored to stand there.

Part V — Community, Prevention & Public Health

21. Health Fair Outreach Worker

Description: Assists with blood-pressure checks, BMI screenings, and health education at community events.

Alignment Preview: Ideal for extroverts who enjoy engaging with the public and promoting wellness.

Pay / Perks: $14–20/hr or volunteer; often short-term.

Springboard Potential: Public health, community outreach, or health education.

Mason's Take: Think of it as healthcare's street team — you're taking prevention to the people. It's sweaty, spontaneous, and incredibly rewarding when someone says, "I didn't know that could save my life."

22. Survey Caller / Patient Experience Rep

Description: Calls patients post-discharge to collect feedback about their hospital or clinic experience.

Alignment Preview: Great for empathetic listeners who can handle both praise and complaints with professionalism.

Pay / Perks: $15–21/hr; often remote.

Springboard Potential: Patient advocacy, quality improvement, or service excellence.

Mason's Take: You'll hear the full spectrum of humanity — from gratitude to frustration. If you can translate emotion into insight, you're already leading change.

23. Telehealth Navigator

Description: Helps patients log in, troubleshoot, and prepare for virtual visits.

Alignment Preview: Perfect for tech-savvy helpers who enjoy guiding others with patience.

Pay / Perks: $16–22/hr; many remote opportunities.

Springboard Potential: Health IT, informatics, or patient-access management.

Mason's Take: If you can get Grandma's iPad camera turned on, you can do anything. You're the bridge between comfort and care in a digital world.

24. EHR Super-User Assistant (Go-Live Support)

Description: Supports staff during new electronic health-record rollouts, answering workflow questions.

Alignment Preview: Best for quick learners who like tech, teamwork, and problem-solving.

Pay / Perks: $18–25/hr; often short-term contracts.

Springboard Potential: Health IT, clinical informatics, or system training.

Mason's Take: You'll learn fast that the most feared word in healthcare isn't "disease" — it's "upgrade." When you help someone master the new system, you reduce burnout in real time.

25. Clinical Research Assistant (Entry Level)

Description: Helps recruit participants, collect data, and manage study documentation under supervision.

Alignment Preview: Great for curious, organized minds who enjoy detail and discovery.

Pay / Perks: $17–24/hr.

Springboard Potential: Research coordinator, clinical trials manager, or graduate study.

Mason's Take: Science doesn't just happen in labs — it happens in clipboards, checklists, and consent forms. Every data point moves medicine forward.

Part VI — Wellness, Movement & Mind-Body Health

26. Fitness Instructor / Group Exercise Leader

Description: Leads group fitness classes in gyms, rehab centers, or community spaces; certification required.

Alignment Preview: Perfect for energetic motivators who thrive on positive feedback and connection.

Pay / Perks: $20–40/class.

Springboard Potential: Wellness coordinator, physical therapy aide, or health coach.

Mason's Take: Movement is medicine — and you're the one writing the prescription. A single upbeat class can shift a patient's entire week.

27. Yoga or Mind-Body Teacher (Therapeutic Focus)

Description: Teaches gentle yoga, mindfulness, or stress-reduction for patients or staff.

Alignment Preview: Ideal for calm, grounded individuals who value balance and presence.

Pay / Perks: $25–50/hr; freelance or contract.

Springboard Potential: Integrative medicine, wellness coaching, or behavioral health.

Mason's Take: You're not just teaching poses — you're teaching peace. When healthcare learns to breathe again, it heals deeper.

28. Nutrition Coach (Entry Certification)

Description: Guides clients on healthy eating through short certification programs; not medical therapy.

Alignment Preview: Great for health enthusiasts who love practical coaching.

Pay / Perks: $20–40/hr; flexible, often remote.

Springboard Potential: Dietitian (RD), public health nutrition, or wellness programs.

Mason's Take: You'll see transformation one grocery list at a time. Nutrition isn't just food — it's empowerment on a plate.

29. Lactation Peer Supporter

Description: Assists new parents with breastfeeding basics; often volunteer or community-based.

Alignment Preview: Perfect for patient, nurturing personalities who advocate for maternal and infant health.

Pay / Perks: $14–20/hr or volunteer.

Springboard Potential: Lactation consultant (IBCLC), maternal health nursing.

Mason's Take: A calm voice in the first week of a baby's life can ripple for decades. You're building confidence one feeding at a time.

30. Occupational Therapy Aide

Description: Supports OTs by setting up therapy spaces, cleaning equipment, and helping patients practice tasks.

Alignment Preview: Good for creative problem-solvers who enjoy helping others regain independence.

Pay / Perks: $15–21/hr; no degree required.

Springboard Potential: OT Assistant, full OT program, or other rehab careers.

Mason's Take: You'll watch people relearn the little things —

tying shoes, holding a spoon, writing their name — and realize those moments are miracles.

Part VII — Therapy & Rehab Pathways

31. Physical Therapy Aide

Description: Helps PTs by preparing equipment, assisting patients with stretches, and keeping therapy areas organized.

Alignment Preview: Perfect for people fascinated by movement, recovery, and human resilience.

Pay / Perks: $15–21/hr; often part-time or student-friendly.

Springboard Potential: PTA (Physical Therapist Assistant), DPT programs, or sports medicine.

Mason's Take: Watching someone take their first unsteady steps after surgery will rewire how you define progress. Motion really is medicine.

32. Rehabilitation Tech (Rehab Aide)

Description: Assists in rehab units — helping transport patients, set up equipment, and monitor safety during exercise.

Alignment Preview: Great for hands-on helpers who want exposure to multiple therapy disciplines.

Pay / Perks: $15–20/hr.

Springboard Potential: Rehab nursing, occupational therapy, speech therapy.

Mason's Take: You're the quiet backbone of rehab. Every transfer, every lap around the unit builds someone else's independence — and your own confidence as a future clinician.

33. Speech Therapy Aide

Description: Prepares therapy materials, helps patients practice communication exercises, and tracks progress.

Alignment Preview: Ideal for patient, creative people interested in language and connection.

Pay / Perks: $15–20/hr.

Springboard Potential: Speech-Language Pathology Assistant (SLPA) or graduate SLP programs.

Mason's Take: Helping someone speak their first clear word after a stroke or injury is unforgettable. Communication isn't just a skill — it's a lifeline.

34. Radiology Transport / Imaging Aide

Description: Escorts patients to radiology, positions them for X-rays or scans, and assists technologists.

Alignment Preview: For those curious about imaging and comfortable around technology.

Pay / Perks: $15–22/hr.

Springboard Potential: Radiologic Technologist (RT[R]), MRI, CT, or ultrasound.

Mason's Take: You'll learn that dignity matters as much as diagnosis. When you gently position a frightened patient for a scan, you set the tone for every image captured.

35. Volunteer Chaplain Assistant

Description: Supports hospital chaplains with rounding, comfort visits, and family support.

Alignment Preview: For compassionate, spiritually grounded individuals who value whole-person care.

Pay / Perks: Volunteer; mentorship and reflection are the rewards.

Springboard Potential: Chaplaincy, social work, or palliative care.

Mason's Take: Healing isn't only clinical — it's spiritual, too. You'll witness moments of grace that charts can't capture.

Part VIII — Heart & Hospitality

36. Environmental Services (EVS) Associate

Description: Maintains cleanliness and infection control in patient rooms and clinical areas.

Alignment Preview: Great for detail-oriented, reliable people who take pride in essential work.

Pay / Perks: $14–20/hr.

Springboard Potential: EVS Supervisor, infection prevention, or facilities management.

Mason's Take: Hospitals can't heal without you — period. You keep pathogens out and patients safe; that's heroism in plain clothes.

37. Dietary Aide / Nutrition Services Assistant

Description: Prepares and delivers patient meals, follows dietary restrictions, and coordinates with clinical staff.

Alignment Preview: Perfect for service-minded individuals who believe food is part of healing.

Pay / Perks: $14–19/hr.

Springboard Potential: Diet Tech, Registered Dietitian, or food-service leadership.

Mason's Take: A warm meal delivered with care can be as therapeutic as any medication. This is compassion served on a tray.

38. Patient Observer / Sitter

Description: Monitors vulnerable patients (fall risk, confused, suicidal) to ensure safety.

Alignment Preview: Perfect for calm, observant people with a steady temperament.

Pay / Perks: $14–20/hr.

Springboard Potential: CNA, psych tech, behavioral health nurse.

Mason's Take: Quiet watchfulness can save a life. You'll discover that true care often looks like simply being there.

39. Volunteer Surgical Waiting Room Liaison

Description: Updates families on surgical progress, provides comfort, and coordinates with OR staff.

Alignment Preview: Ideal for empathetic communicators who can balance urgency and reassurance.

Pay / Perks: Volunteer; valuable exposure to perioperative care.

Springboard Potential: Patient advocacy, surgical services, nurse navigation.

Mason's Take: You'll learn the art of presence — sometimes families don't need answers, they just need you to stay seated beside them.

40. Hospital Concierge / Guest Services

Description: Provides directions, comfort items, and support for patients and families navigating the hospital.

Alignment Preview: For those who thrive on solving problems and brightening stressful days.

Pay / Perks: $15–22/hr.

Springboard Potential: Patient relations, hospitality management in healthcare.

Mason's Take: Hospitals can feel like airports without flight boards — you're the guide who gets people where they need to be, emotionally and physically.

Part IX — Support & Service Foundations

41. Hospital Volunteer (General Services)

Description: Provides support wherever needed — delivering mail, escorting families, stocking supplies, or lending a steady hand.

Alignment Preview: Ideal for those who want broad exposure before choosing a focus.

Pay / Perks: Unpaid; flexible hours and priceless experience.

Springboard Potential: Any healthcare pathway — this is the sampler platter.

Mason's Take: Sometimes the smallest tasks — like delivering a newspaper — become the brightest moment in someone's day. You're proof that kindness is still the best credential in healthcare.

42. Pharmacy Runner / Delivery Assistant

Description: Delivers medications from the central pharmacy to hospital units or directly to patients' homes.

Alignment Preview: Good for dependable people who value accuracy and timeliness.

Pay / Perks: $14–20/hr.

Springboard Potential: Pharmacy Technician, hospital pharmacy support roles.

Mason's Take: Timing matters. A dose delayed can change a day — or a life. You're the heartbeat that keeps medicine moving.

43. Lab Specimen Courier

Description: Transports lab samples between clinics, hospitals, and testing centers while maintaining chain-of-custody integrity.

Alignment Preview: Great for reliable, detail-driven workers comfortable handling sensitive materials.

Pay / Perks: $15–21/hr.

Springboard Potential: Lab Technician, pathology, courier supervision.

Mason's Take: You're not just carrying a box — you're carrying someone's answers. Every mile matters when results determine relief.

44. Patient Equipment Aide

Description: Cleans, restocks, and delivers medical equipment (wheelchairs, IV poles, monitors) throughout the hospital.

Alignment Preview: Perfect for organized self-starters who like working independently but making a visible difference.

Pay / Perks: $15–20/hr.

Springboard Potential: Biomedical Equipment Tech, supply-chain management.

Mason's Take: You'll learn fast that readiness saves lives. When equipment flows smoothly, so does care. You keep the whole system breathing.

45. Biomedical Equipment Cleaning / Prep Assistant

Description: Assists biomedical teams with cleaning, labeling, and organizing devices before clinical use.

Alignment Preview: Great for tech-curious learners who want exposure to medical devices without needing a degree first.

Pay / Perks: $16–22/hr.

Springboard Potential: Biomedical engineering, clinical technology support.

Mason's Take: Every machine has a story — and you're writing its prologue. Keep it clean, keep it calibrated, and you'll keep people safe.

Part X — Communication, Creativity & Advocacy

46. Patient Experience Volunteer (Rounding Assistant)

Description: Visits patients, asks about comfort and care, and escalates concerns to staff.

Alignment Preview: Great for extroverts who thrive on conversation and compassion.

Pay / Perks: Volunteer; unmatched skill-building in empathy and listening.

Springboard Potential: Patient advocacy, quality improvement, hospital leadership.

Mason's Take: Listening is a superpower. When you treat feedback as a gift, you help the system heal itself.

47. Child Life Volunteer / Playroom Assistant

Description: Engages pediatric patients in play, reading, and creative activities during hospital stays.

Alignment Preview: For imaginative, patient individuals who love working with children.

Pay / Perks: Volunteer; some paid aide roles.

Springboard Potential: Child Life Specialist, pediatric nursing, counseling.

Mason's Take: Play heals in ways medicine can't. You'll learn that laughter has measurable outcomes — and infinite value.

48. Social Media Assistant for a Health Nonprofit

Description: Creates posts, photos, or campaigns for organizations promoting wellness and awareness.

Alignment Preview: Perfect for digital storytellers who want to merge creativity with impact.

Pay / Perks: $15–25/hr; freelance or remote.

Springboard Potential: Health communications, public relations, nonprofit leadership.

Mason's Take: A single post can educate hundreds. You're shaping healthcare's narrative in real time — make it true, make it kind, make it count.

49. Health Blogger / Content Writer

Description: Writes articles or newsletters on wellness, careers, or patient stories.

Alignment Preview: Great for writers who enjoy research and storytelling.

Pay / Perks: $25–100/article; freelance flexibility.

Springboard Potential: Medical writing, journalism, health education.

Mason's Take: Words are medicine too — delivered one paragraph at a time. Your perspective can heal confusion as powerfully as a prescription.

50. Podcaster / Interview Host (Healthcare Focus)

Description: Hosts conversations with patients, clinicians, or innovators to share insight and inspiration.

Alignment Preview: Ideal for curious, conversational personalities comfortable with tech and empathy.

Pay / Perks: Income varies (ads, sponsorships); priceless networking.

Springboard Potential: Health media, communications, advocacy.

Mason's Take: Sometimes the best way to heal the system is to give it a microphone. You're archiving the heart of healthcare — one story at a time.

Your First Step

Fifty side hustles later, you can see that healthcare isn't just one door — it's a hallway with many entrances. Some roles are quiet and behind the scenes. Others put you face-to-face with patients and families at their most vulnerable. Some pay well, some pay in experience, and a few will simply confirm whether healthcare is — or isn't — for you.

Remember: side hustles aren't about settling. They're about sampling. Every patient transported, every chart scanned, every late-night call answered — it all counts as forward motion. What matters most isn't the size of the role, but whether it moves you closer to alignment.

So dip your toe in. Try a hustle. Listen closely to yourself as you do. If you find your values, your strengths, and your energy lining up in these small roles, imagine how it will feel when you find the full-time calling that's been waiting for you.

Enjoy your journey — and your experiment!

Chapter 57
The Pivot Playbook™

Pivoting Without Panic: How to Reweave Your Work Back to Who You Are

Part One: Understanding the Dread Thread

Needing to pivot doesn't mean you're failing. It means you're listening.

Misalignment rarely explodes all at once. It drips. It seeps. It threads itself quietly into your days until something that once felt tolerable starts to feel heavy. You still go to work. You still do your job. You still care. But somewhere underneath all of it, something has shifted.

You wake up tired before you even start the day. You scroll longer at night. You fantasize about quitting during traffic. You tell yourself, "It's just a rough patch."

And sometimes it is.

But sometimes it's the Dread Thread.

The Dread Thread: Recognizing Misalignment

The Dread Thread doesn't show up screaming. It whispers.

It's the way your stomach tightens on Sunday afternoon. It's the way Monday feels heavier than it used to. It's the way you stop talking in the break room and start checking job boards in the bathroom.

At first, you explain it away.

It was a rough shift. A difficult patient. A new manager. A staffing shortage.

But the feeling stays.

A nurse once told me she knew something was wrong when she stopped unpacking her lunch at work. She would bring it... but leave it closed. Eating meant settling in. And she didn't want to settle in anymore.

Another clinician joked that he had become "Dr. Dread." He was still competent. Still respected. Still getting paid. But he was no longer himself. His spouse finally asked, quietly, "Do you even like who you are at work anymore?"

That's when the truth landed.

The Dread Thread is not weakness. It is information.

It is your identity brushing up against an environment that no longer fits. It is your nervous system telling the truth before your résumé does. It shows up as burnout, but it starts as misalignment.

And the most dangerous mistake people make is thinking the only solution is to blow up their lives.

You don't have to.

You just have to start reweaving.

Part Two: The Diagnostic Tools

The Sunday Scan: Your Weekly Alignment Check

Once a week—ideally on Sunday—pause.

Not to plan. Not to panic. Just to feel.

Ask yourself:

1 Did I end this week with more energy than I started?

2 Did I feel proud of at least one thing I did?

3 Did I feel respected by the people I worked with?

4 Did I laugh or feel joy at work?

5 Did I learn something or stretch in some way?

6 Did I avoid people or tasks because I just couldn't care?

7 Did I find myself scanning job boards?

8 Do I dread Monday more than I look forward to anything next week?

9 Did work leak into my home in a way that hurt my relationships?

10 Am I more myself outside of work than inside it?

Now count the yeses.

• **7–10 = GREEN ZONE** You're aligned. Keep building. Invest in deepening expertise, mentoring others, or exploring adjacent opportunities that excite you.

- **4-6 = YELLOW ZONE** Something's off. Time to start experimenting. A pivot may be coming, but first, test the water.

- **0-3 = RED ZONE** You're not broken—you're misaligned. It's time to make a plan.

The power isn't in one week. It's in the pattern.

Track your score for 4 weeks. Look for trends. Are you trending down? Up? Stuck? This isn't about perfection—it's about honest information.

The Alignment Audit: Going Deeper

If your Sunday Scan revealed Yellow or Red, dig deeper. This tool helps you identify *exactly* what's misaligned.

Rate each area 1-10 (1 = completely misaligned, 10 = perfectly aligned):

Identity & Values

- Does this work reflect who I am at my core?

- Are my personal values aligned with what this role demands?

- Do I feel proud telling people what I do?

Impact & Meaning

- Do I feel like my work matters?

- Can I see the difference I make?

- Does this role connect to my larger life purpose?

Growth & Learning

- Am I developing skills I care about?

- Does this role challenge me in good ways?

- Is there a future I'm building toward, or am I stuck?

Relationships & Culture

- Do I respect the people I work with?

- Do they respect me?

- Is the workplace culture toxic, neutral, or nourishing?

Sustainability

- Can I maintain this pace without sacrificing my health?

- Is the schedule manageable with my life outside work?

- Am I burning out, or am I energized?

Compensation & Security

- Am I fairly compensated for my work?

- Do I have the security I need?

- Does money align with my other values here, or am I trading too much?

Now look at your lowest scores. Those are your pressure points. A pivot doesn't have to fix everything—but it should address your most critical misalignments.

The Pivot Readiness Scale: Are You Ready to Move?

Not every misalignment requires a pivot. Sometimes it requires a conversation with your manager. Sometimes it requires a boundary. Sometimes it requires a shift in perspective.

Use this scale to determine if you're ready for change:

Score yourself 1-5 on each (5 = completely agree):

• I've identified specifically what's misaligned (not just "I'm unhappy").

• I understand what I need from my next role.

• I have the financial runway for a transition (3-6 months of expenses).

• I've explored quick shifts or medium moves first, or I'm confident they won't help.

• I have support—mentors, friends, or family who believe in me.

• I'm making this choice *toward* something, not just *away* from something.

• I have a realistic timeline in mind.

Score 30+: You're ready. Move forward with confidence.

Score 20-29: You're close. Use the next month to shore up what's missing (especially financial runway and support systems).

Score below 20: Slow down. You may be running from burnout rather than running toward alignment. Take time to rebuild before you pivot.

Part Three: The Pivot Pathways

Quick Shifts (0-6 Months)

Small moves that create breathing room

Quick Shifts aren't escapes. They're test drives. They let you feel your way back to yourself without burning bridges or detonating your income.

A nurse volunteers at a recruitment fair and suddenly realizes she loves talking to students more than taking vitals. A respiratory therapist shadows someone in informatics for half a day and can't stop thinking about it. A tech goes to a one-day conference and leaves with five business cards and a different sense of what's possible.

These are not accidents.

They are alignment signals.

Sometimes a road trip, a volunteer shift, or a single conversation does more to reset your nervous system than three weeks of vacation—because it gives your identity something new to hold.

Quick Shift Ideas by Role:

For Nurses:

• Shadow in clinic settings, operating rooms, informatics, education, or leadership

• Volunteer for a committee or project outside your typical unit

• Attend a specialty conference in an area that intrigues you

• Mentor new nurses or students (tests your teaching instinct)

• Join a professional organization in your state (opens doors)

• Teach a CPR or first aid class (might reveal teaching passion)

For Allied Health (PT, OT, Rad Tech, Lab, etc.):

• Cross-train in a related specialty

• Volunteer at a clinic or community health event

• Present at a departmental meeting or local conference

• Join a quality improvement or research project

• Explore telehealth opportunities

• Shadow in a different setting (hospital vs. clinic vs. home care)

For Physicians:

• Spend a day with a colleague in an adjacent specialty

• Volunteer with an underserved population or global health initiative

• Teach a class or Grand Rounds

• Explore a side interest through a small project

• Attend a conference focused on a different area

• Work with a mentor in an area you're curious about

For High School Students Exploring Healthcare:

• Volunteer at a hospital, clinic, or care facility

• Shadow a healthcare provider (ask your school or local hospital)

• Join health professions clubs at school

- Attend a health careers fair

- Take an online course in an area of interest

- Informational interviews with professionals (even 15 minutes counts)

The Quick Shift Template:

What are you testing? (Be specific: "Do I enjoy patient education more than direct patient care?" or "Do I want to work in tech?")

How will you test it? (The specific Quick Shift you'll do)

Timeline: (When will you do this? Ideally within 6 months)

What will tell you if this is a signal? (What will you feel, see, or learn that indicates alignment?)

Who needs to know? (Your manager? A mentor? Anyone who might help you access this?)

Next step if the signal is strong: (Will you move to a Medium Move? Pursue more education? Have a conversation with your manager?)

Medium Moves (6–24 Months)

Stretching toward a better fit

Medium Moves are where confidence starts to grow.

This is where you rotate into a specialty. Get a certification. Join a quality project. Submit a poster. Say yes to a committee. Lead something. Teach something. Build something.

You're not leaving yet. You're changing how visible, how valuable, and how connected you are.

You stop feeling trapped—because now you have options.

Medium Move Examples:

Certifications & Credentials:

- CEN (Certified Emergency Nurse)

- CNOR (Certified Perioperative Nurse)

- CCRN (Critical Care Registered Nurse)

- CNL (Clinical Nurse Leader)

- RN to BSN degree

- Informatics certifications

- Project management (PMP, CSM)

- Health coaching certification

- Specialty certifications in your field

Lateral Moves Within Your Organization:

- Transfer to a different unit or department

- Move from bedside to clinic

- Move from direct care to education

- Move from bedside to leadership track

- Move from hospital to ambulatory

- Explore telehealth roles

Building Visibility & Value:

- Lead a quality improvement project

- Chair or join a committee (patient safety, culture, education, etc.)

- Present at conferences or departmental meetings

- Publish or write (articles, case studies, blog posts)

- Mentor new staff or students

- Develop a new protocol or workflow

- Join a professional organization and get involved

Education & Development:

- Pursue a bachelor's degree (if you have an associate's)

- Take on a teaching role in nursing school

- Develop an online course in your specialty

- Become a preceptor or clinical instructor

- Pursue a business or MBA certificate

- Get trained in a new technology or system

Entrepreneurial Moves:

- Start a health coaching practice (part-time or full- time)

- Develop a digital health tool or app

- Create educational content (YouTube, podcasts, courses)

- Consult for healthcare organizations

- Write a book (yes, like this one!)

The Medium Move Template:

What specifically do you want to develop or explore? (A skill, a specialty, a role, a network?)

Why does this matter to you? (How does it align with who you want to be?)

What's the concrete action? (Apply for the rotation? Enroll in the program? Talk to your manager?)

Timeline: (When will you start? When will you complete it?)

What support do you need? (Financial? Mentorship? Time? Permission from your manager?)

How will you measure success? (What will change in your confidence, your options, or your daily work experience?)

Exit ramp or entry point? (Is this a stepping stone to something bigger, or does it feel like home?)

Big Transitions (2+ Years)

When you're ready to cross the bridge

Some alignments require a new landscape.

A degree. A new system. A leadership track. A specialty pivot. A complete career change.

But notice what's happening now.

You're not panicking. You're planning.

You're choosing.

Big Transition Pathways:

Advanced Degrees:

- MSN (Master of Science in Nursing) with various specializations

- MBA or MHA (Master of Health Administration)

- PhD or DNP (Doctor of Nursing Practice)

- PA-C (Physician Assistant) program

- Specialized Master's degrees (Public Health, Health Informatics, etc.)

Major Role Changes:

- Clinical nurse → Nurse educator

- Bedside nurse → Nurse leader/manager/director

- Clinician → Healthcare executive

- Clinician → Informatics specialist

- Clinician → Researcher

- Clinician → Policy advocate

- Clinician → Entrepreneur

Specialty Pivots:

- Medical to surgical to ICU to palliative care (or any nursing specialty)

- Hospital to home care to hospice

- Emergency medicine to occupational health

- Acute care to mental health

- Traditional roles to emerging fields (telehealth, global health, preventive medicine)

Complete Career Pivots:

- Healthcare professional → Healthcare entrepreneur

- Clinician → Healthcare technology

- Clinician → Healthcare consulting

- Clinician → Medical writing

- Clinician → Wellness/coaching industry

- Clinician → Nonprofit leadership

The Big Transition Planning Template:

What is the transition? (Be very specific)

Why do you want this? (Connect it back to your Alignment Audit. What misalignments does this fix?)

What's required? (Degrees? Certifications? Years of experience? Financial investment?)

Timeline: (Realistic, with milestones)

Financial runway: (Can you do this while working? Do you need time off? Cost of education?)

Support system: (Mentors in this field? Programs? Communities?)

Plan B: (What if this doesn't work out? How is it not a dead end?)

Hardest part: (Be honest. What will be the biggest challenge? How will you handle it?)

First step: (What happens this month?)

Part Four: Case Studies

Case Study 1: From Bedside Burnout to Nurse Educator

Marcus, RN | 12 years in ICU → Nursing Education

The Dread: Marcus loved the intensity of ICU nursing. He was good at it—really good. But after 12 years, something shifted. New graduates kept coming through, and he found himself dreading direct patient care while lighting up during teaching moments. His Sunday Scan scores dropped to 3. He was sleeping poorly, his marriage was strained, and he caught himself filling out residency applications (for no particular reason) at 2 AM.

The misalignment wasn't with nursing. It was with *how* he was nursing.

The Quick Shift: Marcus volunteered to mentor a new grad. He thought it would feel like more work. Instead, it felt like coming home. For six months, he leaned into this—officially taking on a preceptor role, which required a certification program.

The Medium Move: His hospital created a position for an Education Coordinator within the ICU. Marcus applied. It was a sideways move, not a promotion—same pay, different responsibilities. Fifty percent direct patient care. Fifty percent education and curriculum development.

He took it.

The Result: After two years in this hybrid role, Marcus realized he wanted to go deeper. He enrolled in an RN-to-MSN program with an education focus. Still working full-time.

Challenging? Yes. But for the first time in five years, he was choosing his challenge.

Today, he's a Clinical Nurse Educator at a major medical center, teaches at a local nursing school, and is considering a doctorate in nursing education. He's not burned out. He's lit up.

Key Insight: Marcus didn't need to leave nursing. He needed to leave bedside nursing. His alignment didn't come from changing professions—it came from changing *how* he practiced the profession.

Case Study 2: From Physician Burnout to Healthcare Entrepreneur

Dr. Sarah Chen, MD | 8 years in Emergency Medicine → Digital Health Founder

The Dread: Sarah was a stellar ER physician. She had the respect of her peers, excellent patient outcomes, and a solid income. But she hated it. The administrative burden, the endless documentation, the feeling of firefighting rather than healing. She found herself researching MBA programs and startup culture—not as casual interest, but as escape fantasy.

Her Sunday Scan: consistently 1–2 yeses. Her Alignment Audit showed deep misalignment in Impact & Meaning, Growth & Learning, and Sustainability.

The Quick Shift: During a week off, Sarah attended a health tech conference. Just to look around. She spent two days listening to people building digital health solutions. By day three, she was having lunch with a healthcare technologist. By the end of the week, she'd committed to a 90-day exploration project: could she identify a real problem in emergency medicine that technology could solve?

The Medium Move: Over the next 18 months, Sarah:

- Took an online innovation course

- Joined a healthcare accelerator as a mentor (to learn the ecosystem)

- Partnered with a tech founder to develop a prototype for documentation automation

- Spent 10% of her time on this project, with her hospital's blessing

- Presented at a health tech conference

Her confidence grew. She had options now. She didn't have to hate her day job—but she also knew it wasn't her future.

The Big Transition: Sarah left her full-time ER position to launch her digital health startup full-time. She took a 50% pay cut initially. Her family thought she was crazy. But she had a prototype, early customers, and a grant from an innovation fund. Three years later, her company is growing, she works with healthcare organizations, and she uses her clinical knowledge every day—but in a way that feels aligned.

Key Insight: Sarah's burnout wasn't about working too hard. It was about her identity being misaligned with her environment. Once she found a vehicle for her gifts—innovation, problem-solving, building—the hard work didn't feel like burnout anymore.

Case Study 3: From Overwhelmed Clinic Tech to Specialized Educator

James, Patient Care Tech | 6 years in primary care clinic → Health Professions Educator

The Dread: James started as a patient care tech to support his family while taking community college classes. Six years later, he had an associate's degree in health sciences, but he was still in the same clinic—doing vitals, rooming patients, filing records. He was good at it. But he felt invisible. No growth. No path. He was tired, underpaid, and starting to resent healthcare.

The Quick Shift: James's clinic partnered with a local high school for a health careers program. The director asked if he'd come speak to students about healthcare careers. He said yes mostly to fill an afternoon. The students asked him questions for 45 minutes. He went home and cried—not from sadness, but from feeling *seen*.

The Medium Move: Over the next year, James:

• Volunteered as a speaker at two more health careers events

• Became an official mentor for health careers students through his clinic

• Took online courses in health professions advising

• Connected with the director of the regional health professions program

The director of the program asked if he'd be interested in working part-time while maintaining his clinic role. James said yes. For eight months, he split his time: four days at the clinic, one day developing curriculum and mentoring students.

The Result: A new opportunity opened at the regional health professions education center—full-time educator and career advisor role. More pay than his clinic job. Aligned with his passion. The clinic director told him to go.

James now works with hundreds of students annually, helping them figure out their healthcare path. He's pursuing an online bachelor's degree in health professions education. He's no longer invisible. He's building something.

Key Insight: James's breakthrough came through doing— through small acts that revealed his authentic self to himself and others. He didn't need to wait for permission or a degree. He needed to step toward the signal.

Case Study 4: High School Student to Nursing (with Built-in Pivoting)

Devon, High School Junior → Nursing School → ???

The Journey: Devon thought he wanted to be a nurse because his mom is a nurse and he wanted to make a difference. He volunteered at a hospital for two summers. He shadow a day in the OR and another in the ED. He loved the intensity but wasn't sure about the bedside.

In nursing school, Devon:

• Rotated through all the major specialties (Med- Surg, OB, Peds, ICU, Psych, Community Health)

• Identified that he loved the systems thinking of critical care but loved the patient *relationship* building of psychiatric nursing

• Joined the student health professions organization

- Worked as a student extern in different units each summer

By graduation, Devon didn't feel locked into "I must be a bedside nurse." He understood his own interests. He chose to start in an ICU with a strong orientation program because he wanted bedside experience. But he also knew he was testing something: is *this* the long-term fit?

Three years in, Devon is exploring nurse leadership and quality improvement—moving toward a medium move without panic, because he's been testing all along.

Key Insight: Devon built exploration into his education. He didn't wait until burnout to ask questions. By the time he graduated, he understood himself, the profession, and what kinds of moves aligned with his values.

Part Five: Exercises & Tools

Exercise 1: The Values Excavation

Time: 30–45 minutes

Your misalignment is often rooted in a values conflict. This exercise reveals what you actually value (not what you *think* you should value).

Step 1: Recall a moment you felt truly proud at work. Write it down. What happened? Who was there? What did you do?

Step 2: What value was being honored in that moment? (Examples: service, autonomy, creativity, excellence, leadership, impact, learning, connection, security, justice)

Step 3: Repeat for three moments you felt proud. Look for patterns. What values show up again and again?

Step 4: Now recall a moment you felt deeply frustrated or drained at work. What happened? What value was being violated?

Step 5: Repeat for three frustrating moments. What values are being stepped on?

Step 6: Make two lists:

• Core values being honored in your best moments

• Core values being violated in your worst moments

Step 7: Now ask the hard question: Is your current role able to honor your core values? What would need to change?

If the answer is "a lot would need to change," that's information. That's a signal.

Exercise 2: The Conversation Map

Time: 20 minutes

Before you make a big move, have a conversation. But with whom, and about what?

This exercise helps you identify who should know what, and when.

Fill in the blanks:

People who need to know about my thinking (but not yet): (Trusted mentors, therapist, spouse, close friend—people who support your growth)

People I need to talk to if I'm making a move: (Manager, HR, mentor within my organization)

People I'm building a relationship with: (Potential mentors in my target field, colleagues in adjacent roles)

What I want to explore: (Be specific and non-threatening: "I'm interested in exploring X" is different from "I'm leaving")

Best timing: (When, where, and how will these conversations go best?)

What I need from them: (Advice? Permission? A shadow opportunity? An introduction?)

What happens after the conversation? (What's your next step? What's their role?)

Exercise 3: The Obstacle Audit

Time: 25 minutes

Every pivot has obstacles. Identifying them isn't pessimism—it's planning.

Fill in for your potential move:

Financial obstacles:

- How much does this cost?

- How long can I sustain myself if my income changes?

- What's my funding plan?

- What's my minimum viable income?

Time obstacles:

- Can I do this while working full-time?

- How much time per week does this require?

- What am I sacrificing to make time?

Knowledge/skill obstacles:

- What do I not know that I need to know?

- How will I learn it?

- Who can help me?

Relational obstacles:

- Who might not support this?

- How will I handle that?

- Who *will* support this?

Practical obstacles:

- Do I need a degree? How long?

- Do I need certifications? Cost and time?

- Do I need connections? How will I build them?

- Do I need to relocate?

Identity obstacles:

- What story am I telling myself about what's possible for me?

- Is that story true?

- Who can help me rewrite it?

Now rank them. Which obstacles are deal-breakers? Which are manageable with planning?

Exercise 4: The 5-Year Backwards Timeline

Time: 30 minutes

Instead of predicting the future, imagine it's five years from now, and you're happy.

Step 1: It's five years in the future. You made a pivot, and it worked. You're aligned. You're proud. You're not burned out. Describe what your typical week looks like. What do you do? Who do you work with? How do you feel?

Step 2: One year before that (4 years from now): What were you doing? What transition were you in the middle of?

Step 3: Two years before that (3 years from now): What medium move had you just completed?

Step 4: Three years before that (2 years from now): What were you doing to build toward that medium move?

Step 5: One year from now: What quick shift or exploration were you doing?

Step 6: Six months from now: What's your first step?

Step 7: This month: What's one small thing you could do this month that moves you toward year-future-you?

Exercise 5: The Mentor Circle Map

Time: 20 minutes

You don't pivot alone. You pivot with people who believe in you and know the path.

Create three circles:

Circle 1: People who believe in me (Not necessarily in healthcare, but people who believe in your potential)

Circle 2: People who know where I want to go (People working in or near my target field)

Circle 3: People who have navigated a pivot successfully (People who've made a career change and can show it's possible)

Now ask:

• Who's in all three circles? (These are gold. Nurture these relationships.)

• Who's missing?

• How will I find them?

• What's one step I can take this month to deepen one of these relationships?

• Who can introduce me to someone I need to know?

Part Six: For Healthcare Leaders

Leading Your Team Through Pivot Culture

If you're a manager, director, or organizational leader, you have unprecedented power to reduce burnout by normalizing career evolution.

Principle 1: Make Exploration Safe

Create room for people to explore without it meaning they're leaving.

What this looks like:

• Offer shadow opportunities (people shadowing other departments)

• Support conference attendance, especially in adjacent specialties

• Encourage cross-training and rotations

• Make mentorship available

• Create committee and project opportunities

• Support professional development that might lead elsewhere

What you're signaling: "I want you here AND I want you to be growing toward who you're meant to be. Those aren't in conflict."

Principle 2: Normalize the Conversation

Help your team do their Sunday Scan. Ask about alignment.

What this looks like:

• In 1:1s, ask: "How are you feeling about your work right now?"

• Notice when someone's score is dropping

• Ask: "What would make this role feel more aligned for you?"

• Listen without defensiveness

• Problem-solve together before you accept their resignation

What you're signaling: "Your wellbeing matters to me. If something's wrong, I want to know so we can fix it together if we can."

Principle 3: Create Pathways, Not Just Positions

Help people see the career lattice, not just the career ladder.

What this looks like:

• Show examples of people who've pivoted within your organization

• Create hybrid roles (like Marcus's education coordinator role)

• Support lateral moves as much as promotions

• Celebrate people who've found alignment, even if they left

• Talk openly about different career paths

What you're signaling: "There's more than one way to have a meaningful career here. And if your way leads elsewhere, I'll support that too."

Principle 4: Notice the Signals Early

You see the Dread Thread before anyone. Watch for it.

Early signals:

• Disengagement in meetings

• Withdraw from social interaction

• Increased absences or "mental health" days

• Shift in quality of work or attitude

• Scanning job boards (yes, people do this at work)

• Increased cynicism or complaints

• Protective behavior around their work

What to do:

• Have a caring conversation

- Listen more than you talk

- Ask: "What would help?" before you assume you know

- Offer exploration before you lose them

Principle 5: Let People Leave Well

If someone decides to pivot out, help them go.

What this looks like:

- Be genuinely happy for them

- Help with transition planning

- Share what they learned with the team

- Stay connected (they might come back, and they'll refer good people)

- Ask for their advice as they leave

What you're signaling: "Your growth matters more than my convenience. And you're always part of this community."

Tool: The Career Conversation Template for Managers

Opening: "I've noticed you've been [quieter/less engaged/frustrated]. I care about you and your growth. How are you really doing?"

Listening: Listen without trying to fix. Ask clarifying questions. Don't defend the organization or your decisions. Just listen.

Naming: "It sounds like you're feeling [disconnected/burned out/unchallenged]. Is that right?"

Exploring: "What would help? What's one thing that would make this role feel more aligned for you?"

Problem-solving: "Here's what I can do... Here's what we'd need from you... What do you think?"

Closing: "I want you here, and I want you to be thriving. Let's figure this out together. And if this isn't the right place for you, I'll support your pivot."

Part Seven: Threads to Remember

The Truth About Healthcare Burnout

You don't burn out because you care too much. You burn out because you care deeply in an environment that no longer fits who you are.

Alignment is not a luxury. It is oxygen.

Burnout often gets treated as an individual problem—as if you need to meditate more, exercise more, or develop better coping skills. Sometimes that helps. But if the fundamental misalignment remains, you're trying to breathe underwater with better technique.

The pivot isn't escape. The pivot is coming home to yourself.

The Threads of Alignment

As you navigate your pivot, remember these truths:

1. Small steps matter. You don't have to see the whole path. You just have to see the next step. Quick Shifts reveal what Medium Moves should be. Medium Moves clarify what Big Transitions are possible.

2. Your instincts are data. The Dread Thread isn't weakness. It's your nervous system telling the truth. Listen to it.

3. You're not broken. Misalignment feels like brokenness. It's not. It's growth. It's your identity evolving. It's you outgrowing a role.

4. You have more options than you think. The 345 healthcare careers in this book aren't just different jobs. They're different ways of showing up in healthcare. There is a fit for you.

5. Timing matters, but starting matters more. You don't have to be perfect. You don't have to have it all figured out. You just have to start paying attention. Do your Sunday Scan. Ask one question. Have one conversation. Take one small step.

6. You're not alone. Healthcare is full of people who've felt what you're feeling. Who've questioned what you're questioning. Who've pivoted. Talk to them. Learn from them. Let their paths inform yours.

7. There is no one right answer. Your pivot might be a specialty change. It might be a role change. It might be staying put but shifting how you approach the work. It might be leaving healthcare entirely. The right answer is the one that brings you back to yourself.

The Weaving Continues

Here's the truth no one tells healthcare workers:

You don't have to blow up your life. You just have to stop ignoring the thread.

And start weaving.

Every small shift you make—every question you ask, every door you peek through, every honest Sunday Scan—is another stitch pulling you back toward yourself.

Part Eight: Your First Steps

This Week

Do your Sunday Scan. Answer the ten questions. Count your yeses. Don't judge the answer. Just notice it.

If you scored Yellow or Red: Schedule 30 minutes to do your Alignment Audit. Identify your pressure points.

Tell one person. Not everyone. One trusted person. Your partner. A mentor. A friend. Say: "I'm thinking about my career. I'm not sure what's next, but something feels off." Notice how it feels to say it out loud.

This Month

Do a Quick Shift. Pick one small exploration from the Quick Shift ideas that appeals to you. Shadow someone. Volunteer. Attend something. Take one small step toward understanding what you might want.

Track your Sunday Scan. Do it four weeks in a row. Look for patterns. Are you trending up, down, or stuck?

Build one mentor relationship. Reach out to someone you admire—someone doing work that intrigues you. Ask for 15 minutes of their time. Ask them one genuine question about their career path. Listen more than you talk.

This Quarter

Evaluate your Quick Shift. Did it reveal something? Did it feel like an alignment signal? Or did it confirm that this isn't your path?

If the signal is strong: Plan your first Medium Move. Enroll in that certification. Apply for that rotation. Start that committee. Make the commitment.

If you need more information: Do another Quick Shift. Or a different one. Keep testing.

Connect with your support system. Check in with your mentor. Talk to your family. Build the circle of people who believe in you and know where you're heading.

CLOSING LETTER

To everyone reading this:

You picked up this book—or this section—because something is off. Maybe it's subtle. Maybe it's screaming. Maybe you're not even sure if it's real, or if you're just being ungrateful.

Let me be clear: **It's real.**

The Dread Thread is real. The misalignment is real. And your instinct to listen to it is not weakness—it's wisdom.

You've spent years—maybe decades—in healthcare. You've cared for people when you were exhausted. You've learned to ignore your own needs so you could meet someone else's. You've been a hero in small moments and large ones. You've earned the right to ask: "Is this still aligned with who I am?"

That question doesn't make you selfish. It makes you honest.

And healthcare—the whole system—needs more honest people. We need people who are doing work that aligns with their souls, because that's the only way you sustain compassion. That's the only way you avoid burning out. That's the only way you show up fully for your patients, your team, and yourself.

Maybe your pivot is a small one. Maybe it's seismic. Maybe it happens in six months. Maybe it takes five years. There's no timeline for coming home to yourself.

But here's what I know: **You don't have to figure it out alone.**

You have mentors—in this book and in your life. You have peers who've felt what you're feeling. You have a profession with 345 different ways to show up. You have more options than you think.

Start small. Do your Sunday Scan. Pay attention to the Dread Thread. Take one step toward something that feels alive.

The weaving doesn't happen all at once. But it happens.

Thread by thread. Week by week. Conversation by conversation.

You're not broken. You're not failing. You're listening.

And that's where every pivot begins.

Welcome home to yourself.

APPENDIX: QUICK REFERENCE TOOLS

The Sunday Scan at a Glance

Weekly Check-In Questions:

1 Did I end this week with more energy than I started?

2 Did I feel proud of at least one thing I did?

3 Did I feel respected by the people I worked with?

4 Did I laugh or feel joy at work?

5 Did I learn something or stretch in some way?

6 Did I avoid people or tasks because I just couldn't care?

7 Did I find myself scanning job boards?

8 Do I dread Monday more than I look forward to anything next week?

9 Did work leak into my home in a way that hurt my relationships?

10 Am I more myself outside of work than inside it?

Score: 7–10 = Green (Aligned) | 4–6 = Yellow (Exploring) | 0–3 = Red (Misaligned)

Quick Reference: Pivot Timeline

Timeframe

What It Is

Example

Goal

0–6 Months

Quick Shifts

Shadow, volunteer, attend conference

Test the water, get alignment signals

6–24 Months

Medium Moves

Get certified, rotate departments, lead project

Build confidence and options

2+ Years

Big Transitions

Pursue degree, change roles significantly

Cross the bridge to a new fit

Quick Shift Ideas Checklist

For Nurses:

- ☐ Shadow in a different department

- ☐ Volunteer for a committee or project

- ☐ Mentor a new nurse or student

- ☐ Attend a specialty conference

- ☐ Join a professional organization

- ☐ Teach a CPR or first aid class

- ☐ Explore telehealth

For Allied Health:

- ☐ Cross-train in related specialty

- ☐ Volunteer at community event

- ☐ Present at meeting or conference

- ☐ Join quality improvement project

- ☐ Explore telehealth opportunities

- ☐ Shadow in different setting

For Physicians:

- ☐ Shadow colleague in adjacent specialty

- ☐ Volunteer with underserved population

- ☐ Teach class or Grand Rounds

- ☐ Small exploratory project

- ☐ Attend focused conference

- ☐ Work with mentor in new area

For High School Students:

- ☐ Volunteer at healthcare facility

- ☐ Shadow a healthcare provider

- ☐ Join health professions club

- ☐ Attend health careers fair

- ☐ Take online course in area of interest

- ☐ Have informational interviews

The Conversation Starters

With a potential mentor: "I really respect your work. I'm exploring [area of interest]. Would you have 15 minutes to tell me about your path?"

With your manager: "I've been thinking about my career growth. I'd like to explore [opportunity]. What do you think?"

With your family: "Something's been on my mind about my work. I want to be honest with you about what I'm thinking."

With yourself: "What would I do if I knew I couldn't fail? And what's really stopping me?"

Resources for Each Pivot Type

For Quick Shifts:

• Professional associations in your specialty

• LinkedIn (follow people in adjacent roles)

• Conferences and webinars

• Volunteer.gov and VolunteerMatch

• Your hospital's education department

• Mentorship programs

For Medium Moves:

• Online course platforms (Coursera, edX, LinkedIn Learning)

• Professional certification programs

• Local colleges and universities

• Employer tuition assistance programs

• Professional organizations with leadership development

• Coaching and mentorship

For Big Transitions:

- Graduate programs (MSN, MBA, MHA, DNP)

- Career counseling services

- Professional coaches

- Mentors who've made the transition

- Online degree programs

- Healthcare consulting firms

Final Reflection Questions

Before you close this book, answer:

1 What was the one thing in this Playbook that resonated most with me?

2 What's one small step I could take this week?

3 Who's one person I trust enough to tell about my thinking?

4 If I could design my ideal work situation (not my ideal job, but my ideal way of working), what would it look like?

5 What story am I telling myself about what's possible for me? Is it true?

6 What would change if I believed that alignment was possible for me?

7 When I imagine myself five years from now, feeling proud and aligned, what am I doing?

8 What's the first action I'm committing to?

Remember:

You don't burn out because you care too much. You burn out because you care deeply in an environment that no longer fits.

Alignment is not a luxury. It is oxygen.

And your pivot—whatever it looks like—is not failure. It's listening.

It's coming home.

Thank you for your years of service. Thank you for the patients you've cared for. And thank you for being brave enough to ask the question: "Is this still aligned with who I am?"

That question is how healthcare gets better. One person. One pivot. One stitch at a time.

Chapter 58
Conclusion
By Quint Studer

I am grateful that Mason asked me to contribute to his work and to *What Color Are Your Scrubs?*.

As I read this book, it reminded me of those classic titles often described as *Everything You Want to Know About [a Subject]—But Are Afraid to Ask*. At times, it is simply human nature not to ask questions — for fear of looking uninformed, assuming we should already know the answer, or believing that everyone else must understand it already.

One of the key responsibilities of leadership is addressing all three. Leaders must know what questions are truly out there, avoid assuming people already know the answers, and ensure that information is genuinely understood — not just communicated.

Mason asked me to address why alignment matters, what the current workforce is telling us, the role of leaders, and to offer a closing reflection and call to action. I am grateful for both the invitation and the opportunity.

Years ago, while working with Dan Evans, former CEO of Indiana Health, he asked a deceptively simple question: *Is there a way to diagnose alignment?* At the time, I could not find a practical method — so I created one. Since then, that tool has been refined, simplified, and expanded with additional diagnostic approaches.

What we consistently find is this: leaders often assume alignment is stronger than it actually is.

By alignment, I mean clarity in desired outcomes, clarity in the actions required to achieve those outcomes, and the accountability people both feel and demonstrate in fulfilling their roles and responsibilities. Alignment must be diagnosed before it can be improved.

Healthcare already understands this principle well. Before surgery, the team pauses to ensure everyone is on the same page — clarifying the situation, confirming roles, and addressing questions or concerns. The same is true of huddles, now commonplace across clinical settings. Teams come together to review what is happening, what needs to occur, recognize good performance, and address concerns.

Why are these practices so effective? Because when people are not aligned, outcomes suffer.

These alignment practices most often occur at the unit or department level. Organizations also use town halls, videos, newsletters, and other tools to support alignment more broadly. Yet when we conduct alignment diagnoses, results frequently show that alignment and urgency are lower than leaders expect — particularly when it comes to future challenges, education needs, and skill development.

A simple — but powerful — diagnostic process begins with listening at scale, often through an anonymous survey. At a minimum, it should include everyone in leadership roles, across all organizational layers. The depth can vary based on the organization.

Using a five-point scale, leaders are asked questions such as:

• Over the past three years, how difficult has the external healthcare environment been?

• Over the next three years, how difficult do you expect it to be?

• If the organization continues as it is today, how will results look over the next three years?

Almost every time, results show less alignment than anticipated — especially regarding future difficulty and the need for change. Senior leaders typically see the road ahead as far more challenging than leaders further down the organization. The final question is often the most revealing: *What questions are you hearing from those you lead?*

This highlights a critical truth. Information may be communicated — but alignment depends on leaders in the middle understanding it, believing it, and conveying it effectively. The greater the alignment, the greater the trust. And trust in an organization is like safety in a community: without it, progress is limited.

So what is the workforce telling us?

People want to feel good about where they work and about the leaders they follow. COVID profoundly disrupted healthcare culture. Leaders became less visible, connections were strained, and many people entered healthcare during a period of extreme pressure.

In *Rewiring Excellence*, the Human Capital Ecosystem includes ways to measure what the workforce is telling us. One key element asks leaders to rate how well skill development supports them in their roles. The consistent response is clear: leaders want more opportunities to learn.

In studies, 92% of nurse leaders and 84% of frontline nurses say they are more likely to stay with an organization that invests in them. The organizations with the strongest middle-management teams consistently achieve the best results. My greatest concern today is the under-investment in leadership and frontline skill development. Buildings and technology matter — but investing in people matters just as much, if not more.

This brings us to the role of leaders.

Leaders must invest in themselves through learning, and they must serve as the chief development officers for those they lead. This means investing in relationships. Technology is powerful, but it will never replace the feeling of being genuinely cared about.

We can learn from precision medicine, which uses data to diagnose and guide treatment while still individualizing care. I call this *Precision Leader Development* — understanding the skills required for a role, how a person learns best, how they solve problems, and how to support them effectively. This creates individualized development plans that build trust, capability, and a sense of being valued.

What lies ahead requires working on ourselves, not just in our roles. Healthcare is busy, and the opportunity for reflection and development is easily lost. Many leadership practices were originally designed to build relationships — to listen and connect. We must be careful not to let speed turn those practices into transactions.

I remain an optimist.

Why? Because I work with people. In my experience, I have met very few people in healthcare who did not want to do their best. And I have met very few leaders who were not committed to helping those they serve. We are human, and we drift at times — but healthcare is deeply values-centered.

People and organizations can find their way back to the main highway: serving with purpose, doing worthwhile work, and making a difference.

And that is exactly what you do.

— **Quint Studer**

About Quint Studer

Quint Studer is one of the most influential voices in modern healthcare leadership. A former hospital executive turned performance-improvement pioneer, he is best known for his work helping healthcare organizations strengthen culture, improve outcomes, and build trust at every level of leadership.

Over the course of four decades, Quint's ideas have reshaped how hospitals think about leadership, accountability, and alignment. He is the founder of Studer Group, whose work has supported thousands of healthcare organizations worldwide in improving patient experience, workforce engagement, financial performance, and quality of care. His approach helped elevate employee engagement and patient experience from "soft" initiatives to essential drivers of organizational success.

Quint is the author of several best-selling books, including *Hardwiring Excellence*, *Results That Last*, *The Busy Leader's Handbook*, and *Rewiring Excellence*. His writing is widely used by healthcare executives, educators, and clinical leaders as practical guidance for leading people well in complex, high-pressure environments.

Beyond healthcare, Quint is a philanthropist and community builder with a deep commitment to education, entrepreneurship, and workforce development. His career has been guided by a simple conviction: when leaders create the right environment, people rise — and when people rise, organizations thrive.

Quint's contribution to *What Color Are Your Scrubs?* reflects his lifelong dedication to helping individuals find meaningful, sustainable work and helping organizations create conditions where people can do their best work — not just today, but for the long term.

Chapter 59

The Never End

The Never End

This is not the end — only **The Never End**.

In healthcare, careers are rarely linear. A nurse who dreamed of pediatrics finds purpose in oncology; a technician discovers leadership; a physician transitions into teaching. Each turn is proof that endings are only beginnings in disguise.

That's why I chose to close this book with **The Never End**. It's a reminder that alignment isn't a one-time discovery — it's a lifelong practice. Careers evolve. Passions shift. The places and people you serve will change. But the heartbeat of why you chose healthcare remains constant.

Before you close this book, I want to speak directly to you — not as a leader, not as a system, not as a profession, but as a person doing real work inside healthcare.

If parts of these pages made you feel seen, relieved, or quietly unsettled, there's a reason. Many people working in healthcare

are not burned out because they lack resilience, commitment, or purpose. They are burned out because they are working in roles, environments, or expectations that no longer fit who they are — or what their lives require now.

Misalignment doesn't always announce itself loudly. Sometimes it shows up as chronic exhaustion that rest doesn't fix. Sometimes it looks like competence without joy, or loyalty mixed with resentment. Sometimes it's the sense that you are good at what you do, but you can't imagine doing it this way forever — and you don't know what that means about you.

It doesn't mean you've failed.

It doesn't mean you chose wrong.

And it certainly doesn't mean you don't belong in healthcare.

Alignment is not about finding the perfect job. It is about understanding yourself well enough to make choices that are sustainable — and having environments that don't punish you for doing so. You are allowed to want work that fits. You are allowed to change lanes without leaving the road. You are allowed to honor the season you're in without apologizing for it.

Years ago, I flew to Venice, Italy, to visit my aunt and uncle — a trip that felt like stepping into a painting. I was on KLM Royal Dutch Airlines, and as the plane rolled to a stop on the tarmac, the flight attendants went through their usual arrival announcements. I can't recall their exact words now. But as the engines settled, the captain's voice came over the intercom — calm, steady, almost melodic.

"Thank you for flying with us," she said.

Then, after a small pause that seemed to stretch through the cabin, she added something I've never forgotten:

"Goodbye for now."

Not goodbye forever — just goodbye for now.

Even then, somewhere between the hum of the engines and the soft shuffle of passengers gathering their belongings, the phrase settled into me. It felt like more than a farewell. It was a quiet truth. Journeys don't really end; they simply change form.

So consider this my own goodbye for now.

May these pages encourage you to see yourself differently, to see healthcare differently, and to step more boldly into alignment with who you are and the care you are called to give.

There's nothing better than alignment — except sharing it, side by side, on this journey together.

Goodbye for now,

Mason Preddy

StaySm:)in'!

About the Author

About the Author

Mason Preddy is an author, entrepreneur, and advocate for purpose-driven healthcare careers. His flagship guide to aligned healthcare careers, *What Color Are Your Scrubs?™*, and the companion ScrubTales™ series help readers discover where they belong in the world of care — not by chance, but by alignment.

For more than two and a half decades, Mason has worked inside high schools, colleges and universities, community hospitals, and health systems at the intersection of clinical workforce development and human potential. He has stood in crowded conference rooms as a voice on a video call announced that a hospital had earned Magnet® recognition, helped prepare staff for unannounced Joint Commission surveys, and built pipelines that connect the right people to the right roles. As a judge for Best Employer Awards, collegiate business and leadership competitions, and award programs in nursing, customer service, and innovation — and as a member of multiple boards and advisory councils — he brings a practiced eye for excellence, ethics, and impact to every conversation about careers and care.

A lifelong believer that joy and excellence go hand in hand, Mason writes to bridge the gap between clinical careers and human connection. His work blends storytelling, mentorship, and modern career science to help readers find the healthcare path that fits who they are — not just what they do.

As the creator of the **SCRUB*fits*™** and the **SCRUBf*it*™ Healthcare Career Assessment**, Mason empowers future professionals to match their values, personality, and strengths with the roles that bring out their best. Through his publishing company, Mason Maison® Publishing, he continues to "rewrite the narrative" for the next generation of healthcare talent — one aligned career at a time.

When he's not writing or mentoring, Mason can be found at the beach, traveling, or spoiling his English Bulldog — always dreaming up new ways to help prepare the healthcare generation of tomorrow.

More from Mason Maison™

Coming Soon from Mason Maison™

ScrubTales™ **— A Cinematic Healthcare Career Series**

ScrubTales™ is where healthcare comes alive — not as job descriptions, but as human stories.

Each volume drops you inside a single profession for one unforgettable day: the hum of early-morning alarms, the pulse of hospital hallways, the quiet conversations that change everything, and the moments where purpose clicks into place.

These aren't textbooks.

They're **cinematic, character-driven journeys** that reveal the identity behind the role — the rhythms, the pressures, the alignment, the hidden wisdom, and the breathtaking meaning found in the work.

Every ScrubTales™ book includes:

• **15 Day- In-The Life arc** written in immersive, scene-by-scene detail

• **Alignment reflections** that help readers understand who thrives in the role

• **Skills, traits, red flags, and burnout signatures** specific to the profession

• **The Mini SCRUB*fit*™ Healthcare Career Assessment**

• **Guided exercises for insight, clarity, and direction**

• **Pros & Cons, What I Wish I Had Known, and Top Specialties**

• **Cinematic storytelling woven with real-world clinical truth**

ScrubTales™ is the bridge between **identity and profession**, created for students, career-changers, educators, advisors, and anyone who's ever wondered:

"What does this job *feel* like — and would I fit here?"

From Nurse Practitioners to Physician Assistants, from Pharmacists to Diagnostic Medical Sonographers, from Registered Nurses to Certified Nursing Assistants, each edition invites you to step into the scrubs, breathe the air, carry the weight, and discover the spark that makes healthcare more than a career — **it's a calling shaped by who you are.**

Welcome to ScrubTales™.

Where purpose finds its profession.

ScrubTales™

1. ScrubTales™ — Nurse Practitioner

A cinematic, identity-driven exploration of advanced practice nursing with Day-in-the-Life chapters, alignment mapping, and the Mini **SCRUB*fit*™** Healthcare Career Assessment.

2. ScrubTales™ — Physician Assistant

The bridge between diagnosis and action. Packed with versatility, interprofessional teamwork, and the alignment science behind PA success.

3. ScrubTales™ — Clinical Pharmacist

Precision, stewardship, and the cognitive command center of care — featuring the world of hospital, clinical, and ambulatory pharmacy through The Med Heads.

4. ScrubTales™ — Diagnostic Medical Sonographer

A cinematic immersion into the role that turns echoes into answers and shadows into clarity.

5. ScrubTales™ — Certified Nursing Assistant

The heartbeat of bedside care — presence, connection, teamwork, and the foundational skills that make patient experience possible.

6. *ScrubTales™ — Registered Nurse*

From floor nursing to specialty practice, this volume highlights adaptability, critical thinking, and the holistic care identity at the core of the RN profession.

7. *ScrubTales™ — Radiologic Technologist*

Where physics meets empathy — capturing the science, art, and alignment of imaging with The Diagnostic Division.

8. *ScrubTales™ — Medical Laboratory Scientist*

Behind every diagnosis stands the scientist who finds the truth. A deep dive into accuracy, vigilance, and unseen lifesaving work.

9. *ScrubTales™ — Occupational Therapist*

Creative, restorative, and identity-reshaping. A journey into rebuilding independence and meaning.

10. *ScrubTales™ — Physical Therapist*

Movement, momentum, and mastery — exploring the Recovery Regimen and the power of restoring strength.

www.ingramcontent.com/pod-product-compliance
Lightning Source LLC
Chambersburg PA
CBHW071643310326
41914CB00123B/591